Advances and Controversies in Prostate Cancer

Guest Editors

WILLIAM K. OH, MD
JIM C. HU, MD, MPH

UROLOGIC CLINICS OF NORTH AMERICA

www.urologic.theclinics.com

February 2010 • Volume 37 • Number 1

SAUNDERS an imprint of ELSEVIER, Inc.

W.B. SAUNDERS COMPANY
A Division of Elsevier Inc.

1600 John F. Kennedy Blvd. • Suite 1800 • Philadelphia, PA 19103-2899

http://www.theclinics.com

UROLOGIC CLINICS OF NORTH AMERICA Volume 37, Number 1
February 2010 ISSN 0094-0143, ISBN-13: 978-1-4377-1916-1

Editor: Kerry Holland

Urologic Clinics of North America (ISSN 0094-0143) is published quarterly by Elsevier Inc., 360 Park Avenue South, New York, NY 10010-1710. Months of issue are February, May, August, and November. Business and Editorial Offices: 1600 John F. Kennedy Blvd., Suite 1800, Philadelphia, PA 19103-2899. Periodicals postage paid at New York, NY and additional mailing offices. Subscription prices are $291.00 per year (US individuals), $463.00 per year (US institutions), $333.00 per year (Canadian individuals), $568.00 per year (Canadian institutions), $414.00 per year (foreign individuals), and $568.00 per year (foreign institutions). Foreign air speed delivery is included in all *Clinics* subscription prices. All prices are subject to change without notice. **POSTMASTER:** Send address changes to *Urologic Clinics of North America*, Elsevier Health Sciences Division, Subscription Customer Service, 3251 Riverport Lane, Maryland Heights, MO 63043. Customer Service: 1-800-654-2452 (US). From outside the United States, call 1-314-447-8871. Fax: 1-314-447-8029. E-mail: JournalsCustomerServiceusa@elsevier.com (for print support) and JournalsOnlineSupport-usa@elsevier.com (for online support).

Reprints. For copies of 100 or more, of articles in this publication, please contact the Commercial Reprints Department, Elsevier Inc., 360 Park Avenue South, New York, New York 10010-1710. Tel.: 212-633-3813; Fax: 212-462-1935; E-mail: reprints@elsevier.com.

Urologic Clinics of North America is covered in MEDLINE/PubMed (*Index Medicus*), *Excerpta Medica, Current Contents/Clinical Medicine, Science Citation Index,* and *ISI/BIOMED.*

Printed and bound in the United Kingdom

Transferred to Digital Print 2011

Contributors

GUEST EDITORS

WILLIAM K. OH, MD
Chief, Division of Hematology and Medical Oncology; Professor of Medicine and Urology; Ezra M. Greenspan, MD Professor in Clinical Cancer Therapeutics, Mount Sinai School of Medicine; Associate Director for Clinical Research, The Tisch Cancer Institute, New York, New York

JIM C. HU, MD, MPH
Assistant Professor of Surgery, Division of Urology, Brigham and Women's Hospital, Harvard Medical School, Boston, Massachusetts

AUTHORS

ROBERT ABOUASSALY, MD
Fellow, Urologic Oncology, Division of Urology, Princess Margaret Hospital, University of Toronto, Toronto, Canada

JALIL AFNAN, MD
Department of Radiology, Brigham and Women's Hospital, Boston, Massachusetts

GERALD L. ANDRIOLE, MD
Professor and Chief of Urologic Surgery; Robert K. Royce Distinguished Professor of Urologic Surgery, Division of Urologic Surgery, Department of Surgery, Washington University School of Medicine; Barnes-Jewish Hospital, Siteman Cancer Center, St Louis, Missouri

ARIE S. BELLDEGRUN, MD, FACS
Roy and Carol Doumani Chair in Urologic Oncology; Professor, Department of Urology; Director, Institute of Urologic Oncology, David Geffen School of Medicine at UCLA, Los Angeles, California

ELISA CAPIZZI, MSc
Laboratory of Molecular Oncologic Pathology, Addarii Institute of Oncology, S.Orsola-Malpighi Hospital, Bologna, Italy

FERNANDO CARVAS, BS
Research Fellow, Division of Urology, Brigham and Women's Hospital, Harvard Medical School, Boston, Massachusetts

KIM N. CHI, MD
Division of Medical Oncology, BC Cancer Agency - Vancouver Cancer Centre; Associate Professor of Medicine, Department of Medicine; Department of Urological Sciences, University of British Columbia, Vancouver, British Columbia, Canada

WESLEY W. CHOI, MD
Clinical Fellow, Division of Urology, Brigham and Women's Hospital, Harvard Medical School, Boston, Massachusetts

E. DAVID CRAWFORD, MD
Professor of Surgery/Urology/Radiation Oncology, and Head, Urologic Oncology, E. David Crawford Endowed Chair in Urologic Oncology, University of Colorado Cancer Center, University of Colorado Anschutz Medical Campus, Aurora, Colorado

CHARLES G. DRAKE, MD, PhD
Associate Professor, Department of Oncology, Immunology, and Urology, Johns Hopkins Sidney Kimmel Comprehensive Cancer Center; The Brady Urological Institute, Johns Hopkins University, Baltimore, Maryland

DAVID S. FINLEY, MD
Fellow, Department of Urology, Institute of Urologic Oncology, David Geffen School of Medicine at UCLA, Los Angeles, California

MICHELANGELO FIORENTINO, MD, PhD
Center for Molecular Oncologic Pathology, Departments of Pathology and Medical Oncology, Dana-Farber Cancer Institute, Brigham and Women's Hospital, Harvard Medical School, Boston, Massachusetts; Laboratory of Molecular Oncologic Pathology, Addarii Institute of Oncology, S.Orsola-Malpighi Hospital, Bologna, Italy

MARCOS P. FREIRE, MD, PhD
Research Fellow, Division of Urology, Brigham & Women's Hospital, Harvard Medical School, Boston, Massachusetts

JIM C. HU, MD, MPH
Assistant Professor of Surgery, Division of Urology, Brigham and Women's Hospital, Harvard Medical School, Boston, Massachusetts

ERIC A. KLEIN, MD
Chairman, Glickman Urological and Kidney Institute, Cleveland Clinic, Cleveland, Ohio

YIN LEI, MD
Research Fellow, Division of Urology, Brigham and Women's Hospital, Harvard Medical School, Boston, Massachusetts

MASSIMO LODA, MD
Center for Molecular Oncologic Pathology, Departments of Pathology and Medical Oncology, Dana-Farber Cancer Institute, Brigham and Women's Hospital, Harvard Medical School, Boston, Massachusetts

STACY LOEB, MD
Johns Hopkins Medical Institution, Brady Urological Institute, Baltimore, Maryland

ROBYN J. MACFARLANE, MD
Medical Oncology Resident, Division of Medical Oncology, BC Cancer Agency-Vancouver Cancer Centre, Vancouver, British Columbia, Canada

EDWARD M. MESSING, MD, FACS
Chairman, W.W. Scott Professor of Urology, Department of Urology, University of Rochester Medical Center, Rochester, New York

DAVID C. MILLER, MD, MPH
Assistant Professor of Urology and Epidemology, Department of Urology; Research Scientist, VA Center for Clinical Management Research, University of Michigan School of Medicine, University of Michigan, Ann Arbor, Michigan

WILLIAM K. OH, MD
Chief, Division of Hematology and Medical Oncology; Professor of Medicine and Urology; Ezra M. Greenspan, MD Professor in Clinical Cancer Therapeutics, Mount Sinai School of Medicine; Associate Director for Clinical Research, The Tisch Cancer Institute, New York, New York

GANESH S. PALAPATTU, MD, FACS
Chief of Urologic Oncology, Department of Urology, The Methodist Hospital, Houston, Texas

FREDERIC POULIOT, MD, PhD
Fellow, Department of Urology, Institute of Urologic Oncology, David Geffen School of Medicine at UCLA, Los Angeles, California

KYLE O. ROVE, MD
Resident, Division of Urology, University of Colorado, Anschutz Medical Campus, Aurora, Colorado

EDWARD M. SCHAEFFER, MD, PhD
Assistant Professor, Johns Hopkins Medical Institution, Brady Urological Institute, Baltimore, Maryland

FABIO A.B. SCHUTZ, MD
Lank Center for Genitourinary Oncology, Dana-Farber Cancer Institute, Boston, Massachusetts

ALEX SHTEYNSHLYUGER, MD
Fellow in Urologic Oncology, Division of Urologic Surgery, Department of Surgery, Washington University School of Medicine, Barnes-Jewish Hospital, Siteman Cancer Center, St Louis, Missouri

ERIC A. SINGER, MD, MA
Clinical Fellow, Urologic Oncology Branch, National Cancer Institute, Bethesda, Maryland

ANDREW J. STEPHENSON, MD
Chief, Urologic Oncology, Glickman Urological and Kidney Institute, Cleveland Clinic, Cleveland, Ohio

RICHARD G. STOCK, MD
Professor and Chairman, Department of Radiation Oncology, Mount Sinai School of Medicine, Mount Sinai Hospital, New York, New York

NELSON N. STONE, MD
Clinical Professor, Department of Urology, Mount Sinai School of Medicine, New York, New York

KATHRYN F. SULLIVAN, MD
Resident, Division of Urology, University of Colorado, Anschutz Medical Campus, Aurora, Colorado

CLARE M. TEMPANY, MD
Department of Radiology, Brigham and Women's Hospital, Boston, Massachusetts

PATRICK C. WALSH, MD
Distinguished Service Professor, Johns Hopkins Medical Institution, Brady Urological Institute, Baltimore, Maryland

Contents

GOAL STATEMENT

The goal of *Urologic Clinics of North America* is to keep practicing urologists and urology residents up to date with current clinical practice in urology by providing timely articles reviewing the state of the art in patient care.

ACCREDITATION

The *Urologic Clinics of North America* is planned and implemented in accordance with the Essential Areas and Policies of the Accreditation Council for Continuing Medical Education (ACCME) through the joint sponsorship of the University of Virginia School of Medicine and Elsevier. The University of Virginia School of Medicine is accredited by the ACCME to provide continuing medical education for physicians.

The University of Virginia School of Medicine designates this educational activity for a maximum of 15 *AMA PRA Category 1 Credits*™ for each issue, 60 credits per year. Physicians should only claim credit commensurate with the extent of their participation in the activity.

The American Medical Association has determined that physicians not licensed in the US who participate in this CME activity are eligible for a maximum of 15 *AMA PRA Category 1 Credits*™ for each issue, 60 credits per year.

Credit can be earned by reading the text material, taking the CME examination online at http://www.theclinics.com/home/cme, and completing the evaluation. After taking the test, you will be required to review any and all incorrect answers. Following completion of the test and evaluation, your credit will be awarded and you may print your certificate.

FACULTY DISCLOSURE/CONFLICT OF INTEREST

The University of Virginia School of Medicine, as an ACCME accredited provider, endorses and strives to comply with the Accreditation Council for Continuing Medical Education (ACCME) Standards of Commercial Support, Commonwealth of Virginia statutes, University of Virginia policies and procedures, and associated federal and private regulations and guidelines on the need for disclosure and monitoring of proprietary and financial interests that may affect the scientific integrity and balance of content delivered in continuing medical education activities under our auspices.

The University of Virginia School of Medicine requires that all CME activities accredited through this institution be developed independently and be scientifically rigorous, balanced and objective in the presentation/discussion of its content, theories and practices.

All authors/editors participating in an accredited CME activity are expected to disclose to the readers relevant financial relationships with commercial entities occurring within the past 12 months (such as grants or research support, employee, consultant, stock holder, member of speakers bureau, etc.). The University of Virginia School of Medicine will employ appropriate mechanisms to resolve potential conflicts of interest to maintain the standards of fair and balanced education to the reader. Questions about specific strategies can be directed to the Office of Continuing Medical Education, University of Virginia School of Medicine, Charlottesville, Virginia.

The faculty and staff of the University of Virginia Office of Continuing Medical Education have no financial affiliations to disclose.

The authors/editors listed below have identified no professional or financial affiliations for themselves or their spouse/partner:
Robert Abouassaly, MD; Jalil Afnan, MD; Arie S. Belldegrun, MD, FACS; Elisa Capizzi, MSc; Fernando Carvas, BS; Kim N. Chi, MD; Wesley W. Choi, MD; David S. Finley, MD; Michelangelo Fiorentino, MD, PhD; Marcos P. Freire, MD, PhD; Kerry K. Holland (Acquisitions Editor); Jim C. Hu, MD, MPH (Guest Editor); Eric A. Klein, MD; Yin Lei, MD; Massimo Loda, MD; Stacy Loeb, MD; Robyn J. Macfarlane, MD; Edward M. Messing, MD, FACS; David C. Miller, MD, MPH; Ganesh S. Palapattu, MD, FACS; Frederic Pouliot, MD, PhD; Kyle O. Rove, MD; Edward M. Schaeffer, MD, PhD; Fabio A.B. Schutz, MD; Alex Shteynshlyuger, MD; Eric A. Singer, MD, MA; William Steers, MD (Test Author); Andrew J. Stephenson, MD; Richard G. Stock, MD; Kathryn F. Sullivan, MD; and Patrick C. Walsh, MD.

The authors/editors listed below identified the following professional or financial affiliations for themselves or their spouse/partner:
Gerald L. Andriole, MD is a consultant for Aeterna Zentaris, Amgen, EMD Serono, Ferring Pharmaceuticals, GenProbe, GlaxoSmithKline, Nema Steba, Onconome, and Veridex; is an industry funded research/investigator for Aeterna Zentaris; is on the Speakers' Bureau for GlaxoSmithKline; and is a stockholder for Cambridge Endo, Envisioneering Medical, and Viking Medical.
E. David Crawford, MD receives compensation as a meeting participant or lecturer for Watson, Endo, GSK, Oncura, Endocare, Ferring, and Sanofi Aventis; is a consultant for Elgen; receives grant support from NIH and the University of Colorado Cancer Center; and has a family member who receives compensation from Ferring.
Charles G. Drake, MD, PhD is a consultant for Amplimmune Inc, Medarex, Inc, Dendreon, Inc, ProTox, Inc, and Sanofi Aventis, Inc; owns stock in Amplimmune Inc; and holds a patent with Medarex, Inc.
William K. Oh, MD (Guest Editor) is an industry funded research/investigator for Sanofi-Aventis and Genentech, and is on the Speakers' Bureau for Sanofi-Aventis.
Nelson N. Stone, MD owns stock in Prologics LLC, is a consultant for Nihon MediPhysics, and is on the Advisory Committee/Board for the Prostate Cancer Education Council.
Clare M. Tempany, MD receives grant support from NIH, and is an industry funded research/investigator and consultant for Insightec Inc.

Disclosure of Discussion of Non-FDA Approved Uses for Pharmaceutical Products and/or Medical Devices.
The University of Virginia School of Medicine, as an ACCME provider, requires that all faculty presenters identify and disclose any off-label uses for pharmaceutical and medical device products. The University of Virginia School of Medicine recommends that each physician fully review all the available data on new products or procedures prior to clinical use.

TO ENROLL

To enroll in the Urologic Clinics of North America Continuing Medical Education program, call customer service at 1-800-654-2452 or visit us online at www.theclinics.com/home/cme. The CME program is available to subscribers for an additional fee of $195.00.

Urologic Clinics of North America

FORTHCOMING ISSUES

May 2010

Pediatrics
Tom Kolon, MD, *Guest Editor*

August 2010

Penile and Urethral Cancer
Jack H. Mydlo, MD, *Guest Editor*

November 2010

Treating the Adult Neurogenic Bladder
John T. Stoffel, MD, and
Edward J. McGuire, MD,
Guest Editors

RECENT ISSUES

November 2009

Benign Prostatic Hyperplasia and Lower Urinary Tract Symptoms
Jerry G. Blaivas, MD and Jeffrey P. Weiss, MD,
Guest Editors

August 2009

Vasectomy and Vasectomy Reversal: Important Issues
Jay I. Sandlow, MD and
Harris M. Nagler, MD, FACS, *Guest Editors*

May 2009

New Technology in Urologic Surgery
Mihir M. Desai, MD, *Guest Editor*

RELATED INTEREST

Hematology/Oncology Clinics of North America, June 2006 (Vol. 20, No. 4)
Prostate Cancer
William K. Oh, MD, *Guest Editor*

Preface

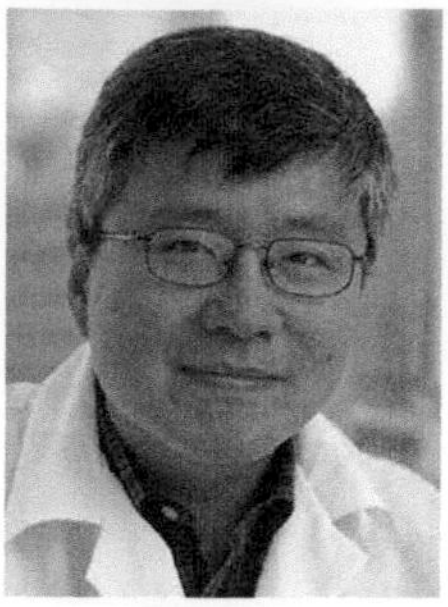
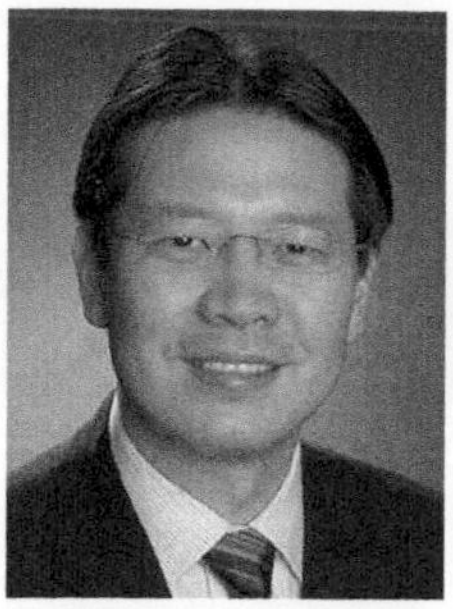

William K. Oh, MD   Jim C. Hu, MD, MPH

Guest Editors

Dilemmas and controversies in the management of prostate cancer continue to present a vexing challenge to physicians and patients dealing with the disease. The past several years have been remarkable for several paradigm shifts in what we have learned about the biology of prostate cancer and how patients are being treated. Some changes represent huge shifts in technology, which have completely altered the landscape in terms of imaging, surgery, and radiation. Other findings have basically reinforced some of the facts we have known for many years, such as the key role of androgen receptor in the biology of prostate cancer.

In this issue of *Urologic Clinics of North America*, our outstanding contributors—all leaders in the field—review landmark studies that have shown that 5-alpha reductase inhibitors indeed are effective in the chemoprevention of prostate cancer. They also review other phase III studies that have raised questions about how aggressively we should screen the general population with prostate-specific antigen tests. Once prostate cancer is diagnosed, newer novel imaging techniques are allowing for better staging and—with some controversy—the possibility of guided and potentially focal therapeutics with cryotherapy and high-intensity focused ultrasound. Moreover, disruptive technologies, such as robotic-assisted laparoscopic surgery and the Internet have toppled traditional word-of-mouth referral patterns, making patients themselves drivers of early adoption of new technology. Moreover, for men opting for surgery, the appropriateness and extent of pelvic lymph node dissection remain unclear. The field of radiation therapy has also rapidly changed, and continued evidence for its efficacy is being evaluated both as primary and adjuvant therapy.

New data on systemic therapies are reviewed, including those given at the time of diagnosis and at the time of relapse, such as hormones and chemotherapy. A new immunotherapy treatment for prostate cancer will likely be commercially available in 2010. Indeed, perhaps the future of prostate cancer can be seen in new advances in the role of biomarkers and novel therapeutics, as molecular medicine begins to demonstrate promise in prostate cancer patients.

We believe we are at a critical juncture in prostate cancer, where new science and new technology will drive us to understand the heterogeneity of the disease better and enable us to treat our patients with the least morbidity and best outcomes.

William K. Oh, MD
Division of Hematology and Medical Oncology
The Tisch Cancer Institute
Mount Sinai School of Medicine
One Gustave L. Levy Place, Box 1079
New York, NY 10029, USA

Jim C. Hu, MD, MPH
Division of Urologic Surgery
Brigham and Women's Hospital
Dana-Farber Cancer Institute and
Harvard Medical School
75 Francis Street
Boston, MA 02115, USA

E-mail addresses:
william.oh@mssm.edu (W.K. Oh)
jhu2@partners.org (J.C. Hu)

Urol Clin N Am 37 (2010) xiii
doi:10.1016/j.ucl.2009.12.001

Prostate Cancer: To Screen or Not to Screen?

Alex Shteynshlyuger, MD, Gerald L. Andriole, MD*

KEYWORDS

- Screening • Prostate cancer • Prostate-specific antigen
- ERSPC trial • PLCO trial

The debate about usefulness of population-based prostate cancer screening has been ongoing for decades, with little consensus among professional medical societies, cancer advocacy groups, or public health professionals.[1–3] There is no doubt clinicians need to know whether screening is effective, as prostate cancer is associated with significant mortality and morbidity that will likely increase as the population ages.

Recent publication of 2 large-scale randomized studies addressing the issues of population screening for prostate cancer with level I evidence did little to resolve the controversy. The Prostate, Lung, Colorectal, Ovarian (PLCO) cancer screening trial and the European Randomized Study of Screening for Prostate Cancer (ERSPC) trial evaluated screening with prostate-specific antigen (PSA) and digital rectal examination (DRE). These studies demonstrate that PSA based screening has led to a significant increase in diagnosis of prostate cancer with uncertain mortality benefits. Both studies have limitations that may have led to divergent results, thus leaving clinicians in a quandary regarding screening.[4,5]

THE BURDEN OF PROSTATE CANCER

In the United States, 192,280 men will be diagnosed with and 27,360 will die of prostate cancer in 2009. A man aged 40 years has a 3% lifetime chance of dying from prostate cancer and 16% chance of lifetime diagnosis of prostate cancer.[6] As medical care and resultant life expectancy improve, the burden of prostate cancer morbidity and the likelihood of prostate-specific mortality are expected to increase because prostate cancer mortality peaks at around age 80 years (**Table 1**).

In the pre-PSA era, approximately 11% of men were diagnosed with clinically symptomatic prostate cancer and 75% died of prostate cancer or with prostate cancer as a contributing cause. The median length from diagnosis to death was 41 months.[7] Among men with clinically detected prostate cancer in the Scandinavian trial of radical prostatectomy (RP) versus watchful waiting (WW), 20% of men died of prostate cancer in the WW group and 26% developed metastasis at 12-year follow-up. Those with extracapsular disease had 14 times the risk of prostate cancer death compared with those with organ-confined tumors.[8]

Whereas before the PSA era only 27% of prostate cancer cases were clinically localized, in the PSA era 97% to 98% of screening-detected prostate cancer is clinically localized.[4,5,7]

Quality of life (QOL) among newly diagnosed men with prostate cancer versus men without prostate cancer is worse, as there are higher rates of depression, anxiety, and worse voiding and bowel function.[9–11] Moreover, all treatment modalities result in temporary or permanent deterioration in QOL, particularly in the domains of sexual function, incontinence, bowel function, and vitality. Whereas side effect severity and frequency vary, all treatments affect the QOL of patients and their spouses.[12,13]

Division of Urologic Surgery, Department of Surgery, Washington University School of Medicine, Barnes-Jewish Hospital, Siteman Cancer Center, 4960 Children's Place, Campus Box 8242, St Louis, MO 63110, USA
* Corresponding author.
E-mail address: andrioleg@wustl.edu (G.L. Andriole).

Urol Clin N Am 37 (2010) 1–9
doi:10.1016/j.ucl.2009.11.004

Table 1
Deaths from prostate cancer by age: United States, 2005

	35–44 Years	45–54 Years	55–64 Years	65–74 Years	75–84 Years	85 Years and Older
Deaths from prostate cancer (n = 28,905)	24	395 (1%)	2154 (7%)	5764 (20%)	11,666 (40%)	8897 (31%)
Overall deaths (men and women, n = 2,448,017)	84,785 (3%)	183,530 (7%)	275,301 (11%)	398,355 (16%)	686,665 (28%)	703,169 (29%)

Data from U.S. Census Bureau, statistical abstract of the United States: 2009 (128th edition). Washington, DC; 2008. Table 103: expectation of life and expected deaths by race, sex, and age: 2005. Available at: http://www.census.gov/compendia/statab/tables/09s0103.pdf. Accessed October 10, 2009.

Foregoing treatment in favor of WW is not optimal. QOL has been evaluated in the Scandinavian trial of RP versus WW. In that study, patients who had RP and who were alive at the time of evaluation had QOL and sense of well being that was better than that among men undergoing WW. Likewise, patients in the RP group had lower rates of anxiety and depressed mood despite the higher frequency of erectile dysfunction (80% vs 55%) and incontinence (42% vs 25%) 6 to 8 years after study enrollment. Men with bone metastases who were receiving androgen deprivation therapy (ADT) had a significantly reduced QOL, mood, and sense of well being if they were in the WW group.[14]

These findings suggest that even in the absence of treatment, a diagnosis of prostate cancer is associated with significant morbidity. Several explanations for the inferior QOL scores in the WW arm of the study have been offered: (1) patients may regret not getting a potentially curative surgical intervention; (2) the expectations of significant surgical morbidity in the RP group might have lowered their threshold for QOL; (3) the WW group might have greater expectations of QOL than realistically possible. It is well known that expectations can alter perception.[14] It is possible that counseling about expectations at the onset differed for the 2 groups of patients, and may have been the determining factor in poor QOL among the WW study arm if their expectations were higher than the QOL that they experienced.

Overall, these considerations reinforce the need for the urological community to do something about prostate cancer.

WHY SCREEN: RATIONALE FOR SCREENING

The goals of population screening for prostate cancer fall into 3 categories:

1. Reduction of prostate cancer mortality
2. Reduction of morbidity associated with prostate cancer
3. Reduction of financial costs associated with symptomatic prostate cancer.

Although these goals seem self-evident, there are 3 biases worth considering. It is well accepted that population screening is associated with overdiagnosis, which is referred to as detection bias. Overdiagnosis refers to identification of disease in patients in whom it would have never become symptomatic during their lifetime. Screening can also lead to lead-time bias with earlier diagnosis but no effect on mortality. Lead-time bias gives the appearance of longer survival because of earlier detection with no overall improvement in life expectancy. Population screening is also more likely to detect less aggressive disease due to the longer interval before it becomes symptomatic. This factor has been referred to as length bias.

LEAD TIMES AND OVERDIAGNOSIS

With high discrepancy rate between clinical diagnosis of prostate cancer and histologic prevalence of prostate cancer, population-screening initiatives carry a significant risk of overdiagnosis of prostate cancer. Overdiagnosis refers to identification of latent disease that would not have otherwise caused symptoms or been identified during the patient's lifetime.

In the case of prostate cancer screening, overdiagnosis of subclinical disease is often associated with significant overtreatment due to the current inability to distinguish between prostate cancers that have a high potential for symptomatic progression during a patient's lifetime and those that are destined to have no clinical manifestations.[15]

Overtreatment leads to unnecessary costs to the health care system, and significant morbidity and possible mortality to some patients exposed to curative treatment.

Estimates for overdiagnosis of screen-detected prostate cancer in the United States range from 23% to 42%. Welch and Albertsen[16] estimated that more than 1 million men were overdiagnosed by PSA-based screening between 1987 and 2005. Modeling of SEER data suggests that uncensored lead time ranges from 7.2 to 10 years whereas nonoverdiagnosed lead time ranges from 5.4 to 6.9 years.[15] Based on reports of 11% prevalence of symptomatic prostate cancer by age 80, with 16% lifetime risk of diagnosis of prostate cancer for a man in the United States, a crude calculation suggests that the overdiagnosis rate of 45% is consistent with Draisma's 42% overdiagnosis rate.[6,7]

PROSTATE CANCER SCREENING TOOLS

Digital Rectal Examination

The sensitivity of DRE for prostate cancer is dependent on the tumor stage and observer bias.[17] At present, the sensitivity of DRE is poor and depends on the degree of DRE abnormality. DRE detects 15% of cancers that would go undetected by PSA screening with a threshold of 4 ng/mL. DRE is likely to detect higher risk tumors than PSA alone; 20% of tumors detected by DRE with PSA less than 2 ng/mL are nonorgan confined.[17] Positive predictive value (PPV) for abnormal DRE can be as high as 50%.[18] Men with abnormal DRE typically have more advanced disease, and cT2 disease is often pathologically upstaged to pT3 disease.[19] Because DRE screening tends to detect nonorgan-confined disease undetected by PSA screening, the opportunity for cure with DRE testing alone is limited.

Prostate-Specific Antigen

The operating test characteristics of PSA depend on several factors, including the PSA threshold used for biopsy and patient age.[20–23] For patients with mean age of 63 years, detection rate of prostate cancer when combined with DRE for PSA of 2.5 to 3.5 ng/mL is 28%; for PSA of 4 to 9.9 ng/mL it is 46%, and for PSA greater than 10 ng/mL, the detection rate is 60% with extended 12-core or saturation biopsy.[22] Specificity improves at higher PSA thresholds while sensitivity declines significantly. Among men with mean age of 70, 46% had prostate cancer at PSA levels of 10 to 20 ng/mL, 76% had prostate cancer with PSA between 20 and 50 ng/mL, and 93% had prostate cancer with PSA greater than 50 ng/mL.[20]

The Prostate Cancer Prevention Trial (PCPT) is unique in that men underwent sextant biopsy irrespective of their PSA level. Prostate cancer was found in 6.6% of men with PSA of less than 0.5 ng/mL (12% high grade), in 10% of men with PSA 0.6 to 1 ng/mL (10% high grade); in 17% of men with PSA 1.1 to 2 ng/mL (12% high grade); in 24% of men with PSA 2.1 to 3 ng/mL (19% high grade); and in 27% of men with PSA 3.1 to 4 ng/mL (25% high grade).[24] PSA sensitivities and specificities vary by age, especially for PSA values less than 4.0 ng/mL (**Table 2**). PSA sensitivity is better for high-grade disease (Gleason ≥7 vs <7 or no cancer) but even at PSA cutoff of 2.1 ng/mL, the sensitivity is only 76%, dropping to 57% at PSA 3.1 ng/mL or more (see **Table 2**).

Table 2
Sensitivity and specificity for prostate cancer by age and PSA level

PSA (ng/mL)	Sensitivity <70 y	Specificity <70 y	Sensitivity >70 y	Specificity >70 y	Sensitivity Gleason ≥7 vs Gleason <7 or No Cancer	Specificity Gleason ≥7 vs Gleason <7 or No Cancer
1.1	82.6	43.2	81.4	37.6	92.9	34.6
2.1	54.8	72.8	53.9	68.5	76.2	65.5
3.1	37.3	85	34.3	85.2	57.6	82.3
4.1	27.7	91.7	21.1	92.9	40.4	90
6.1	5.7	97.5	5.0	98.6	13.2	97.8
8.1	2.5	99.1	1.5	99.1	4.8	99
10.1	1.3	99.4	0.7	99.7	2.4	99.5

Data from Thompson IM, Ankerst DP, Chi C, et al. Operating characteristics of prostate-specific antigen in men with an initial PSA level of 3.0 ng/ml or lower. JAMA 2005;294(1):66–70.

Prostate Biopsy

Prostate biopsy has some characteristics of a good screening test. Extended 12-core biopsy has sensitivity close to 80% to 90% (with 10%–20% false negative rate based on re-biopsy detection of prostate cancer) for prostate cancer, and 100% specificity with no false positives. Prostate biopsy is associated with a reasonable safety profile and a relatively low risk of significant complications.[25,26] However, the true histologic false negative rate may be as high as 48% based on comparison of biopsy detected and step-section detected prostate cancer in autopsy series among men with no prior diagnosis of prostate cancer.[27] Moreover, data obtained from prostate biopsy (Gleason score, volume and burden of disease as measured by % of positive cores and linear length) has a high predictive value for assessment of risk of clinical progression of prostate cancer. However, due to the invasive nature of prostate biopsy, its acceptance as a screening test is not likely to become widespread. The use of invasive procedures as a screening tool is well accepted in population screening. For example, in screening for colon cancer, sigmoidoscopy and colonoscopy, which have similar test characteristics to prostate biopsy, are well accepted for screening due to availability of highly effective treatment with significant reduction in mortality, morbidity, and cost effectiveness. Colonoscopy has slightly higher risks associated with it than does a prostate biopsy and is more invasive, but allows for therapeutic removal of small premalignant lesions. Acceptance of prostate biopsy as a screening tool will await advances in knowledge that would allow separation with a high degree of certainty of overdiagnosed tumors from those that are likely to become symptomatic.

Transrectal Ultrasound

Transrectal Ultrasound (TRUS) suffers from poor sensitivity and specificity for prostate cancer. In a study of patients with previously diagnosed prostate cancer, B-mode TRUS detected 45% of cancers with a specificity of 75%. Contrast-enhanced TRUS has better characteristics, with a sensitivity of 71% among patients with established prostate cancer and specificity of 50%.[28] The performance characteristics of TRUS in populations with low prevalence of prostate cancer are not conducive to its use for screening. TRUS is an invasive test that also suffers from operator-dependent variability. Various modifications such as power Doppler TRUS have not attained significant improvement in sensitivity to justify its use as a screening tool.

Magnetic Resonance Imaging

Magnetic Resonance Imaging (MRI) is a promising modality in evaluation of prostate cancer. In a small study of patients with diagnosed prostate cancer, T2-weighted MR had 41% sensitivity and diffusion-weighted MR had 57% sensitivity for detection of prostate cancer foci detected on whole-mount section histopathology of RP specimens. Prostate biopsy detected 92% of prostate cancer foci in this study.[29] The performance of MR in population setting has not been studied. At this time the operating test characteristics of MRI are not favorable for use in prostate cancer screening.

TO SCREEN OR NOT TO SCREEN USING PSA: THE PLCO AND ERSPC STUDIES

The PLCO study enrolled men between the ages of 55 and 74 years for annual screening with PSA for 6 years and DRE for 4 years. PSA of 4 ng/mL was used as a cutoff for abnormal value. There was a significant contamination rate (>50%) in the nonscreened study arm. The study protocol did not specify a mandatory evaluation protocol for patients with elevated PSA nor did it use a predefined treatment protocol for patients who were diagnosed with prostate cancer. Both were defined as "community standard" so that it would be similar to the approaches to biopsy and treatment that were offered to control patients. At 7 years, men in the screening arm were 22% more likely to be diagnosed with prostate cancer. At 10 years of follow-up, no survival advantage could be shown in the actively screened arm.[4]

The study findings are preliminary and based on relatively few deaths. These findings suggest that patients with less than 10-year life expectancy are not expected to benefit from PSA screening. Moreover, high contamination rates in the control arm may make the PLCO a study of more intense screening compared with less intense screening in the control arm.[30]

The ERSPC study is a combination of multiple studies with slightly different protocols in terms of PSA cutoffs, as well as inclusion and exclusion criteria for enrollment. Men were enrolled at the mean age of 61, and a mean PSA cutoff of 3.0 ng/mL was used. The ERSPC study demonstrated that the risk of death from prostate cancer was reduced by 20% in men aged 55 to 69 years who underwent PSA screening. This figure corresponds to absolute reduction in mortality of 0.6% from 3% to 2.4%. The number needed to treat (NNT) to prevent one prostate death was 48 in this study, while 1410 men had to be serially screened to prevent 1 prostate cancer mortality. There was no mandatory treatment protocol for men diagnosed with prostate cancer, and the mortality benefit may have been due to treatment differences between the arms. Men in the screening group were less likely to have Gleason ≥7 (27% vs 45% in control group), which might contribute to the observed survival advantage in the screening group. Of note, no overall survival benefit was shown in this study. Moreover, most of the prostate cancer mortality benefit was derived from countries with historically higher prostate cancer mortality rates. While the core group compared men aged 55 to 69 years, those in the 60 to 64 stratum derived no benefit, nor did those in the 50 to 54 or 70 to 74 age groups.[5]

These studies demonstrate that whereas population screening for prostate cancer may be effective in decreasing mortality using particular screening protocols, it is associated with significant overdiagnosis and overtreatment. It is not clear that using contemporary PSA screening protocols in the United States and Europe leads to overall favorable risk/benefit ratio. Whereas relative reduction in mortality may be as high as 20%, the absolute decrease in mortality is about 0.6%. The associated treatment morbidity and costs are not insignificant. In addition, many cancers miss detection and treatment; most men (80%) with prostate cancer who are destined to die from prostate cancer or to develop morbidity attributable to the disease did not benefit from screening and treatment protocol used in the ERSPC trial. Lack of overall survival benefit in the ERSPC trial is a significant red flag for screening. Understanding the effect of screening and treatment on morbidity, QOL, and costs is essential to fully evaluate whether the 20% relative reduction in cancer-specific mortality is sufficiently beneficial to recommend screening.

There are several explanations for the discrepancies between the PLCO and the ERSPC studies. The ERSPC study may have had less contamination in the control arm. Other differences were that the PLCO used PSA of 4 ng/mL and the ERSPC used PSA of 3 ng/mL as the screening cutoffs, which may have led to the differences in outcomes (**Table 3**). With PSA cutoff of 3 ng/mL, 57% of high-risk tumors (Gleason ≥7) are detected. Using PSA cutoff of 4 ng/mL, the overall detection of prostate cancer was higher in the PLCO, presumably due to annual screening with detection of more low-risk tumors; only 40% of detected tumors were high risk (see **Table 2**). This figure corresponds to a 43% greater risk of detecting high-risk tumors in the ERSPC study. The lower detection of high-risk tumors in the PLCO may contribute to its inability to demonstrate survival benefit, if any, from screening.

Neither study mandated predefined treatment protocols. The ERSPC study used mostly sextant core biopsy schemes, which is now known to be suboptimal for diagnosis of significant prostate cancer. The PLCO used "community standard" for biopsy and treatments, so it is likely that contemporary biopsy schemes and treatments were applied equally in both arms.

Based on these trials, one cannot state that population screening with PSA is either effective or ineffective. The most rational conclusion is that the PLCO trial did not demonstrate benefit at 10 years, with more intense compared with less intense PSA screening combined with community standards of care during the study period. Lengthier follow-up may change this conclusion. The take-home message from the ERSPC trial is that PSA screening with a cutoff of 3 ng/mL in certain age groups, from regions with relatively high cancer death rates, led to 20% relative risk reduction in mortality. However, the trade-offs in morbidity, costs, and QOL required to capture a small improvement in cancer-specific mortality without improvement in overall survival remain unknown.

EFFECT OF SCREENING FOR PROSTATE CANCER ON QUALITY OF LIFE

No study directly compares the QOL of men undergoing prostate cancer screening with a control population; however, diagnosis of prostate cancer affects QOL. WW is sometimes more detrimental than surgery to QOL. Whether it is driven by expectations is unknown.[14] Stratification of low-risk patients into active surveillance may be associated with an adverse affect on QOL due to increased levels of anxiety. Whether this detrimental effect can be modulated by education through recalibrating expectations remains unknown. Thus, overdetection itself is expected to have a detrimental effect on QOL even if patients are substratified into risk groups with avoidance of consequences of active treatment (RP or radiotherapy [RT]) in the low-risk groups. However, data on morbidity and complications of screening with PSA and DRE are available. Approximately 90% of men diagnosed with prostate cancer choose definitive therapy while 10% choose active surveillance, WW, or no treatment at all. Estimates from screening intervention studies suggest that 18 to 48 men must be treated to prevent 1 prostate cancer-specific death.[5,16]

Table 3
Summary table: PLCO versus ERSCP

	PLCO	ERSCP
Inclusion criteria	Age 55–74 Multi-institutional trial: US	Age 55–69 Collection of 7 European trials with different screening protocols, different ages of entry, controls
Exclusion criteria	History of prostate, lung, colon or ovarian cancer More than 1 PSA test in the previous 3 years	History of prostate cancer
Study design	Enrollment 1993–2001 Annual PSA for 6 years; DRE for 4 years—intervention arm; community standard of care or no screening for control group PSA >4 ng/mL cutoff value Primary care physicians notified of the screening test (PSA and DRE) results. Management based on community standard of care. No protocol for biopsy or treatment of prostate cancer—community standard of care	Enrollment 1991–2003 PSA screening once every 4 years—intervention arm; control—no screening PSA >3 ng/mL cutoff value No protocol for treatment of prostate cancer—community standard of care
Results	No difference in survival between screened and nonscreened arms at 7–10 years. No reduction in incidence of advanced cancer	20% reduction in prostate cancer–specific death in the screened group (27% in men actually screened) at 9 years of follow-up. No overall survival difference between the screened and control groups. Reduction in incidence of advanced cancer by screening 1410 men screened and 48 men treated to prevent 1 mortality from prostate cancer False-positive PSA accounted for 75.9% of biopsies. PPV of biopsy = 24.1% 8.2% in the screening group and 4.8 in control group were diagnosed with prostate cancer
Limitations	High rate of "contamination" in the control group leads to decreased statistical power; would require more events to attain significance	Suboptimal treatment with low dose RT Screened men were 2.77 times more likely to undergo RP vs controls

The effect of prostate cancer treatment on the QOL of patients and their spouses has been studied in a prospective multi-institutional study.[13] Most patients experience some deterioration in the QOL as measured by sexual function, urinary incontinence, urinary irritation or obstruction, bowel or rectal function, and vitality. Effects are domain dependent based on treatment received. Overall, at least 50% to 83% of men after RP, 31% to 78% of men after external RT, and 30% to 78% of men after brachytherapy experience moderate to severe distress due to deterioration in QOL across all domains. In addition, 44% to 69% of partners or spouses of RP patients experience distress; 22% to 48% of partners of men who underwent external RT experience distress; and 13% to 41% of spouses of those who underwent brachytherapy experienced distress.[13] Considering the morbidity of treatment as evidenced by deterioration of QOL for patients and their spouses and the significant overtreatment associated with prostate cancer, the overall benefit of PSA screening is uncertain.

WHO SHOULD BE SCREENED?

Screening for prostate cancer should be offered to men expected to benefit from treatment for prostate cancer if detected. The benefits of screening and treatment for prostate cancer should outweigh risks. The screening intervention should be cost effective to be applied to the population. In the absence of demonstrable reduction in morbidity, costs or overall mortality in the ERSPC trial, there is insufficient evidence to warrant population-based screening for prostate cancer.

It is well established by the Scandinavian study of RP versus WW that only men younger than 65 years experienced survival benefit from RP. Moreover, prostate cancer-specific mortality was concentrated among men with extracapsular disease at RP. Men older than versus younger than 65 years were more likely to have extracapsular disease (54% vs 39%) and Gleason greater than 6 (71% vs 66%). Survival benefits became evident as early as 6 years after enrollment.[8] With estimates of PSA screening lead-time bias of 6 to 10 years, it may take 12 to 16 years to demonstrate PSA screening survival benefit.[15] Based on findings, one can extrapolate that only men younger than 55 to 60 years (accounting for the 6–10 year lead-time bias) may benefit from PSA screening.

The US Preventive Services Task Force issued a recommendation against screening for prostate cancer in men 75 years or older. However, the peak morbidity and mortality from prostate cancer occurs in men aged 75 to 85 years (see **Table 1**).[3] At age 75 years, a man in the United States has a life expectancy of 10 years.[31] In a subgroup analysis of a randomized study of RT compared with RT plus 6 months of ADT in men with high-risk localized prostate cancer, healthy men with a mean age of 75 experienced a significantly lower overall mortality at 7.6 years of 16.5% compared with 41.4% for those receiving combined treatment. This benefit was not noted in men with significant comorbidities. In men with significant comorbidities, addition of ADT was associated with significantly increased risk of overall mortality. This fact suggests that healthy men over the age of 75 can derive similar benefit to younger men from treatment.[32]

There are no data to support treatment benefit for men with asymptomatic prostate cancer with life expectancy of less than 5 to 7 years. With a mean follow-up of 7.7 years, men with a mean age of 73 years on active surveillance for low-risk prostate cancer had no increased risk of metastasis or prostate cancer–specific mortality compared with similar men who underwent immediate treatment.[33]

WHAT IS A CLINICIAN TO DO?

Current evidence shows limited benefit of population screening for prostate cancer and significant psychological, physical, and financial morbidity of screening and diagnosis of prostate cancer. Yet, studies demonstrating marginal benefit of PSA screening were performed in an era characterized by arguably obsolete treatment protocols. Effectiveness of a population-screening program to reduce mortality, morbidity, and costs is intimately dependent on the receiver characteristics of the screening test and the effectiveness of the treatment modalities.

The final chapter on population screening for prostate cancer has yet to be written. Screening effectiveness can be improved by use of better screening tests or through use of targeted, more effective treatment. It is conceivable that as screening tests with improved characteristics for detecting aggressive cancers become available (and with good negative predictive value for clinical progression), the risk/benefit ratio will become more favorable. Finally, knowledge of optimal patient selection for disease-stage specific treatment modalities for prostate cancer may be enhanced by results from the Prostate Testing for Cancer and Treatment (ProtecT) study and longer follow-up of the PLCO and ERSPC trials.

SUMMARY

There is no demonstrable overall survival benefit from screening, while significant overtreatment and treatment morbidity have been demonstrated. Future efforts should focus on improvement in screening methodology to identify a greater proportion of cancers that are destined to become symptomatic. Prognostication and substratification of cancers into more precise management categories is necessary. Finally, clinicians need to manage patients based on their individual risk stratification to minimize overtreatment and to deliver optimal therapy to those who will benefit from treatment.

REFERENCES

1. Barry MJ. Screening for prostate cancer—the controversy that refuses to die. N Engl J Med 2009;360(13):1351–4.
2. Holmberg L. Prostate cancer screening: the need for problem-solving that puts men's interests first. Eur Urol 2009;56(1):34–7.
3. U.S. Preventive Services Task Force. Screening for prostate cancer: U.S. preventive services task force recommendation statement. Ann Intern Med 2008; 149(3):185–91.

4. Andriole GL, Crawford ED, Grubb RL 3rd, et al. PLCO Project Team. Mortality results from a randomized prostate-cancer screening trial. N Engl J Med 2009;360(13):1310–9. Erratum in: N Engl J Med 2009 Apr 23;360(17):1797.
5. Schröder FH, Hugosson J, Roobol MJ, et al. ERSPC Investigators. Screening and prostate-cancer mortality in a randomized European study. N Engl J Med 2009;360(13):1320–8.
6. Horner MJ, Ries LAG, Krapcho M, et al, editors. SEER Cancer statistics review, 1975–2006. Bethesda (MD): National Cancer Institute. Table 23.9: cancer of the prostate. Available at: http://seer.cancer.gov/csr/1975_2006/index.html. Accessed October 15, 2009.
7. Hugosson J, Aus G, Becker C, et al. Would prostate cancer detected by screening with prostate-specific antigen develop into clinical cancer if left undiagnosed? A comparison of two population-based studies in Sweden. BJU Int 2000;85(9):1078–84.
8. Bill-Axelson A, Holmberg L, Filén F, et al. Radical prostatectomy versus watchful waiting in localized prostate cancer: the Scandinavian prostate cancer group-4 randomized trial. J Natl Cancer Inst 2008; 100(16):1144–54.
9. Lev EL, Eller LS, Gejerman G, et al. Quality of life of men treated for localized prostate cancer: outcomes at 6 and 12 months. Support Care Cancer 2009; 17(5):509–17.
10. Couper JW, Love AW, Dunai JV, et al. The psychological aftermath of prostate cancer treatment choices: a comparison of depression, anxiety and quality of life outcomes over the 12 months following diagnosis. Med J Aust 2009;190(suppl 7):S86–9.
11. Litwin MS, Hays RD, Fink A, et al. Quality-of-life outcomes in men treated for localized prostate cancer. JAMA 1995;273(2):129–35.
12. Litwin MS, Gore JL, Kwan L, et al. Quality of life after surgery, external beam irradiation, or brachytherapy for early-stage prostate cancer. Cancer 2007; 109(11):2239–47.
13. Sanda MG, Dunn RL, Michalski J, et al. Quality of life and satisfaction with outcome among prostate-cancer survivors. N Engl J Med 2008;358(12): 1250–61.
14. Johansson E, Bill-Axelson A, Holmberg L, et al. Time, symptom burden, androgen deprivation, and self-assessed quality of life after radical prostatectomy or watchful waiting: the Randomized Scandinavian Prostate Cancer Group Study Number 4 (SPCG-4) clinical trial. Eur Urol 2009;55(2):422–30.
15. Draisma G, Etzioni R, Tsodikov A, et al. Lead time and overdiagnosis in prostate-specific antigen screening: importance of methods and context. J Natl Cancer Inst 2009;101(6):374–83.
16. Welch HG, Albertsen PC. Prostate cancer diagnosis and treatment after the introduction of prostate-specific antigen screening: 1986–2005. J Natl Cancer Inst 2009;101(19):1325–9.
17. Okotie OT, Roehl KA, Han M, et al. Characteristics of prostate cancer detected by digital rectal examination only. Urology 2007;70(6):1117–20.
18. Gosselaar C, Roobol MJ, Roemeling S, et al. The role of the digital rectal examination in subsequent screening visits in the European randomized study of screening for prostate cancer (ERSPC), Rotterdam. Eur Urol 2008;54(3):581–8.
19. Thompson IM, Ernst JJ, Gangai MP, et al. Adenocarcinoma of the prostate: results of routine urological screening. J Urol 1984;132(4):690–2.
20. Philip J, Hanchanale V, Foster CS, et al. Importance of peripheral biopsies in maximizing the detection of early prostate cancer in repeat 12-core biopsy protocols. BJU Int 2006;98(3):559–62.
21. Pepe P, Aragona F. Saturation prostate needle biopsy and prostate cancer detection at initial and repeat evaluation. Urology 2007;70(6):1131–5.
22. Jones JS, Patel A, Schoenfield L, et al. Saturation technique does not improve cancer detection as an initial prostate biopsy strategy. J Urol 2006; 175(2):485–8.
23. Thompson IM, Ankerst DP, Chi C, et al. Operating characteristics of prostate-specific antigen in men with an initial PSA level of 3.0 ng/ml or lower. JAMA 2005;294(1):66–70.
24. Thompson IM, Pauler DK, Goodman PJ, et al. Prevalence of prostate cancer among men with a prostate-specific antigen level < or = 4.0 ng per milliliter. N Engl J Med 2004;350(22):2239–46.
25. Raaijmakers R, Kirkels WJ, Roobol MJ, et al. Complication rates and risk factors of 5802 transrectal ultrasound-guided sextant biopsies of the prostate within a population-based screening program. Urology 2002;60(5):826–30.
26. Djavan B, Waldert M, Zlotta A, et al. Safety and morbidity of first and repeat transrectal ultrasound guided prostate needle biopsies: results of a prospective European prostate cancer detection study [review]. J Urol 2001;166(3):856–60.
27. Haas GP, Delongchamps NB, Jones RF, et al. Needle biopsies on autopsy prostates: sensitivity of cancer detection based on true prevalence. J Natl Cancer Inst 2007;99(19):1484–9.
28. Seitz M, Gratzke C, Schlenker B, et al. Contrast-enhanced transrectal ultrasound (CE-TRUS) with cadence-contrast pulse sequence (CPS) technology for the identification of prostate cancer. Urol Oncol 2009. [Epub ahead of print].
29. Shimizu T, Nishie A, Ro T, et al. Prostate cancer detection: the value of performing an MRI before a biopsy. Acta Radiol 2009;50(9):1080–8.
30. Boyle P, Brawley OW. Prostate cancer: current evidence weighs against population screening. CA Cancer J Clin 2009;59(4):220–4.

31. U.S. Census Bureau, statistical abstract of the United States: 2009 (128th edition). Washington, DC; 2008. Table 103: expectation of life and expected deaths by race, sex, and age: 2005. Available at: http://www.census.gov/compendia/statab/tables/09s0103.pdf. Accessed October 10, 2009.
32. Nguyen PL, Chen MH, Renshaw AA, et al. Survival following radiation and androgen suppression therapy for prostate cancer in healthy older men: implications for screening recommendations. Int J Radiat Oncol Biol Phys 2009. [Epub ahead of print].
33. Shappley WV 3rd, Kenfield SA, Kasperzyk JL, et al. Prospective study of determinants and outcomes of deferred treatment or watchful waiting among men with prostate cancer in a nationwide cohort. J Clin Oncol 2009;27(30):4980–5.

Chemoprevention of Prostate Cancer

Andrew J. Stephenson, MD[a,*], Robert Abouassaly, MD[b], Eric A. Klein, MD[a]

KEYWORDS

- Chemoprevention • Prostatic neoplasms
- Testosterone 5α-reductase • Finasteride
- Dutasteride • Micronutrients • Vitamins
- Hydroxymethylglutaryl-CoA reductase inhibitors

In 2009, an estimated 192,000 men will be diagnosed with prostate cancer and over 27,000 will die from this disease.[1] The ubiquity and mortality of prostate cancer make it an attractive and appropriate target for primary chemoprevention. Numerous observations in the epidemiologic literature suggest associations between various dietary and lifestyle factors and the risk for developing prostate cancer. However, many of the risk factors for prostate cancer (age, ethnicity, and genetic factors) are not modifiable, and as much as 40% of the risk of the disease is estimated to be genetic. Given the incidence, prevalence, disease-related mortality, substantial cost of treatment, and treatment-related morbidity of prostate cancer, chemoprevention has become an important public health approach to reduce the mortality and burden of therapy for this disease.

Chemoprevention is defined as the use of specific natural or synthetic agents to reverse, suppress, or prevent the carcinogenic process thereby preventing the development of clinically evident cancer. Primary chemoprevention targets the general population of healthy individuals at risk to prevent the development of prostate cancer. Secondary prevention strategies target individuals with premalignant lesions (eg, high-grade prostate epithelial neoplasia [HGPIN]) with the goal of preventing progression to frank cancer. Tertiary prevention aims to prevent the development of a second primary cancer in an affected individual. The challenge of primary chemoprevention is finding an effective intervention that has acceptable toxicity and cost as well as identifying a population of individuals at sufficiently increased risk for developing prostate cancer for which chemoprevention is appropriate and cost-effective.

Enthusiasm for chemoprevention of prostate cancer has heightened in recent years with the publication of several large, randomized trials (namely the Prostate Cancer Prevention Trial [PCPT]), demonstrating that this disease may be prevented by a relatively nontoxic oral agent.[2] However, the failure to alter the incidence of prostate cancer using selenium and vitamin E in the Selenium and Vitamin E Cancer Prevention Trial (SELECT) is a reminder that chemopreventive strategies supported by strong epidemiologic and biologic rationale may not always be effective.[3] A listing of the completed and ongoing primary and secondary chemoprevention trials is listed in **Table 1**. Epidemiologic evidence suggests the existence of several other pharmacologic agents and nutritional supplements that appear promising for large-scale studies. It is conceivable that these agents may be useful in different populations.

[a] Glickman Urological and Kidney Institute, Cleveland Clinic, 9500 Euclid Avenue, Desk Q10-1, Cleveland, OH 44195-0001, USA
[b] Division of Urology, Princess Margaret Hospital, University of Toronto, 610 University Avenue, Toronto, ON M5G 2M9, Canada
* Corresponding author.
E-mail address: stephea2@ccf.org (A.J. Stephenson).

Urol Clin N Am 37 (2010) 11–21
doi:10.1016/j.ucl.2009.11.003
0094-0143/10/$ – see front matter

Table 1
Completed and ongoing primary and secondary chemoprevention trials in prostate cancer

Trial	Risk Group	Agent	Target	Results
Prostate Cancer Prevention Trial	Low (PSA level <3.0 ng/mL)	Finasteride	Type I 5α-reductase	Updated 2008
Selenium and Vitamin E Cancer Prevention Trial	Low (PSA level <4.0 ng/mL)	Selenium, vitamin E	Oxidative stress	Reported 2008
Reduction by Dutasteride of Prostate Cancer Events Trial	Intermediate (PSA level, 2.5–10 ng/mL)	Dutasteride	Type I and II 5α-reductase	Reported 2009
Southwest Oncology Group 9917	High (HGPIN)	Selenium	Selenium-mediated effects	2010
Toremifene	High (HGPIN)	Toremifene	Estrogen receptor	2010
National Cancer Institute of Canada	High (HGPIN)	Selenium, vitamin E, soy protein	Oxidative stress	

RATIONALE FOR CHEMOPREVENTION OF PROSTATE CANCER

Biologic Rationale

The molecular pathogenesis of prostate cancer lends itself to a primary prevention strategy. Prostate carcinogenesis is a multistep process induced by genetic and epigenetic changes that disrupt molecular pathways involved in cell proliferation, differentiation, apoptosis, and senescence. Several precursor lesions for prostate cancer have been described (HGPIN, proliferative inflammatory atrophy, and atypical small acinar neoplasia), which possess many genetic changes that are present in prostate cancer and represent intermediate stages between normal and malignant epithelium.[4] These lesions may appear as early as 20 years before the appearance of clinically evident cancer, suggesting that the development of prostate cancer occurs over a protracted time interval. In theory, the prolonged carcinogenesis of prostate cancer provides an opportunity to intervene before a malignancy is established.

Clinical Rationale

Mortality from prostate cancer may be reduced through early detection, prevention, and improvements in local and systemic therapy. The limitations of screening for prostate cancer were highlighted with the publication of 2 randomized trials in the United States (Prostate Lung Colorectal and Ovarian Cancer Screening Trial [PLCO]) and Europe (European Randomized Study of Screening for Prostate Cancer [ERSPC]).[5,6] ERSPC randomized 162,433 men from 7 countries to screening at 4-year intervals versus no screening and reported a significant increase in the incidence of prostate cancer (8.2% vs 4.8%) and a 20% relative risk reduction in prostate cancer–specific mortality at 10 years.[6] However, the investigators highlighted the problem of overdiagnosis with mass screening, as they estimated 48 men would need to be treated to prevent 1 death from prostate cancer at 10 years. In the PLCO trial, 76,693 men were randomized to annual screening versus no screening, and no significant difference in prostate cancer–specific mortality was reported.[5] The PLCO trial has been criticized for substantial contamination of screening in the control, the low rate of prostate biopsy in men with indications for biopsy, and the low-risk nature of both populations at the time of randomization.[5,7]

The risk of overdiagnosis has been estimated using cancer incidence rates from ERSPC and Surveillance, Epidemiology and End Results (SEER) Program registry. In these studies, overdiagnosis is defined as detection of cancers that would have otherwise remained undetected throughout a man's lifetime in the absence of screening. Assuming annual screening beginning at age 55 years, the overdiagnosis rate of prostate cancer has been reported to be 30% to 50%.[8–10] If overdiagnosis is defined as the detection of nonlethal prostate cancer, an estimated 84% of detected cancers would represent overdiagnosis.[11] Based on these studies and the 2 randomized trials, prostate-specific antigen (PSA) screening is associated with (at best) a slight reduction in prostate cancer–specific mortality with a substantial risk of overdiagnosis.

Whereas the urologic community recognizes the overdiagnosis of prostate cancer at the population level, a diagnosis of prostate cancer in the United States generally leads to radical therapy of some form. The safety and feasibility of active surveillance has been demonstrated in several cohorts with low reported overall and cause-specific mortality with 10 years of follow-up.[12] However, it is not widely embraced because of concerns that clinical staging and grading will underestimate the threat posed by cancers. In the United States, only 5% of low-risk patients choose active surveillance (including only 9% of men meeting the Epstein criteria for insignificant cancer),[13] and an estimated 73% of those who do ultimately opt for radical therapy within 4 years.[14–16] More than 70% of elderly men aged 65 to 80 years with low- and intermediate-risk prostate cancer received some form of therapy (surgery, radiation, or hormonal therapy) in a recent population-based study.[17] Given the protracted natural history of screen-detected cancers, it is unlikely that many of these men benefited from treatment in terms of preventing metastasis and death from prostate cancer.

The burden of therapy for prostate cancer can also be measured by the effect of treatments on health-related quality of life (HRQOL). A recent study of complications after surgical therapy for localized disease in an unselected population-based cohort reported that at more than 18 months after radical prostatectomy, 8.4% of men were incontinent and 42% reported that their sexual performance was a moderate-to-large problem.[18] In a prospective cohort study that compared outcomes in patients 5 years after radiation or surgery with those in age-matched controls, the authors concluded that "declines in urinary and sexual function domains after diagnosis and treatment of localized cancer far exceeded any effects from aging…."[19] A multicenter, prospective, longitudinal study assessing HRQOL after local therapy found that all treatments had a significant effect on urinary, sexual, bowel, and/or hormonal function.[20]

Two randomized trials have demonstrated that radical therapy (radical prostatectomy and external-beam radiotherapy) can significantly alter the natural history of prostate cancer in men diagnosed in the absence of screening.[21,22] In an update of the Scandinavian Prostate Cancer Group-4 randomized trial of radical prostatectomy versus watchful waiting, a 5.4% absolute reduction in prostate cancer–specific mortality at 12 years was observed with radical prostatectomy (12.5% vs 17.9%).[21] However, this study demonstrates that 70% of men with a lethal form of prostate cancer will ultimately die from prostate cancer despite radical local therapy.

It seems self-evident that an effective prevention strategy would spare many men the burden of diagnosis and cure and reduce the overdiagnosis problem associated with widespread opportunistic PSA screening. When combined with aggressive early detection and treatment, chemoprevention also has the potential to reduce the mortality from prostate cancer, which remains the second leading cause of cancer deaths among men in the United States.

CHEMOPREVENTION TRIALS IN PROSTATE CANCER

5α-Reductase Inhibitors

Prostate Cancer Prevention Trial

PCPT was the first large-scale primary chemoprevention trial in men at risk for prostate cancer.[2] The study randomized 18,882 men aged 55 years or older with a normal digital rectal examination (DRE) and a PSA level of 3.0 ng/mL or less to finasteride, 5 mg/d, or placebo for 7 years. The rationale for finasteride (a selective type II 5α-reductase inhibitor [5ARI]) as a chemopreventive agent is based on the absence of prostate cancer in men with congenital deficiency of 5α-reductase (the enzyme that converts testosterone to dihydrotestosterone) and the critical role of androgens in the development of prostate cancer. In PCPT, prostate biopsy was recommended at the end of study for all participants or for those "on-trial" if men had a PSA level of 4 ng/mL or more (adjusted for the effect of finasteride) or an abnormal DRE. The primary end point was the prevalence of prostate cancer during the 7 years of the study, as diagnosed by biopsy for-cause or end-of-study biopsy. Ultimately, 9060 participants (48%) were evaluable for the primary endpoint.

The main finding of PCPT was a 25% (95% confidence interval [CI], 19–31) reduction in the period prevalence of prostate cancer in men randomized to daily finasteride (18.4%) compared with placebo (24.4%). The relative benefit of finasteride versus placebo in reducing the risk of prostate cancer was apparent across all groups defined by age (55–59, 60–64, and ≥65 years at randomization), ethnicity (white, black, Hispanic, other), family history of prostate cancer, and PSA level at the beginning of the study (≤1, 1.1–2, and 2.1–3 ng/mL), with hazard ratios (HRs) between 0.66 and 0.81. The risk reduction in the finasteride arm was seen in both clinically apparent tumors (those diagnosed "for cause" because of an elevated PSA or abnormal DRE) and end-of-study biopsies (men with PSA level <4.0 ng/mL and normal DRE at study termination). Finasteride also reduced the risk of HGPIN (without associated prostate cancer) compared with placebo (HR, 0.85; 95% CI, 0.73–0.99; P = .04).[23] However, a significant increase in the prevalence biopsy Gleason score 7 to 10 cancers was observed in men receiving finasteride (280 [37%]) compared with placebo (237 [22%]), particularly for biopsy Gleason score 8 to 10 cancers (90 [12%] in the finasteride arm vs 53 [5%] in the placebo arm). There were an equal number of deaths resulting from prostate cancer (5) in each study arm. Sexual side effects were also more common with finasteride, whereas urinary symptoms were more common with placebo.

Several relevant observations can be made about the results of the trial. Most surprising was the 24.4% prevalence of prostate cancer in the placebo arm, 4 times higher than the 6% assumed for the trial design. This discrepancy can be explained by the fact that the 6% assumption was based on SEER incidence estimates, which are derived from clinically evident cases, and not on the prevalence in men with PSA level less than 4 ng/mL and normal DRE who underwent biopsy. The incidence of clinically evident cancers detected "for cause" by elevations in PSA levels or abnormal PSA was 7.2% at 7 years, similar to the incidence of cancer in the screening arms of ERSPC (8.2%) and PLCO (7.4%).[5,6] Another observation was a marked effect of finasteride on the prevalence of biopsy Gleason score 2 to 6 tumors, no effect on the prevalence of biopsy Gleason score 7 tumors, and a slight increase in the prevalence of biopsy Gleason score 8 to 10 tumors. The higher incidence of biopsy Gleason score 8 to 10 tumors was restricted to those men undergoing for-cause biopsy, although this is partly explained by the low prevalence of these high-grade cancers in men with PSA level less than 4.0 ng/mL and with normal DRE (20 of 3652 in finasteride arm vs 8 of 3820 in placebo arm).

Secondary analyses of the PCPT have demonstrated an overall improved sensitivity of DRE and a higher accuracy of PSA for the diagnosis of prostate cancer in the finasteride arm.[24,25] Finasteride-treated glands were also 28% smaller on average compared with those in the placebo arm.[2] Data suggest that having a smaller prostate enhanced the detection of cancer and proportionately more diagnosed cancers are high-grade.[26] These effects of finasteride on the detection of prostate cancer should bias PCPT in favor of the placebo arm and lead to a greater detection of all grades of prostate cancer with finasteride, further strengthening the results of the trial.

Following the original publication of PCPT, there were 2 areas of intense debate over the trial's findings. The first was that critics argue that finasteride prevents insignificant cancers and does little to prevent potentially lethal cancers. This criticism was based on the fact that the incidence of cancers in control arm (24.4%) was significantly higher than a man's lifetime risk of developing prostate cancer (18%) and 4 times higher than the cancer incidence in screening trials over a similar period. Finasteride also reduced the prevalence of low-grade cancers and did not appear to reduce the risk of high-grade cancers. However, in a secondary analysis of 93.4% of biopsy specimens that were subject to central pathology review, the rate of insignificant cancers (as defined by the Epstein criteria[13]) among the biopsy Gleason 2 to 6 cancers detected in the finasteride (38%) and placebo arms (36%) was not significantly different.[27] Most of the cancers detected in PCPT were clinically significant (80% in finasteride arm and 72% in the placebo arm). Viewed in the context of clinical relevance as defined by current urologic practice, preventing biopsy Gleason 2 to 6 cancers by finasteride also prevents the anxiety, cost, and morbidity associated with their treatment. From a public health perspective, preventing the burden of cure in newly diagnosed patients should be added as a positive to the 25% reduction in risk of diagnosis and significant reduction in urinary symptoms associated with finasteride use.

The second question raised by PCPT was whether finasteride induces the development of high-grade or aggressive cancers. Androgen deprivation therapy is known to change the appearance of prostatic epithelium in a way that could bias interpretation.[28] Thus, the apparent increase in high-grade cancers in men treated with finasteride may be an artifact of these morphologic changes. However, when this was examined in PCPT, there appeared to be no morphologic effect of finasteride on prostate cancer grading when specimens were reviewed by a panel of expert pathologists blinded to treatment arm.[29] Another potential explanation for the observed increase in high-grade tumors in the finasteride group is ascertainment bias. As stated earlier, finasteride has been shown to increase the sensitivity of PSA and DRE and to decrease prostate volume by 28%, leading to a higher probability of finding the high-grade component of cancer (among men with pathologic Gleason 7–10 cancer) on biopsy. Indeed, the rate of upgrading from biopsy Gleason score 2 to 6 to pathologic Gleason score 7 to 10 among men treated by radical prostatectomy was higher in the placebo arm compared with the finasteride arm.[27]

If finasteride induces high-grade cancers, one would expect a higher proportion of cancers with adverse features by biopsy criteria or at radical prostatectomy in the finasteride arm. No significant difference in the proportion of cancers with perineural invasion, length of cancer in biopsy specimens, and bilaterality of cancer on biopsy was identified between the arms, and men on finasteride with biopsy Gleason 2 to 7 cancers had fewer positive biopsy scores compared with men on placebo.[27,29] Among the 528 men who were treated by radical prostatectomy, no significant difference in the rate of extraprostatic extension, seminal vesicle invasion, or lymph node metastasis was observed between the 2 arms, and there were fewer pathologic Gleason 7 to 10 cancers among men treated with finasteride versus placebo (89 vs 105).

In a secondary analysis of PCPT that adjusted for the effects of finasteride on the detection of prostate cancer, the adjusted prostate cancer rates were estimated to be 21.1% in the placebo group and 14.7% in the finasteride group, a 30% risk reduction for all cancers (HR, 0.70; 95% CI, 0.64–0.76) and a nonstatistically significant 14% increase in high-grade cancer.[30] Accounting for the increased probability of upgrading to pathologic Gleason 7 to 10 cancer at radical prostatectomy among men with biopsy Gleason 2 to 6 cancers in the placebo arm, the investigators estimated the rate of true high-grade cancer to be 6% in the finasteride arm and 8.2% in the placebo arm, representing a 27% relative risk reduction in the rate of true high-grade cancers in men treated with finasteride (HR, 0.73; 95% CI, 0.56–0.96). Using different methodology in an independent analysis, Pinsky and colleagues[31] concurred that the rate of true high-grade disease may have been lower in the finasteride group compared with the placebo group.

Although the concerns raised by the original publication of PCPT regarding the apparent increased risk of high-grade cancer in men receiving finasteride were valid,[32] these subsequent studies indicate that finasteride does not induce the development of Gleason 7 to 10 cancers and may reduce a man's risk of high-grade cancer. In March 2009, the American Urological Association and the American Society of Clinical Oncology jointly published guidelines based on expert review of the available evidence stating that use of finasteride for the prevention of cancer should be discussed with at-risk men.[33]

In addition to the prevention of prostate cancer, 5ARIs have other benefits that need to be considered. As mentioned earlier, finasteride improves the sensitivity of PSA and DRE for prostate cancer detection.[24,25] Furthermore, randomized, placebo-controlled trials of men with symptomatic benign prostatic hyperplasia (BPH) have demonstrated that finasteride reduces the severity of lower urinary tract symptoms, risk of acute urinary retention, and need for surgical intervention.[34,35]

On the other hand, adverse effects more common with finasteride than placebo include impaired sexual or erectile function and endocrine effects. Pooled data from randomized trials indicate absolute differences of 2% (95% CI, 1–2) for gynecomastia, 3% (95% CI, 1–6) for decreased libido, 4% (95% CI, 1%–8%) for erectile dysfunction, and 4% (95% CI, 8–17) for reduced volume of ejaculate.[36] Sexual dysfunction was also assessed in the PCPT participants during the 7-year trial period using the Sexual Activity Scale. Compared with baseline scores, over the course of 7 years finasteride was associated with a slight increase in sexual dysfunction relative to placebo, equivalent to about half the effect of being 6.5 years older at randomization.[37]

Reduction by Dutasteride of Prostate Cancer Events Trial

The REDUCE (Reduction by Dutasteride of Prostate Cancer Events) trial is another large-scale, randomized, placebo-controlled primary chemoprevention trial using a different 5ARI called dutasteride, which is an inhibitor of both type 1 and type 2 isoforms of 5ARI. Dutasteride has been shown to reduce the risk of prostate cancer in men treated for lower urinary tract symptoms related to BPH compared with placebo.[38] The REDUCE trial completed accrual in 2005, and the initial results have been presented in abstract form only at this time.[39] Eligibility for REDUCE included men with a prior negative prostate biopsy within 6 months of enrollment who were aged 50 to 75 years and had baseline PSA levels of 2.5 to 10 ng/mL and prostate volume of 80 cm^3 or less. The primary endpoint of REDUCE is the prevalence of cancer on study-mandated prostate biopsies performed at 2 and 4 years after randomization.

The trial accrued 8231 men, of which 6726 (82.6%) underwent at least 1 biopsy and 1516 (22.5%) were diagnosed with prostate cancer. Dutasteride reduced the risk of prostate cancer during 4 years by 23% (857 in the placebo arm vs 659 in the dutasteride arm, $P<.001$). Interestingly, no significant increase in biopsy Gleason 8 to 10 cancers was observed in the study (19 in placebo vs 29 in dutasteride, $P = .15$). As with finasteride in PCPT, the benefit of dutasteride in prostate cancer risk versus placebo was apparent across all subgroups, including age (<65 vs ≥65 years), family history, and PSA level at study entry (relative risk reduction, 22%–32%). Dutasteride also demonstrated beneficial effects on BPH outcomes (acute urinary retention and BPH-related surgery) and was generally well tolerated (15% drug-related adverse events in placebo vs 22% in dutasteride arm).

PCPT and REDUCE confirm the consistency of the effect of 5ARI at reducing the risk of prostate cancer, with a similar magnitude of risk reduction across all subgroups without any apparent increase in the risk of high-grade cancers. The fact that the results of the REDUCE trial were congruent with those of the PCPT with respect to the magnitude of risk reduction, benefits on BPH endpoints, minimal toxicity, and absence of issues related to tumor grade suggest that 5ARIs represent an effective primary prevention strategy and these agents should be used more liberally for prevention of prostate cancer. However, deciding whether or not the advantages outweigh the potential disadvantages of 5ARI for prostate cancer chemoprevention is not a simple task (**Table 2**). A recently published decision analysis model for 5ARIs as chemopreventive agents found that widespread use of these agents are unlikely to be cost-effective because of the usually indolent natural history of treated prostate cancer, but these agents may be cost-effective in high-risk populations.[40]

Vitamins and Micronutrients

Selenium and Vitamin E Cancer Prevention Trial

SELECT was a randomized, placebo-controlled, population-based primary chemoprevention trial designed to test the efficacy of selenium and vitamin E alone and in combination in the prevention of prostate cancer.[41] The rationale for selenium was based on a secondary analysis of the Nutritional Prevention of Cancer Trial of oral selenized yeast for nonmelanoma skin cancer, in which men randomized to selenium versus placebo had a 65% reduction in the prostate cancer incidence during a mean follow-up of 4.5 years.[42] Selenium is an essential trace element occurring in both organic and inorganic forms, with marked geographic variability of selenium in food related to local soil content.

The rationale for vitamin E as chemopreventive agent for prostate cancer was based on the Alpha-Tocopherol, Beta-Carotene Cancer Prevention (ATBC) trial for lung cancer incidence and mortality, in which male smokers were randomized to alpha-tocopherol (50 mg/d) and beta carotene (20 mg/d) alone or in combination versus placebo.[43] On secondary analysis, the ATBC trial found a statistically significant 32% reduction in prostate cancer incidence in those receiving alpha-tocopherol.[44] Vitamin E is a family of naturally occurring, essential, fat-soluble vitamin compounds, which functions as the major lipid-soluble antioxidant in cell membranes. The most active form of vitamin E is alpha-tocopherol; it is also among the most abundant, is widely distributed in nature, and the predominant form in human tissues. Alpha-tocopherol may influence the development of cancer through several mechanisms, including induction of cell cycle arrest and through direct antiandrogen activity.

The SELECT was the largest cancer prevention trial ever performed, and it randomized 35,533 men to 4 treatment arms (selenium + placebo, vitamin E + placebo, selenium + vitamin E, and placebo + placebo).[3] Eligibility criteria included age 50 years or more for African Americans, 55

Table 2
Outline of advantages and disadvantages of the use of 5ARIs for the chemoprevention of prostate cancer

Advantages	Disadvantages
23%–30% reduction in risk of prostate cancer	No proven effect on mortality
May reduce risk of Gleason 7–10 cancers	May increase risk of Gleason 7–10 cancers
Reduction of overdiagnosis and overtreatment (burden of cure)	Increased sexual side effects
20% reduction in risk of HGPIN	Cost
Improves the performance of PSA and DRE for early detection of prostate cancer	
Reduces symptoms, complications, surgical interventions for BPH	

years or more for Caucasians, a DRE not suspicious for cancer, serum PSA level of 4 ng/mL or less, and normal blood pressure. The primary endpoint was biopsy-confirmed prostate cancer, although the indications for biopsy were not dictated by protocol. Although the study duration was planned for 12 years, the independent data and safety monitoring committee recommended discontinuation of the study after the second interim analysis at 7 years because the data convincingly demonstrated no effect on the risk of prostate cancer by either agent alone or in combination and no chance of a beneficial effect of the hypothesized magnitude with continued supplementation.[3] HRs for prostate cancer were 1.13 (99% CI, 0.95–1.13) for vitamin E, 1.04 (99% CI, 0.87–1.24) for selenium, and 1.05 (99% CI, 0.88–1.25) for selenium and vitamin E. Secondary analyses also showed no effect on the risks of lung, colorectal, or overall cancer incidence, no effect on cardiovascular events, and no effect on overall survival.

Null results for the effect of vitamin E on prostate cancer risk were also reported in the Physicians' Health Study II, a randomized trial of vitamin E (400 IU every other day) and vitamin C (500 mg/d) versus placebo in the prevention of prostate and other cancers.[45] Together, these results suggest that neither selenium nor vitamin E should be used in the hope of preventing prostate or other cancers.

Other Agents

Selective estrogen receptor modulators

Selective estrogen receptor modulators (SERMs) possess both agonistic and antagonistic estrogen-like activity and have been shown to repress prostate cancer growth in several transgenic mouse models. In the transgenic adenocarcinoma of mouse prostate (TRAMP) model, toremifene reduces the incidence of HGPIN and cancer in an estrogen-dependent, androgen-independent mechanism. Toremifene is currently approved for the management of breast cancer and was tested in a phase 2b trial for decreasing the prostate cancer risk in which 514 men with HGPIN were randomized to toremifene, 20, 40, or 60 mg/d, or placebo.[46] Although the 40- and 60-mg doses did not affect the risk of prostate cancer, the 20-mg dose was associated with a 48% decrease in the risk of prostate cancer at 12 months. A phase 3 trial is currently ongoing to assess toremifene's activity against HGPIN and prostate cancer incidence.

Soy

Legumes play an important role in the traditional diets of Asian countries where the incidence of prostate cancer is low, but they play only a minor role in diet of the West where the incidence is highest worldwide. Soybeans are unique among the legumes because they are a concentrated source of isoflavones, which have weak estrogenic activity. The major isoflavone components of soy, including genistein, daidzein, and their metabolites, inhibit benign and malignant prostatic epithelial cell growth, downregulate androgen-regulated genes, and reduce tumor growth in animals. Migration studies and lower prostate cancer rates in Asian men with higher soy intake also support the role of soy as an anticancer agent. A combination of vitamin E, selenium, and soy protein is being investigated in a randomized phase 2, placebo-controlled secondary chemoprevention trial in men with HGPIN, and this study is funded by the National Cancer Institute of Canada.

Lycopene

Lycopene is a red-orange carotenoid found primarily in tomatoes and tomato-derived products and other red fruits and vegetables. Lycopene is a highly unsaturated acyclic isomer of beta carotene, is the predominant carotenoid in human plasma, and possesses potent antioxidant activity. There is mixed epidemiologic evidence that lycopene consumption is associated with a lower risk of prostate cancer.[47] A nested case-control study in PLCO prospectively examined the intake of more than 25 tomato-containing foods by 29,361 men and found no correlation with the incidence of prostate cancer.[48] Currently, no phase 3 trials examining the role of lycopene in prostate cancer prevention are being conducted.

Green tea (Camellia sinensis)

Green tea has been suggested to prevent prostate cancer based on epidemiologic observations of a low incidence of prostate cancer among Asians with a high dietary intake. Previous work has focused on the effects of polyphenols (ie, flavanols, also know as catechins), which account for 30% to 40% of extractable solids from dried green tea leaves. In vitro studies of (−)-epigallocatechin-3-gallate (the major polyphenolic constituent of green tea) have shown that it induces apoptosis, cell-growth inhibition, and cell cycle dysregulation of prostate cancer. In a small randomized, placebo-controlled, secondary chemoprevention trial of green tea catechin tablets in 60 men with HGPIN, 9 men in the placebo arm were diagnosed with prostate cancer at 1 year compared with only 1 in the treatment group.[49] Confirmatory trials are needed to better assess the role of green tea consumption in the prevention of prostate cancer.

Statins

Statins are widely used cholesterol-lowering drugs given for the treatment and prevention of atherosclerotic cardiovascular disease. They inhibit 3-hydroxy-3-methylglutaryl coenzyme A (HMG-CoA), the rate-limiting enzyme in cholesterol biosynthesis. Statins may prevent the development of prostate cancer through anti-inflammatory effects, inhibiting angiogenesis, altering steroid hormone biosynthesis or metabolism, cell cycle regulation, or promoting apoptosis.[50] Several observational studies have shown an inverse association between statin use and risk of prostate cancer,[51–53] although others found no association,[54,55] and 2 studies showed an increase in overall prostate cancer risk.[56,57] Randomized trials of the use of statin to prevent cardiovascular disease reported no association with prostate cancer incidence, although such trials were limited by short durations of statin use, brief follow-up periods, and relatively young participants who develop few cancers.[58–60] A meta-analysis of 6 randomized clinical trials, 6 cohort studies, and 7 case-control studies found no association between statin use and overall prostate cancer incidence but did find a protective association with advanced prostate cancer (HR, 0.77; 95% CI, 0.64–0.93).[61] This finding suggests an effect of statins at a late stage in carcinogenesis (eg, tumor progression). Long-term statin users are generally healthier and more adherent to therapy and to screening for disease (and possibly earlier prostate cancer detection) than nonusers. Long-term statin users are generally healthier and more adherent to therapy and screening (leading to possibly earlier detection of prostate cancer) than non-users. Statin users have been shown to have lower serum PSA levels than nonusers.[62] Although this result suggests an anticancer effect, decreased PSA levels could reduce the apparent incidence of prostate cancer in statin users, as there would be fewer individuals with elevated PSA levels to prompt prostate biopsy. Further research is needed to help determine the role, if any, of statins in the prevention of prostate cancer. The unexpected, nonstatistically significant increase in prostate cancer risk in men taking vitamin E in SELECT should caution against the use of statins as chemopreventive agents until there is evidence of a benefit from randomized trials.

CHEMOPREVENTION AND PROSTATE CANCER RISK

A framework for the implementation of preventive strategies for prostate cancer based on an individual's risk and the preventive treatment used is illustrated in **Fig. 1**. For men at low risk of prostate cancer, lifestyle modification, dietary changes, and/or administration of vitamins and micronutrients are appropriate interventions because of the low cost and risk. However, no specific lifestyle modification, vitamin, or micronutrient has been proven to reduce a man's risk of prostate cancer. For higher-risk patients, chemoprevention with pharmacologic agents may be appropriate, as the risk of prostate cancer may justify the cost and potential side effects of these agents. Currently, there is no group at sufficiently increased risk of prostate cancer to justify definitive local therapy as a prophylactic measure.

Patients with HGPIN are at a sufficiently increased risk of prostate cancer to justify chemoprevention with 5ARIs,[23] although the prognostic significance of HGPIN for prostate cancer detection in heavily screened populations has been questioned.[63] Other high-risk groups include those with elevated PSA levels, rapid PSA velocity, sub-Saharan African ethnicity, or family history of prostate cancer. The risk of prostate cancer and high-grade cancer can be accurately calculated for the individual patient based on his age, ethnicity, family history, baseline PSA level, DRE findings, prior prostate biopsy history, and use of 5ARIs.[64] Changes in PSA levels early in life may be prognostic for the long-term risk of prostate cancer and may be used to identify a cohort at sufficiently increased risk to justify pharmacologic chemoprevention. In a population-based study from Malmö, Sweden, of 21,277 men younger than 50 years enrolled from 1974 to 1986, a PSA level of more than 1 ng/mL at age 44 to 50 years was associated with a 3.7 times increased risk of prostate cancer and 7 to 22 times increased risk of advanced disease (clinical stage T3 or greater or bone metastasis) by age 75 years.[65,66] In an

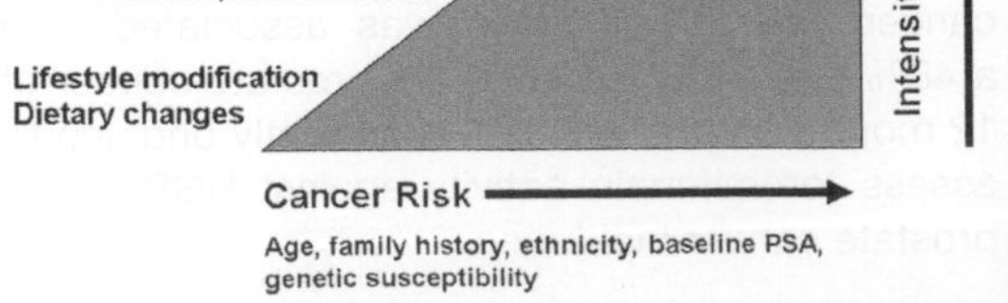

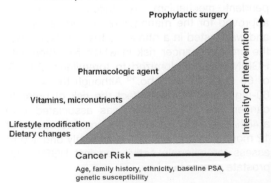

Fig. 1. Framework for the prevention of prostate cancer based on a man's risk of developing the disease and the intensity of the chemopreventive strategy.

update of its clinical practice guidelines for PSA, the American Urological Association now recommends a baseline PSA level at age 40 years.[67] Genome-wide association studies have also identified allelic variants associated with prostate cancer risk that may be used to identify appropriate candidates for chemoprevention. Zheng and colleagues[68] used 5 single-nucleotide polymorphisms (SNPs) in 5 chromosomal regions (3 at 8q24, 17q12, 17q24.3) to build a multivariable model for prostate cancer that included age, geographic region, and family history. The relative risk of prostate cancer in men with all 5 SNPs was 4.5 and 9.5, respectively, in men without and with a family history of prostate cancer. The cumulative effect of these genetic variants and family history was independent of PSA levels at diagnosis.

SUMMARY

Prostate cancer is an attractive target for chemoprevention because of its ubiquity, potential lethality, treatment-related morbidity, long latency between premalignant lesions and clinically evident cancer, and defined molecular pathogenesis. The PCPT and REDUCE trials represent the first firm evidence that this cancer can be prevented by a relatively nontoxic oral agent. 5ARIs represent an effective primary prevention strategy, and these agents should be used more liberally for prevention of prostate cancer, particularly in high-risk patients. The current body of evidence argues against routine recommendation of any nutritional supplement for the prevention of prostate cancer. The dietary factors that may contribute to the development of prostate cancer are complex, and there is currently little evidence that specific dietary manipulations may significantly alter a man's risk for this cancer.[69]

REFERENCES

1. Jemal A, Siegel R, Ward E, et al. Cancer statistics, 2009. CA Cancer J Clin 2009;59(4):225–49.
2. Thompson IM, Goodman PJ, Tangen CM, et al. The influence of finasteride on the development of prostate cancer. N Engl J Med 2003;349(3):215–24.
3. Lippman SM, Klein EA, Goodman PJ, et al. Effect of selenium and vitamin E on risk of prostate cancer and other cancers: the selenium and vitamin E cancer prevention trial (SELECT). JAMA 2009; 301(1):39–51.
4. Nelson WG, De Marzo AM, Isaacs WB. Prostate cancer. N Engl J Med 2003;349(4):366–81.
5. Andriole GL, Grubb RL 3rd, Buys SS, et al. Mortality results from a randomized prostate-cancer screening trial. N Engl J Med 2009;260(13):1310–9.
6. Schroder FH, Hugosson J, Roobol MJ, et al. Screening and prostate-cancer mortality in a randomized European study. N Engl J Med 2009;360(13):1320–8.
7. Andriole GL, Levin DL, Crawford ED, et al. Prostate cancer screening in the prostate, lung, colorectal and ovarian (PLCO) cancer screening trial: findings from the initial screening round of a randomized trial. J Natl Cancer Inst 2005;97(6):433–8.
8. Draisma G, Boer R, Otto SJ, et al. Lead times and overdetection due to prostate-specific antigen screening: estimates from the European randomized study of screening for prostate cancer. J Natl Cancer Inst 2003;95(12):868–78.
9. Draisma G, Etzioni R, Tsodikov A, et al. Lead time and overdiagnosis in prostate-specific antigen screening: importance of methods and context. J Natl Cancer Inst 2009;101(6):374–83.
10. Etzioni R, Penson DF, Legler JM, et al. Overdiagnosis due to prostate-specific antigen screening: lessons from U.S. prostate cancer incidence trends. J Natl Cancer Inst 2002;94(13):981–90.
11. McGregor M, Hanley JA, Boivin JF, et al. Screening for prostate cancer: estimating the magnitude of overdetection. CMAJ 1998;159(11):1368–72.
12. Klotz L. Active surveillance for prostate cancer: for whom? J Clin Oncol 2005;23(32):8165–9.
13. Epstein JI, Walsh PC, Carmichael M, et al. Pathologic and clinical findings to predict tumor extent of nonpalpable (stage T1c) prostate cancer. JAMA 1994;271(5):368–74.
14. Harlan SR, Cooperberg MR, Elkin EP, et al. Time trends and characteristics of men choosing watchful waiting for initial treatment of localized prostate cancer: results from CaPSURE. J Urol 2003;170(5): 1804–7.
15. Barocas DA, Cowan JE, Smith JA Jr, et al. What percentage of patients with newly diagnosed carcinoma of the prostate are candidates for surveillance? An analysis of the CaPSURE database. J Urol 2008;180(4):1330–4 [discussion: 1334–5].
16. Carter CA, Donahue T, Sun L, et al. Temporarily deferred therapy (watchful waiting) for men younger than 70 years and with low-risk localized prostate cancer in the prostate-specific antigen era. J Clin Oncol 2003;21(21):4001–8.
17. Wong YN, Mitra N, Hudes G, et al. Survival associated with treatment vs observation of localized prostate cancer in elderly men. JAMA 2006;296(22): 2683–93.
18. Stanford JL, Feng Z, Hamilton AS, et al. Urinary and sexual function after radical prostatectomy for clinically localized prostate cancer: the Prostate Cancer Outcomes Study. JAMA 2000;283(3):354–60.
19. Hoffman RM, Gilliland FD, Penson DF, et al. Cross-sectional and longitudinal comparisons of health-related quality of life between patients with prostate

carcinoma and matched controls. Cancer 2004; 101(9):2011–9.
20. Sanda MG, Dunn RL, Michalski J, et al. Quality of life and satisfaction with outcome among prostate-cancer survivors. N Engl J Med 2008;358(12): 1250–61.
21. Bill-Axelson A, Holmberg L, Filen F, et al. Radical prostatectomy versus watchful waiting in localized prostate cancer: the Scandinavian prostate cancer group-4 randomized trial. J Natl Cancer Inst 2008; 100(16):1144–54.
22. Widmark A, Klepp O, Solberg A, et al. Endocrine treatment, with or without radiotherapy, in locally advanced prostate cancer (SPCG-7/SFUO-3): an open randomised phase III trial. Lancet 2009; 373(9660):301–8.
23. Thompson IM, Lucia MS, Redman MW, et al. Finasteride decreases the risk of prostatic intraepithelial neoplasia. J Urol 2007;178(1):107–9 [discussion: 110].
24. Thompson IM, Chi C, Ankerst DP, et al. Effect of finasteride on the sensitivity of PSA for detecting prostate cancer. J Natl Cancer Inst 2006;98(16): 1128–33.
25. Thompson IM, Tangen CM, Goodman PJ, et al. Finasteride improves the sensitivity of digital rectal examination for prostate cancer detection. J Urol 2007;177(5):1749–52.
26. Kulkarni GS, Al-Azab R, Lockwood G, et al. Evidence for a biopsy derived grade artifact among larger prostate glands. J Urol 2006;175(2):505–9.
27. Lucia MS, Darke AK, Goodman PJ, et al. Pathologic characteristics of cancers detected in the Prostate Cancer Prevention Trial: implications for prostate cancer detection and chemoprevention. Cancer Prev Res 2008;1(3):167–73.
28. Civantos F, Soloway MS, Pinto JE. Histopathological effects of androgen deprivation in prostatic cancer. Semin Urol Oncol 1996;14(2 Suppl 2):22–31.
29. Lucia MS, Epstein JI, Goodman PJ, et al. Finasteride and high-grade prostate cancer in the Prostate Cancer Prevention Trial. J Natl Cancer Inst 2007; 99(18):1375–83.
30. Redman MW, Tangen CM, Goodman PJ, et al. Finasteride does not increase the risk of high-grade prostate cancer: a bias-adjusted modeling approach. Cancer Prev Res 2008;1(3):174–81.
31. Pinsky P, Parnes H, Ford L. Estimating rates of true high-grade disease in the prostate cancer prevention trial. Cancer Prev Res (Phila Pa) 2008;1(3):182–6.
32. Scardino PT. The prevention of prostate cancer–the dilemma continues. N Engl J Med 2003;349(3): 297–9.
33. Kramer BS, Hagerty KL, Justman S, et al. Use of 5-alpha-reductase inhibitors for prostate cancer chemoprevention: American Society of Clinical Oncology/American Urological Association 2008 Clinical Practice Guideline. J Clin Oncol 2009; 27(9):1502–16.
34. McConnell JD, Bruskewitz R, Walsh P, et al. The effect of finasteride on the risk of acute urinary retention and the need for surgical treatment among men with benign prostatic hyperplasia. Finasteride long-term efficacy and safety study group. N Engl J Med 1998;338(9):557–63.
35. McConnell JD, Roehrborn CG, Bautista OM, et al. The long-term effect of doxazosin, finasteride, and combination therapy on the clinical progression of benign prostatic hyperplasia. N Engl J Med 2003; 349(25):2387–98.
36. Wilt TJ, MacDonald R, Hagerty K, et al. Five-alpha-reductase Inhibitors for prostate cancer prevention. Cochrane Database Syst Rev 2008;(2):CD007091.
37. Moinpour CM, Darke AK, Donaldson GW, et al. Longitudinal analysis of sexual function reported by men in the Prostate Cancer Prevention Trial. J Natl Cancer Inst 2007;99(13):1025–35.
38. Andriole GL, Roehrborn C, Schulman C, et al. Effect of dutasteride on the detection of prostate cancer in men with benign prostatic hyperplasia. Urology 2004;64(3):537–41 [discussion: 542–3].
39. Andriole G, Bostwick D, Brawley O, et al. The effect of dutasteride on prostate cancer risk reduction. J Urol 2009;181(Suppl 4) [Abstract LBA1:555].
40. Svatek RS, Lee JJ, Roehrborn CG, et al. Cost-effectiveness of prostate cancer chemoprevention: a quality of life-years analysis. Cancer 2008;112(5): 1058–65.
41. Lippman SM, Goodman PJ, Klein EA, et al. Designing the selenium and vitamin E cancer prevention trial (SELECT). J Natl Cancer Inst 2005; 97(2):94–102.
42. Clark LC, Combs GF Jr, Turnbull BW, et al. Effects of selenium supplementation for cancer prevention in patients with carcinoma of the skin. A randomized controlled trial. Nutritional prevention of cancer study group. JAMA 1996;276(24):1957–63.
43. The effect of vitamin E and beta carotene on the incidence of lung cancer and other cancers in male smokers. The alpha-tocopherol, beta carotene cancer prevention study group. N Engl J Med 1994;330(15):1029–35.
44. Albanes D, Heinonen OP, Huttunen JK, et al. Effects of alpha-tocopherol and beta-carotene supplements on cancer incidence in the alpha-tocopherol beta-carotene cancer prevention study. Am J Clin Nutr 1995;62(Suppl 6):1427S–30S.
45. Gaziano JM, Glynn RJ, Christen WG, et al. Vitamins E and C in the prevention of prostate and total cancer in men: the Physicians' Health Study II randomized controlled trial. JAMA 2009;301(1): 52–62.
46. Price D, Stein B, Sieber P, et al. Toremifene for the prevention of prostate cancer in men with high grade

prostatic intraepithelial neoplasia: results of a double-blind, placebo controlled, phase IIB clinical trial. J Urol 2006;176(3):965–70 [discussion: 970–1].
47. Giovannucci E. Tomatoes, tomato-based products, lycopene, and cancer: review of the epidemiologic literature. J Natl Cancer Inst 1999;91(4):317–31.
48. Peters U, Leitzmann MF, Chatterjee N, et al. Serum lycopene, other carotenoids, and prostate cancer risk: a nested case-control study in the prostate, lung, colorectal, and ovarian cancer screening trial. Cancer Epidemiol Biomarkers Prev 2007;16(5):962–8.
49. Bettuzzi S, Brausi M, Rizzi F, et al. Chemoprevention of human prostate cancer by oral administration of green tea catechins in volunteers with high-grade prostate intraepithelial neoplasia: a preliminary report from a one-year proof-of-principle study. Cancer Res 2006;66(2):1234–40.
50. Murtola TJ, Visakorpi T, Lahtela J, et al. Statins and prostate cancer prevention: where we are now, and future directions. Nat Clin Pract Urol 2008; 5(7):376–87.
51. Graaf MR, Beiderbeck AB, Egberts AC, et al. The risk of cancer in users of statins. J Clin Oncol 2004;22(12):2388–94.
52. Platz EA, Leitzmann MF, Visvanathan K, et al. Statin drugs and risk of advanced prostate cancer. J Natl Cancer Inst 2006;98(24):1819–25.
53. Shannon J, Tewoderos S, Garzotto M, et al. Statins and prostate cancer risk: a case-control study. Am J Epidemiol 2005;162(4):318–25.
54. Agalliu I, Salinas CA, Hansten PD, et al. Statin use and risk of prostate cancer: results from a population-based epidemiologic study. Am J Epidemiol 2008;168(3):250–60.
55. Flick ED, Habel LA, Chan KA, et al. Statin use and risk of prostate cancer in the California men's health study cohort. Cancer Epidemiol Biomarkers Prev 2007;16(11):2218–25.
56. Kaye JA, Jick H. Statin use and cancer risk in the general practice research database. Br J Cancer 2004;90(3):635–7.
57. Murtola TJ, Tammela TL, Lahtela J, et al. Cholesterol-lowering drugs and prostate cancer risk: a population-based case-control study. Cancer Epidemiol Biomarkers Prev 2007;16(11):2226–32.
58. Baigent C, Keech A, Kearney PM, et al. Efficacy and safety of cholesterol-lowering treatment: prospective meta-analysis of data from 90,056 participants in 14 randomised trials of statins. Lancet 2005;366(9493): 1267–78.
59. Browning DR, Martin RM. Statins and risk of cancer: a systematic review and metaanalysis. Int J Cancer 2007;120(4):833–43.
60. Dale KM, Coleman CI, Henyan NN, et al. Statins and cancer risk: a meta-analysis. JAMA 2006;295(1): 74–80.
61. Bonovas S, Filioussi K, Sitaras NM. Statin use and the risk of prostate cancer: a metaanalysis of 6 randomized clinical trials and 13 observational studies. Int J Cancer 2008;123(4):899–904.
62. Hamilton RJ, Goldberg KC, Platz EA, et al. The influence of statin medications on prostate-specific antigen levels. J Natl Cancer Inst 2008;100(21): 1511–8.
63. Epstein JI, Herawi M. Prostate needle biopsies containing prostatic intraepithelial neoplasia or atypical foci suspicious for carcinoma: implications for patient care. J Urol 2006;175(3 Pt 1):820–34.
64. Thompson IM, Ankerst DP, Chi C, et al. Assessing prostate cancer risk: results from the prostate cancer prevention trial. J Natl Cancer Inst 2006; 98(8):529–34.
65. Lilja H, Ulmert D, Bjork T, et al. Long-term prediction of prostate cancer up to 25 years before diagnosis of prostate cancer using prostate kallikreins measured at age 44 to 50 years. J Clin Oncol 2007;25(4):431–6.
66. Ulmert D, Cronin AM, Bjork T, et al. Prostate-specific antigen at or before age 50 as a predictor of advanced prostate cancer diagnosed up to 25 years later: a case-control study. BMC Med 2008;6:6.
67. Greene KL, Albertsen PC, Babaian RJ, et al. Prostate specific antigen best practice statement: 2009 update. J Urol 2009;182(5):2232–41.
68. Zheng SL, Sun J, Wiklund F, et al. Cumulative association of five genetic variants with prostate cancer. N Engl J Med 2008;358(9):910–9.
69. Freedland SJ, Aronson WJ. Dietary intervention strategies to modulate prostate cancer risk and prognosis. Curr Opin Urol 2009;19(3):263–7.

Update on Prostate Imaging

Jalil Afnan, MD, Clare M. Tempany, MD*

KEYWORDS

• MRI • DCE • DWI • Spectroscopy • Biomarkers

Successful and accurate imaging of prostate cancer is integral to its clinical management from detection and staging to subsequent monitoring. Various modalities are used including ultrasound, computed tomography, and magnetic resonance imaging, with the greatest advances seen in the field of magnetic resonance.

ULTRASOUND

Since the introduction of grayscale transrectal ultrasound imaging for prostate cancer in the late 1960s,[1] technical developments have improved image quality. However, in conjunction with biopsy, it remains a test with widely variable sensitivity and specificity, ranging from 50% to 92% and from 46% to 91%, respectively.[2,3] Furthermore, it has been shown that the positive predictive value of transrectal ultrasound-guided biopsies may be as low as 15.2%, compared with 28% for digital rectal examination.[4] This is attributed to variable tumor echogenicity, the multifocal nature of disease, concomitant inflammatory or pathologic processes, and operator inexperience.

Although three-dimensional ultrasonography, color Doppler, and microbubble contrast agents have been shown to improve sensitivity, specificity, and accuracy to varying degrees,[5–7] ultrasound remains primarily a cost-effective imaging modality to guide transrectal biopsy. Ultrasound has an adjunct role during seed placement in brachytherapy, and targeted therapies such as magnetic resonance imaging (MRI)-guided focused ultrasound[8] and cryoablation of focal lesions.

Elastography relies on detecting variance in tissue compliance, generated by compression and relaxation, used in conjunction with an imaging modality such as ultrasound or MRI. With ultrasound, Elastography has a sensitivity and specificity of more than 75%, and a positive predictive value of up to 88%.[9–11]

COMPUTED TOMOGRAPHY

Although computed tomography (CT) has a limited role in the detection of prostate cancer, in patients with highly elevated prostate-specific antigen (PSA) levels, it may be a useful modality to assess nodal involvement, capable of scanning the entire body in a short period of time. However, MRI and dedicated bone scans have been shown to be superior in their assessment of both nodes and bone metastases.[12]

Positron emission tomography (PET) relies on increased cellular metabolism of radiotracer by tumor cells,to identify loci of tumor or recurrence. PET has not been widely used in prostate cancer, however a potential role is emerging for locoregional nodal staging, detection of recurrent and metastatic disease in biochemical relapse, and assessment of tumor response to therapy.[13]

MAGNETIC RESONANCE IMAGING

Since its introduction into clinical practice, MRI has provided a previously unparalleled opportunity to visualize prostate tissue detail without patient exposure to ionizing radiation. The myriad of refinements that have been necessary to increase signal-to-noise ratio and achieve higher spatial, spectral, and temporal resolution are beyond the

Disclosures: None.
Department of Radiology, Brigham and Women's Hospital, 75 Francis Street, Boston, MA 02115, USA
* Corresponding author.
E-mail address: ctempany@bwh.harvard.edu (C.M. Tempany).

Urol Clin N Am 37 (2010) 23–25
doi:10.1016/j.ucl.2009.11.009
0094-0143/10/$ – see front matter

scope of this article, however consensus is being reached within the literature that a 3-Tesla strength magnetic field, and use of a pelvic phased-array coil and/or endorectal pelvic phased-array coil represent the current gold standard.[14–16]

MRI encompasses various sequences, each suited to expose a particular anatomic or pathophysiologic feature of disease. Multiparametric imaging is therefore necessary to fully use the potential of MR and to accurately stage and monitor disease.[17–19] Standard T1- and T2-weighted images are used in concert to define morphology and distinguish between areas of signal drop arising from foci of cancer as opposed to artifact related to hemorrhage or inflammatory change from recent biopsy.

Additional functional sequences such as dynamic contrast enhanced (DCE), diffusion-weighted imaging (DWI) and magnetic resonance spectroscopy (MRS) are used, each of which provides unique information on tissue characteristics.[20–22] DCE acquires data on tissue perfusion characteristics and tumor wash-in and wash-out contrast. These rely on pathophysiologic principles that tumors display increased angiogenesis, thus are expected to show early and increased enhancement. Graphic representations of the data are generated, from which computer-assisted quantitative analysis is derived.

DWI records the microscopic motion of water molecules within tissue, based on the theory that poorly differentiated cancers show marked tissue heterogeneity and decreased water movement. An apparent diffusion coefficient (ADC) map is generated, and ADC values then acquired, assisting in detection of foci of disease. Spectroscopy examines cellular metabolism within single or multiple voxels, using high levels of choline and low levels of citrate as likely areas of cancer. Meta-analyses have shown in certain patient populations that MRS has high specificity, but low sensitivity, suggesting a role as a rule-in test for low-risk patients.[23]

Various novel radiotracers and positron-emitting radioisotopes have been proposed, including [^{11}C]choline, [^{18}F]fluorocholine and [^{11}C]acetate, and [^{18}F]fluoride, [^{11}C]methionine and [^{11}C]tyrosine, respectively. These together with radiolabeled monoclonal antibodies against specific cancer cell surface antigens, may represent more sensitive means of tumor detection, either for staging purposes or evaluating biochemical recurrence.[24,25]

Currently, state of the art imaging of prostate cancer involves multiparametric MRI at either 3-Tesla or 1.5 Tesla, incorporating T1- and T2-weighted sequences, together with DWI and DCE. It has been proposed that prebiopsy MRI may obfuscate the potential confusion generated by residual blood products, potential distortion of native tissue, and local inflammation.[26,27] However, given the increasing frequency of this disease and the potential cost burden of obtaining an MRI because of increased PSA levels and/or abnormal prostate digital examination, it is unlikely to be a viable solution. However, increasing evidence suggests an important role for MRI prior to, or during, a biopsy can be very useful, allowing targeted biopsies. This should lead to increased accuracy and assist in therapy planning. Ongoing research will attempt to better delineate foci of disease and achieve greater sensitivity and specificity, with the use of more sophisticated imaging techniques, postprocessing software, and novel biomolecular markers.

ACKNOWLEDGMENTS

This work was supported in part by the following NIH grants: R01 CA-109246 and U41-RR 019703.

REFERENCES

1. Wantanabe H, Kato H, Kato T, et al. Diagnostic application of ultrasonotomography for the prostate. Jpn J Urol 1968;59:273–9.
2. Lorentzen T, Nerstrom H, Iversen P, et al. Local staging of prostate cancer with transrectal ultrasound: a literature review. Prostate Suppl 1992;4: 11–6.
3. Scherr DS, Eastham J, Ohori M, et al. Prostate biopsy techniques and indications: when, where, and how? Semin Urol Oncol 2002;20(1):18–31.
4. Mettlin C, Lee F, Drago J, et al. The American Cancer Society National Prostate Cancer Detection Project. Findings on the detection of early prostate cancer in 2425 men. Cancer 1991;67(12):2949–58.
5. Hricak H, Choyke PL, Eberhardt SC, et al. Imaging prostate cancer: a multidisciplinary perspective. Radiology 2007;243(1):28–53.
6. Wink M, Frauscher F, Cosgrove D, et al. Contrast-enhanced ultrasound and prostate cancer; a multicentre European research coordination project. Eur Urol 2008;54(5):982–92.
7. Tang J, Yang JC, Luo Y, et al. Enhancement characteristics of benign and malignant focal peripheral nodules in the peripheral zone of the prostate gland studied using contrast-enhanced transrectal ultrasound. Clin Radiol 2008;63(10):1086–91.
8. Jolesz FA. MRI-guided focused ultrasound surgery. Annu Rev Med 2009;60:417–30.
9. Zhang M, Nigwekar P, Castaneda B, et al. Quantitative characterization of viscoelastic properties of

human prostate correlated with histology. Ultrasound Med Biol 2008;34(7):1033–42.
10. Salomon G, Köllerman J, Thederan I, et al. Evaluation of prostate cancer detection with ultrasound real-time elastography: a comparison with step section pathological analysis after radical prostatectomy. Eur Urol 2008;54(6):1354–62.
11. Sumura M, Shigeno K, Hyuga T, et al. Initial evaluation of prostate cancer with real-time elastography based on step-section pathologic analysis after radical prostatectomy: a preliminary study. Int J Urol 2007;14(9):811–6.
12. Dotan ZA. Bone imaging in prostate cancer. Nat Clin Pract Urol 2008;5(8):434–44.
13. Jadvar H. Molecular imaging of prostate cancer with ^{18}F-fluorodeoxyglucose PET. Nat Rev Urol 2009; 6(6):317–23.
14. Cornfeld DM, Weinreb JC. MR imaging of the prostate: 1.5T versus 3T. Magn Reson Imaging Clin N Am 2007;15(3):433–48, viii.
15. Fütterer JJ, Barentsz JO, Heijmink SW. Value of 3-T magnetic resonance imaging in local staging of prostate cancer. Top Magn Reson Imaging 2008; 19(6):285–9.
16. Villers A, Lemaitre L, Haffner J, et al. Current status of MRI for the diagnosis, staging and prognosis of prostate cancer: implications for focal therapy and active surveillance. Curr Opin Urol 2009;19(3): 274–82.
17. Kurhanewicz J, Vigneron D, Carroll P, et al. Multiparametric magnetic resonance imaging in prostate cancer: present and future. Curr Opin Urol 2008; 18(1):71–7.
18. Macura KJ. Multiparametric magnetic resonance imaging of the prostate: current status in prostate cancer detection, localization, and staging. Semin Roentgenol 2008;43(4):303–13.
19. Puech P, Huglo D, Petyt G, et al. Imaging of organ-confined prostate cancer: functional ultrasound, MRI and PET/computed tomography. Curr Opin Urol 2009;19(2):168–76.
20. Mazaheri Y, Shukla-Dave A, Muellner A, et al. MR imaging of the prostate in clinical practice. MAGMA 2008;21(6):379–92.
21. McMahon CJ, Bloch BN, Lenkinski RE, et al. Dynamic contrast-enhanced MR imaging in the evaluation of patients with prostate cancer. Magn Reson Imaging Clin N Am 2009;17(2):363–83.
22. Tanimoto A, Nakashima J, Kohno H, et al. Prostate cancer screening: the clinical value of diffusion-weighted imaging and dynamic MR imaging in combination with T2-weighted imaging. J Magn Reson Imaging 2007;25(1):146–52.
23. Umbehr M, Bachmann LM, Held U, et al. Combined magnetic resonance imaging and magnetic resonance spectroscopy imaging in the diagnosis of prostate cancer: a systematic review and meta-analysis. Eur Urol 2009;55(3):575–90.
24. Ravizzini G, Turkbey B, Kurdziela K, et al. New horizons in prostate cancer imaging. Eur J Radiol 2009; 70(2):212–26.
25. Apolo AB, Pandit-Taskar N, Morris MJ. Novel tracers and their development for the imaging of metastatic prostate cancer. J Nucl Med 2008;49(12):2031–41.
26. Ahmed HU, Kirkham A, Arya M, et al. Is it time to consider a role for MRI before prostate biopsy? Nat Rev Clin Oncol 2009;6(4):197–206.
27. Shimizu T, Nishie A, Ro T, et al. Prostate cancer detection: the value of performing an MRI before a biopsy. Acta Radiol 2009;50(9):1080–8.

High-intensity Focused Ultrasound: Ready for Primetime

Kyle O. Rove, MD[a], Kathryn F. Sullivan, MD[b], E. David Crawford, MD[c,d,e,*]

KEYWORDS

- Prostate cancer • High-intensity focused ultrasound
- HIFU • PSA • Biochemical recurrence

Prostate cancer (CaP) is the second most common cause of cancer deaths in the United States, and the incidence of CaP has remained constant at 165 cases per 100,000 men.[1] Since 1990, the age-adjusted death rate has decreased by 31%. The decrease in death rate is most likely due to early detection and treatment.[1] The decrease in mortality has not been as significant as expected compared with the increase in diagnosis of CaP. The discrepancy between incidence and mortality has been attributed to increasing detection of clinically insignificant tumors.

Furthermore, prostate screening (ie, digital rectal examination [DRE] and prostate specific antigen [PSA]) may identify clinically insignificant cancers and result in over diagnosis and over treatment of prostate cancer. CaP screening may result in over treatment of prostate cancer by at least 30%.[2] Since the beginning of the PSA era, CaP screening has shifted the disease burden to organ-confined and lower-grade disease.[3] Etzioni and colleagues[4] estimated that 10% of men with low-grade prostate cancer are over treated with radical surgery, and 45% are over treated with radiation therapy.

Some of the side effects of radical prostatectomy and radiation therapy include urinary incontinence and impotence. The incidence of these morbidities has decreased with improved technique; however, these morbidities are significant for individuals who may be over treated for their otherwise indolent CaP.[3]

Once diagnosed with CaP, a patient must make an informed decision on which mode of treatment to pursue. This decision is made more difficult by the varied modalities, invasiveness, outcomes, and return to baseline function after treatment. Moreover, treatment type depends on clinical stage, Gleason grade, patient preference, and other comorbid conditions.[3] Treatment types include active surveillance, radical prostatectomy, cryotherapy, and radiation therapy (either brachytherapy or external-beam radiation).[3] In addition, several new and innovative therapies such as high-intensity ultrasound (HIFU) are being studied.

HIFU was introduced 15 years ago for the treatment of benign prostatic hypertrophy.[5] In 1996,

[a] Division of Urology, University of Colorado Anschutz Medical Campus, 12631 East 17th Avenue, Mailstop C302, Aurora, CO 80045, USA
[b] Division of Urology, University of Colorado Anschutz Medical Campus, 12631 East 17th Avenue, Mailstop C319, Aurora, CO 80045, USA
[c] Department of Surgery, University of Colorado Cancer Center, University of Colorado Anschutz Medical Campus, 12631 East 17th Avenue, Mailstop C319, Aurora, CO 80045, USA
[d] Division of Urology, University of Colorado Cancer Center, University of Colorado Anschutz Medical Campus, 12631 East 17th Avenue, Mailstop C319, Aurora, CO 80045, USA
[e] Department of Radiation Oncology, University of Colorado Cancer Center, University of Colorado Anschutz Medical Campus, 12631 East 17th Avenue, Mailstop C319, Aurora, CO 80045, USA
* Corresponding author. Department of Surgery, University of Colorado Cancer Center, University of Colorado Anschutz Medical Campus, 12631 East 17th Avenue, Mailstop C319, Aurora, CO 80045.
E-mail address: david.crawford@ucdenver.edu (E.D. Crawford).

Urol Clin N Am 37 (2010) 27–35
doi:10.1016/j.ucl.2009.11.010

Gelet and colleagues[6] used HIFU for the treatment of localized low-grade CaP. Many studies have been performed to evaluate the use of HIFU for low-grade, localized prostate cancer. HIFU has also been used as salvage therapy after radiation. The National Institute for Clinical Excellence (NICE) in the UK evaluated HIFU in 2005 and found that there was sufficient evidence to recommend its use for the treatment of CaP.[7] However, in 2008, NICE only recommended the use of HIFU in controlled clinical trials or when patients are entered into a registry and closely followed.[8,9] The French Association of Urology (FAU) and the Association of Italian Urologists (AURO) now recommend HIFU as standard treatment for patients with localized disease, who are unsuitable for or who failed radiation, or who are unsuitable for surgery.[7] The European Association of Urology guidelines, however, state HIFU is "investigational or experimental."[10] In the United States, HIFU is currently not approved for treatment of CaP outside ongoing investigational trials. As more studies elucidate long-term disease-free rates, it is expected that consensus recommendations on the use of HIFU for localized CaP will soon emerge.

Recent response to the over diagnosis of CaP and over treatment of CaP by urologists has led to the need to consider other forms of therapy that have less morbid side effects and are less invasive. HIFU is a minimally invasive treatment of CaP and needs to be evaluated for efficacy that is similar to or exceeds other modalities of treatment, minimum side effects, quicker recovery from treatment, and hopefully reduced treatment costs. HIFU uses ultrasound energy to cause mechanical and thermal injury to the target tissue. In this article, the authors review the current literature on the experimental therapy for HIFU. The HIFU technique, its mechanism of action, patient selection, current efficacy studies, complications, follow-up after HIFU treatment, and future developments are discussed.

HIFU TECHNIQUE

HIFU, when used for the treatment of localized prostate cancer, uses an ultrasound transducer placed in the rectum to generate acoustic energy that is focused on the tissue target, creating high temperatures and irreversible coagulative necrosis. HIFU uses a trackless principle, whereby tissue outside the focal plane is not damaged; the transrectal probe sits on the rectal mucosa and sends acoustic energy through the intervening tissues, only heating the tissue volume targeted by the probe.[11] The probe is repositioned mechanically as needed to target the entire prostate. This technique is minimally invasive, requires less anesthesia and involves a shorter recovery period than surgery, and can be performed in a day surgery setting.

HIFU is generally performed with the patient under spinal or general anesthesia. The operation can last from 1 to 4 hours, and should not be performed with prostate volumes greater than 40 mL. Often, a limited transurethral resection of the prostate (TURP) is performed before application of HIFU to reduce the risk of postoperative urinary retention.[12] (Notably, study protocols of US trials do not permit the use of TURP before HIFU.) The patient is placed in the lithotomy position. The ultrasound probe is covered with a condom and inserted gently into the rectum using lubricating jelly. Once inserted, an articulating arm aids in maintaining the position of the probe. Cool water (17–18°C) is circulated through the condom to protect adjacent tissues from thermal damage throughout the procedure.[13] The prostate is visualized using real-time diagnostic images generated by the probe using lower, nondestructive acoustic energies (0.1–100 mW/cm^2). Once the target areas are identified, the prostate tissue is ablated with high energies (1300–2200 W/cm^2) focused in a small 1- to 3-mm-wide by 5- to 26-mm-long focal plane. Each pulse heats the tissue to 80 to 98°C over a 3-second period. The gland is revisualized with lower ultrasound energies between ablative pulses. The probe is then moved and rotated in a semi-automated manner (device-dependent) using lower-energy diagnostic images to target adjacent prostate tissue. The end goal is to create overlapping lesions until the whole gland is treated. Patients often require a urethral or suprapubic catheter for several days.

Body movement and breathing pose continued challenges to the application of this technology.[14] In addition, the small target volumes make it more difficult to achieve homogeneous treatment of the entire gland. Because the HIFU device settings are based on animal models with presumed uniform tissue characteristics, further difficulty arises from uneven absorption of the acoustic energy influenced by possible heat-resistant tumor cells, prostatic calcifications, and differences in local blood perfusion.[15,16]

CURRENT MARKET PRODUCTS

Two commercially-available ultrasound-guided transrectal devices are currently used for the treatment of prostate cancer: the Ablatherm (EDAP TMS, Lyon, France) and the Sonablate 500 (Focus Surgery, IN, USA). While these devices are approved in the treatment of localized prostate cancer in Asia and Europe, their use in the United States is currently limited to investigational, phase III trials only. Both HIFU devices are trackless, in that no tissue is damaged between the probe and the targeted area of tissue in the focal plane. The original Ablatherm employs two probes each with piezoceramic transducers, has fixed-power settings, and requires a transurethral resection of the prostate (TURP) to be performed preoperatively due to limitations in depth of treatment. A newer version uses a single probe with two transducers. One transducer is dedicated to imaging and the other to treatment, enabling real-time visualization during treatment. Additionally, the newer Ablatherm device has three dedicated treatment parameters for the different clinical scenarios, including primary treatment, repeat HIFU, and salvage therapy. The Sonablate 500 device offers greater mobility and customization of treatment settings, allowing for more surgeon control over the HIFU beam characteristics, including adjustment of focal length, energy and power delivered to the target. The device enables users to tailor treatment to the particular characteristics of a patient's prostate and disease burden through transverse and sagittal low-energy, real-time imaging and software monitoring of tissue changes. The Sonablate 500 also incorporates imaging of blood flow around the neurovascular bundles; a clinician can alter treatment based on this visual feedback. Because the volume of tissue targeted by the Sonablate 500 is smaller than that of the more automated Ablatherm device, more manual manipulation of the transrectal probe is required.[17]

MECHANISM OF ACTION

The application of high-intensity ultrasound in medicine began with studies in 1954 by Lindstrom and Fry, who were investigating the possibility of its use in the treatment of neurologic disorders.[18,19] Fry and colleagues[20] also discovered that in focusing these high-energy acoustic waves, they could be used safely in vivo. Attempts were made to apply its use in tumors of various organs throughout the 1970s, but at lower energies for long durations. Without any method to measure target tissue temperatures noninvasively, however, this investigational treatment modality fell out of favor. In the 1980s, extracorporeal shockwave lithotripsy came to the forefront with its approval for use by the Food and Drug Administration (FDA) in 1984, allowing for the noninvasive treatment of kidney stones.[21] In the 1990s, HIFU as a treatment of soft-tissue tumors was revived after advancements in the underlying technology, namely with the introduction of noninvasive tissue temperature monitoring. Its origination in the treatment of prostate cancer came from the canine prostate experiments by Gelet,[22] Bihrle,[23] and Kincaide and colleagues.[24]

HIFU destroys target tissue through the thermal and mechanical effects of nonionizing, acoustic radiation (ie, sound waves) delivered to target tissues after focusing by an acoustic lens, bowl-shaped transducer, or electronic phased array (**Fig. 1**). Because HIFU uses nonionizing radiation, it can be repeated one or more times in multiple sessions. The thermal effects are achieved by heating tissues to 60°C or higher, resulting in near-instantaneous coagulative necrosis and cell death.[25] By focusing the energy, more destruction occurs within the focal plane, but tissues outside the target area are spared damage, as energy intensities are far lower.

Mechanical Effects of HIFU

The use of high-frequency sound waves results in various, significant mechanical effects on the tissues in addition to the thermal effects just mentioned. These include cavitation, microstreaming, and radiation forces. Cavitation is the creation or movement of gas in an acoustic field. As the tissue compresses and expands with exposure to the acoustic waves, gas is extracted creating bubbles. These bubbles interact with the acoustic field and begin to oscillate violently. The bubbles collapse and create high-velocity jets that disrupt cell membranes.[26] Microstreaming refers to the rapid movement of liquid outside an oscillating bubble generated through cavitation forces.

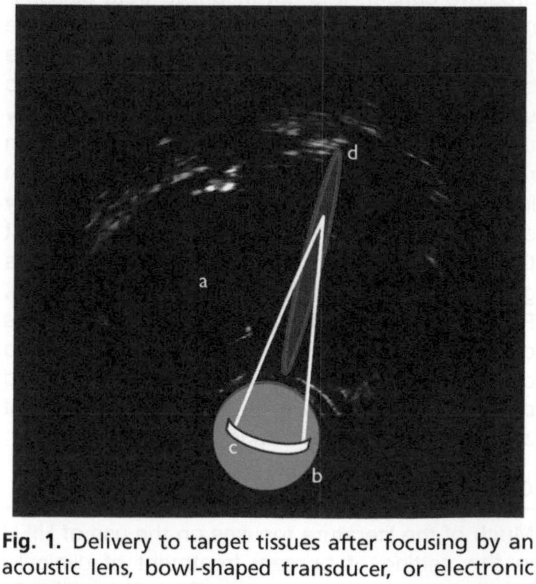

Fig. 1. Delivery to target tissues after focusing by an acoustic lens, bowl-shaped transducer, or electronic phased array.

When the bubbles oscillate, nearby tissues are subjected to shearing forces that can also disrupt cell membranes.[27] Radiation forces are the pressures tissues endure when either absorbing or reflecting sound waves. Because tissues and solids respond differently from liquid media, movement of liquids can create streaming and shearing effects that disrupt cell membrane integrity.[28] Overall, the primary mechanism of cell death in HIFU therapy is coagulative necrosis, but the sum contribution of thermal and mechanical effects is ultimately responsible for ablation of target tissues.

It has been hypothesized that these mechanical effects might contribute to local spread of tumor cells, limiting the clinical efficacy of HIFU. Several studies have refuted this claim in vitro and in vivo.[29,30]

Other Effects

The high temperatures also induce the creation and release of chemically reactive free radicals. These have direct and indirect activity on surviving cells, namely in the induction of apoptosis and activity on nuclear DNA. Nearby tissues are also believed to undergo apoptosis induced by the lower levels of acoustic radiation and heat experienced during HIFU treatment. Necrosis and cavitation take days to months to peak and are believed to correlate with PSA nadir.

Limitations

Despite being a noninvasive modality in the treatment of prostate cancer, it is not without any untoward side effects. Because HIFU works best in contiguous tissues, its use is limited to localized prostate cancer; it is not meant to treat disseminated, widespread, or otherwise inoperable cancers. In addition, because ultrasound is the basis of HIFU, unwanted effects of diagnostic ultrasound imaging also apply to its higher-energy use: shadowing and refraction. Shadowing can result from large prostatic calcifications (>10 mm in diameter), which can interfere with the delivery of acoustic energy. This could potentially impact the ability to completely ablate larger glands greater than 40 mL, limiting clinical efficacy. Reflection of sound waves into nearby tissues outside the focal plane, although normally of no consequence in diagnostic imaging, could produce burns in tissues adjacent to the treatment zone (rectum, bowel, bladder).

Clinical Use of HIFU

Much of the literature focuses on the use of HIFU in the setting of primary treatment of clinically localized prostate cancer (T1c–T2a). The minimally invasive characteristics of HIFU also make it suitable as a salvage treatment option for patients with biochemical failure after other types of primary treatment, namely after radical prostatectomy or external-beam radiotherapy. HIFU does not preclude the use of other future treatment modalities; that is, prostatectomy[31] and radiotherapy[32] have been safely performed following HIFU treatment.

PATIENT SELECTION

Criteria for individuals who qualify for HIFU have not been clearly defined. In general, they are individuals with localized disease and who do not want or do not qualify for surgical or radiation treatment. Several HIFU studies have included individuals more than 70 years-old and who were not candidates for prostatectomy or radiation or who did not desire these treatment options.[7,33–35]

The prostate size of individuals receiving HIFU treatment must be less than or equal to 40 mL[7,34]; however, the anterior-posterior diameter of the prostate should not exceed 45 mm using the Sonablate device and should be no longer than 25 mm with the Ablatherm instrument. Greater prostate volume is one of the primary contraindications for HIFU. Prostate volumes larger than 40 mL may lead to incomplete treatment of the gland. HIFU waves do not penetrate beyond 19 to 26 mm, which in larger prostates would make reaching the anterior and anterobasal regions of the prostate impossible. However, these regions of the prostate have low incidence of CaP and size may not be as important a factor; improved HIFU technology may overcome the size limitation.[36] Some studies have used transurethral resection of the prostate (TURP) or 5α-reductase inhibitors to decrease the size of the prostate before HIFU treatment.

Other criteria for HIFU treatment include clinical stage and PSA level. Most studies include only individuals with clinical stage T1 to T2 or localized CaP.[7,12,13,34,35,37,38] The clinical stage is independent of the Gleason score. The criteria for PSA level of candidates enrolled in multiple studies are variable. Study criteria for PSA include PSA level less than 10 ng/mL, PSA level less than 15 ng/mL,[12,13] PSA level less than 20 ng/mL. Several studies have set a PSA level of less than 15 ng/mL as their PSA criteria, however, there are no clear data on an absolute maximum PSA level.[7] Several clinical trials in the United States have set a PSA level less than 10ng/mL and Gleason score of less than or equal to 6.

Other relative contraindications for HIFU treatment include high volume of intraprostatic calcifications, as mentioned previously. These calcifications can lead to scattering of the ultrasound waves, which may decrease the safety and efficacy of the treatment. Anatomic or pathologic conditions of the rectum that may interfere with the placement of the HIFU probe into the rectum are contraindications for HIFU therapy.

TREATMENT OUTCOMES

Studies

Initial studies of HIFU in the treatment of localized CaP are nearing completion in the United States, and several international trials with longer-term outcomes have been published showing positive clinical outcomes with low morbidity. Most studies reveal that PSA nadirs are reached within 3 to 4 months.[7] In a systematic review of the French literature on primary HIFU using the Ablatherm device, negative biopsy rates after 3 months ranged from 80% to 90% in most studies (51%–96% in all studies). Negative biopsy rates for the Sonablate device ranged from 64% to 87% (**Fig. 2**). Long-term disease-free rates with HIFU for the 2 devices are shown in **Fig. 3**. PSA nadirs of 0.5 ng/mL or less were achieved in 42% to 84% of patients treated with the Ablatherm device. A study in the United Kingdom found that PSA nadirs of 0.2 ng/mL or less and 0.5 ng/mL or less were achieved in 80% and 60%, respectively, for the Sonablate device. The data are similar to several trials demonstrating biochemical or pathologic disease-free rates after 5 years, ranging from 66% to 78%.[37]

Follow-up data on the Ablatherm device are more extensive than the Sonablate device. In a series by Blana and colleagues[39] with the longest follow-up to date (mean 6.4 years), the actuarial disease-free survival was 59% after 6 years. Eight-year cancer-specific and overall survival were 98% and 83%, respectively. Even with longer follow-up time, the authors cannot state whether HIFU improves survival over active surveillance; longer follow-up periods are needed.

Important Markers

Pretreatment PSA level has been shown to correlate with biochemical disease-free survival (BDFS).[38,40,41] More recently, more focus has been brought to the intuitive relationship between PSA nadir and clinical outcomes, specifically BDFS and negative biopsy rate. Ganzer and colleagues[42] demonstrated that a PSA nadir of 0.2 ng/mL or less is associated with improved disease-free survival, based on analysis of data for 103 men who underwent HIFU as primary treatment of localized CaP.

Lack of Appropriate HIFU-Specific Biochemical Failure Definition

Unfortunately, no standard definition of BDFS exists specific to primary treatment of clinically localized CaP with HIFU, a point of often contentious debate. In addition, among the various studies reporting long-term results, there is no consensus on which definition is the most appropriate and valid. Many studies cite the definitions used for primary radiation treatment, that is, the American Society for Therapeutic Radiology and Oncology (ASTRO) definitions. The original definition (3 consecutive increases in PSA after reaching nadir) is cited in studies from the late 1990s and early 2000s. Unfortunately, this definition is flawed on the premise that it precludes early biochemical

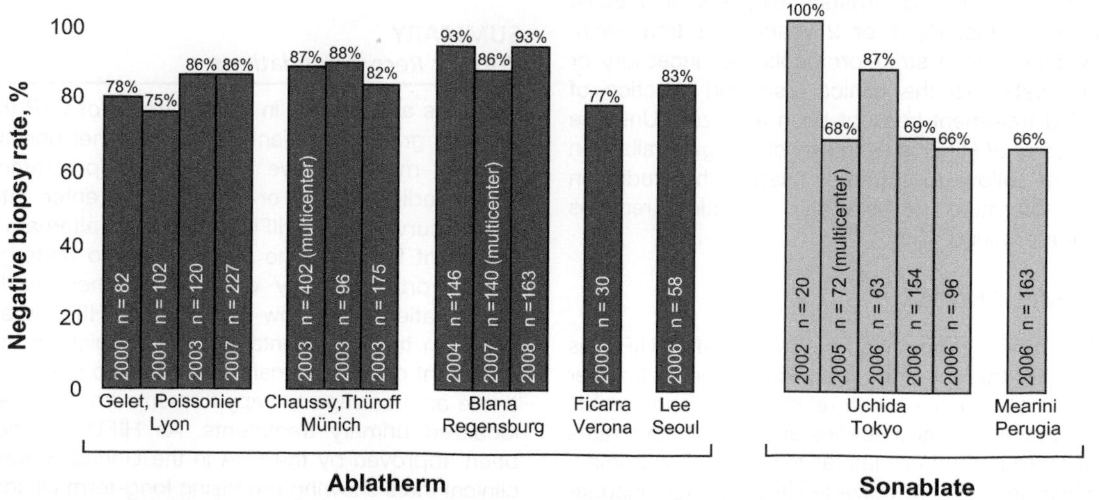

Fig. 2. Negative biopsy rates with HIFU for the Ablatherm and Sonablate devices.

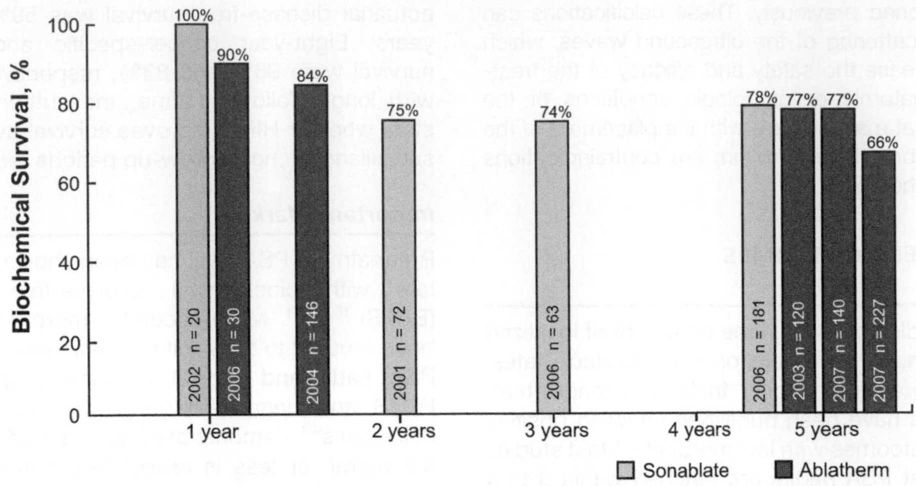

Fig. 3. Long-term disease-free rates with HIFU for the Ablatherm and Sonablate devices.

reoccurrence. More recent studies have cited the ASTRO Phoenix criteria for BDFS: PSA nadir + 2 ng/mL constitutes biochemical failure.[43] Other end points cited in HIFU studies include PSA nadir, negative biopsy rates after a specific interval after treatment, and changes from baseline in International Prostate Symptom Score (IPSS) scores. The relationship between BDFS and overall survival, however, remains elusive. It is hoped that more long-term study results will resolve this unanswered question.

FOLLOW-UP

Follow-up after primary or salvage HIFU therapy is not well defined outside the research protocols used by clinical studies. Most studies use a combination of serum PSA checked every 3 to 4 months for the first 2 years after treatment and transrectal ultrasound-guided prostate biopsies at specific intervals (usually 1 or 2 years after treatment). Whether these strict protocols are necessary or applicable to the clinical use and practice of HIFU treatment has not been analyzed. Until the efficacy of HIFU is better resolved, generalization of the follow-up schemes used in the studies in the literature to standard practice remains undetermined.

COMPLICATIONS

The most common complications after HIFU as primary therapy are urinary incontinence, bladder outlet obstruction, urethral strictures, and erectile dysfunction. Many studies also report (low) rates of rectourethral fistulas (as low as <1% in primary HIFU and <3% in salvage HIFU). Urinary incontinence has been observed in 8% to 25% of patients undergoing primary treatment by HIFU without preoperative TURP, and 6% to 13% of patients who underwent primary HIFU with TURP.[7] Rates of urinary stricture also favor primary HIFU with TURP as only 8% of patients developed stricture when TURP was performed beforehand as opposed to 30% in patients who underwent HIFU without TURP. Although TURP has no bearing on disease control (as measured by PSA nadir, negative biopsy rate, or biochemical failure), it is indicated to reduce rates of incontinence, stricture, and bladder outlet obstruction.[12] The rate of impotence varies from 20% to 77% of patients treated with HIFU, depending on patient selection and device used, with several Italian and French studies showing moderate erectile dysfunction after treatment.[40,44]

SUMMARY

Current Recommendations

HIFU fills a niche role in the treatment of CaP for a select group of patients who are either unsuitable for more invasive interventions (prostatectomy, radiotherapy), or unwilling to enter into active surveillance. HIFU is also an alternative treatment for men who do not want to undergo radical prostatectomy or radiation therapy. In some patients with low-risk disease, HIFU is an option in the armamentarium of urologists in the treatment of prostate cancer. HIFU also may play a role as a salvage therapy in men who fail other localized primary treatments. As HIFU has not been approved by the FDA in the United States, clinical trials showing promising long-term clinical outcomes are currently underway.

Ongoing Studies

In a multicenter, nonrandomized phase III study for clinically localized CaP (T1c–T2a) in the United States, HIFU (Sonablate 500) is being compared with brachytherapy with target enrollment of 466 men between the ages of 45 and 75 years, Gleason score less than or equal to 6, and PSA less than or equal to 10 ng/mL. Absence of biochemical recurrence, defined by the ASTRO Phoenix criteria in addition to negative biopsy at 24 months, is the primary end point.

A phase III, multicenter, single-arm study investigating the safety and efficacy of salvage HIFU (Sonablate) for recurrent localized prostate cancer after external-beam radiation failure is currently underway. Target enrollment is 212 men between the ages of 40 and 85 years, with a PSA level between 0.5 ng/mL and 10 ng/mL, who received electron beam radiation therapy 2 or more years prior, and have biopsy-confirmed prostate cancer.

Another nonrandomized phase II/III trial will compare primary HIFU (Ablatherm) to cryoablation. Target enrollment is 446 men aged 60 years or more with Gleason score of 6 or less, and PSA level 10 ng/mL or less, and T2a or lower grade disease. The primary outcome is PSA nadir less than 0.5 ng/mL, stable PSA, and negative biopsy at 24 months. These end points are far more stringent than many previous trial definitions of biochemical and pathologic disease-free states. Secondary end points will include PSA nadir less than 0.5 ng/mL at 6 months, disease-specific and overall survival, change from baseline UCLA Prostate Cancer Index and IPSS.

Future

Imaging techniques continue to improve in the setting of HIFU treatment. Doppler or blood-flow ultrasound guidance and magnetic resonance-guided HIFU are currently under investigation in the treatment of hepatic masses and uterine fibroids, and may improve precision of treatment. In addition to technical improvements, longer-term clinical trials with standard measures of clinical efficacy are needed to bring HIFU into the fold of accepted treatments for men with localized prostate cancer.

Overview

- HIFU is an investigational treatment modality for prostate cancer in the United States. Several phase III trials are ongoing.
- HIFU technology is well understood in its effect on tissues, the resulting coagulative necrosis, and mechanical disruption of cell membranes.
- HIFU is generally well tolerated, and the most common side effect is acute urinary retention.
- The guidelines for PSA and transrectal ultrasound-guided biopsy of the prostate after treatment are not well elucidated outside clinical trials. Interpretation of PSA after HIFU treatment is still not well understood.
- HIFU therapy for low-risk clinically localized prostate cancer seems increasingly attractive for men who turn down the option of active surveillance but who are also poor surgical candidates.

REFERENCES

1. Jemal A, Siegel R, Ward E, et al. Cancer statistics 2007. CA Cancer J Clin 2007;57:43–66.
2. Scattoni V, Zlotta A, Montironi R, et al. Extended and saturation prostatic biopsy in the diagnosis and characterization of prostate cancer: a critical analysis of the literature. Eur Urol 2007;52:1309–22.
3. Crawford ED, Barqawi A. Targeted focal therapy: a minimally invasive ablation technique for early prostate cancer. Oncology 2007;21:27–32.
4. Etzioni R, Penson DF, Legler JM, et al. Overdiagnosis due to prostate-specific antigen screening: lessons from U.S. prostate cancer incidence trends. J Natl Cancer Inst 2002;94:981–90.
5. Hou A, Sullivan K, Crawford ED. Targeted focal therapy for prostate cancer: a review. Curr Opin Urol 2009;19:283–9.
6. Gelet A, Chapelon JY, Bouvier R, et al. Local control of prostate cancer by transrectal HIFU therapy: preliminary results. J Urol 1999;161:156–62.
7. Rebillard X, Soulie M, Chartier-Kastler E, et al. High-intensity focused ultrasound in prostate cancer: a systematic literature review of the French Association of Urology. BJU Int 2008;101:1205–13.
8. Challacombe BJ, Murphy DG, Zakri R, et al. High-intensity focused ultrasound for localized prostate cancer: initial experience with a 2-year follow up. BJU Int 2009;104:200–4.
9. Association of Italian Urologists. Guidelines on prostate cancer: diagnosis, staging and therapy. Pietra Ligure (Italy): Association of Italian Urologists; 2008. Available at: http://www.auro.it/wp-content/uploads/al10.pdf.
10. Heidenreich A, Aus G, Bolla M, et al. EAU guidelines on prostate cancer. Eur Urol 2008;53:68–80.
11. Warwick R, Pond J. Trackless lesions in nervous tissues produced by high intensity focused ultrasound (high-frequency mechanical waves). J Anat 1968;102:387–405.

12. Chaussy C, Thuroff S. The status of high-intensity focused ultrasound in the treatment of localized prostate cancer and the impact of a combined resection. Curr Urol Rep 2003;4:248–52.
13. Blana A, Walter B, Rogenhofer S, et al. High-intensity focused ultrasound for the treatment of localized prostate cancer: 5-year experience. Urology 2004; 63:297–300.
14. Tanter M, Pernot M, Aubry FJ, et al. Compensating for bone interfaces and respiratory motion in high-intensity focused ultrasound. Int J Hyperthermia 2007;23:141–51.
15. Watkin NA, ter Haar GR, Rivens I. The intensity dependence of the site of maximal energy deposition in focused ultrasound surgery. Ultrasoud Med Biol 1996;22:483–91.
16. Chen L, ter Haar GR, Hill CR, et al. Effect of blood perfusion on the ablation of liver parenchyma with high-intensity focused ultrasound. Phys Med Biol 1994;38:1661–73.
17. Illing RO, Leslie TA, Kennedy JE, et al. Visually directed HIFU for organ confined prostate cancer—a proposed standard for the conduct of therapy. BJU Int 2006;98:1187–92.
18. Lindstrom PA. Prefrontal ultrasonic irradiation: a substitute for lobotomy. AMA Arch Neurol Psychiatry 1954;72:399–425.
19. Ballentine HT Jr, Bell E, Manlapaz J. Progress and problems in the neurological applications of focused ultrasound. J Neurosurg 1960;17:858–76.
20. Fry W, Barnard K, Fry F, et al. Ultrasonic lesions in the mammalian central nervous system with ultrasound. Science 1955;122:517–8.
21. Chassy C, Brendel W, Schmiedt E. Extracorporeally induced destruction of kidney stones by shock waves. Lancet 1980;2:1265–8.
22. Gelet A, Chapelon JY, Margonari J, et al. Prostatic tissue destruction by high-intensity focused ultrasound: experimentation on canine prostate. J Endourol 1993;7:249–53.
23. Bihrle R, Foster RS, Sanghvi NT, et al. High-intensity focused ultrasound in the treatment of prostatic tissue. Urology 1994;43:21–6.
24. Kincaide LF, Sanghvi NT, Cummings O, et al. Noninvasive ultrasonic subtotal ablation of the prostate in dogs. Am J Vet Res 1995;57:1225–7.
25. Dewhirst MW, Viglianti BL, Lora-Michiels M, et al. Basic principles of thermal dosimetry and thermal thresholds for tissue damage from hyperthermia. Int J Hyperthermia 2003;19:267–94.
26. Coussios CC, Farny CH, Haar GT, et al. Role of acoustic cavitation in the delivery and monitoring of cancer treatment by high-intensity focused ultrasound (HIFU). Int J Hyperthermia 2007;23: 105–20.
27. Holland CK, Apfel RE. Thresholds for transient cavitation produced by pulsed ultrasound in a controlled nuclei environment. J Acoust Soc Am 1990;88: 2059–69.
28. Vaezy S, Shi X, Martin R, et al. Real-time visualization of high intensity focused ultrasound treatment using ultrasound imaging. Ultrasound Med Biol 2001;27:33–42.
29. Kennedy JE, ter Haar GR, Wu F, et al. Contrast-enhanced ultrasound assessment of tissue response to high-intensity focused ultrasound. Ultrasound Med Biol 2004;30:851–4.
30. Kennedy JE. High-intensity focused ultrasound in the treatment of solid tumours. Nature Rev 2005; 10:1039.
31. Liatsikos E, Bynens B, Rabenalt R, et al. Treatment of patients after failed high intensity focused ultrasound and radiotherapy for localized prostate cancer: salvage laparoscopic extraperitoneal radical prostatectomy. J Endourol 2008;22:2295–8.
32. Pasticier G, Chapet O, Badet L, et al. Salvage radiotherapy after high-intensity focused ultrasound for localized prostate cancer: early clinical results. Urology 2008;72:1305–9.
33. Archer PL, Hodgson KJ, Murphy DG, et al. High-intensity focused ultrasound for treating prostate cancer. BJU Int 2006;99:28–32.
34. Murat FJ, Poissonnier L, Pasticier G, et al. High-intensity focused ultrasound for prostate cancer. Cancer Control 2007;14:244–9.
35. Tsakiris P, Thuroff S, Rosette J, et al. Transrectal high-intensity focused ultrasound devices: a critical appraisal of the available evidence. J Endourol 2008;22:221–9.
36. Barqawi A, Crawford ED. Emerging role of HIFU as a noninvasive ablative method to treat localized prostate cancer. Oncology 2008;22:123.
37. Uchida T, Ohkusa H, Yamashita H, et al. Five years experience of transrectal high-intensity focused ultrasound using the Sonablate device in the treatment of localized prostate cancer. Int J Urol 2006; 13:228–33.
38. Lee HM, Hong JH, Choi HY. High-intensity focused ultrasound therapy for clinically localized prostate cancer. Prostate Cancer Prostatic Dis 2006;9: 439–43.
39. Blana A, Thüroff S, Murat FJ, et al. First analysis of the long-term results with transrectal HIFU in patients with localised prostate cancer. Eur Urol 2008;53:1194–203.
40. Poissonnier L, Chapelon JY, Rouvière O, et al. Control of prostate cancer by transrectal IFU in 227 patients. Eur Urol 2007;51:381–7.
41. Gelet A, Chapelon JY, Murat FJ, et al. Prostate cancer control with transrectal HIFU in 124 patients: 7-years' actuarial results. Eur Urol Suppl 2005;5:133
42. Ganzer R, Rogenhofer S, Walter B, et al. PSA nadir is a significant predictor of treatment failure after

high-intensity focused ultrasound (HIFU) treatment of localised prostate cancer. Eur Urol 2008;53: 547–53.

43. Roach M III, Hangks G, Thames H Jr, et al. Defining biochemical failure following radiotherapy with or without hormonal therapy in men with clinically localized prostate cancer: recommendations of the RTOG-ASTRO Phoenix Consensus Conference. Int J Radiat Oncol Biol Phys 2006;65:965–74.
44. Mearini L, D'Urso L, Collura D, et al. Visually directed transrectal high intensity focused ultrasound for the treatment of prostate cancer: a preliminary report on the Italian experience. J Urol 2009;181:105–11 [discussion: 111–2].

Overcoming the Learning Curve for Robotic-assisted Laparoscopic Radical Prostatectomy

Marcos P. Freire, MD, PhD[1], Wesley W. Choi, MD[1], Yin Lei, MD, Fernando Carvas, BS, Jim C. Hu, MD, MPH*

KEYWORDS

- Radical prostatectomy • Robotic surgical technique
- Prostate cancer • Learning curve

For 70 years following Hugh Hampton Young's perineal radical prostatectomy series, there were surprisingly few alterations to the surgical technique and approach.[1] However, advances in pelvic anatomy and surgical technique to control bleeding from the dorsal venous complex (DVC) coupled with preservation of the neurovascular bundles (NVBs) decreased morbidity and led to a conversion from the perineal to the retropubic open approach.[2] The advent of prostate-specific antigen (PSA) afforded a measure of the completeness of surgical resection and led to additional technical modifications and a drop in the acceptable postprostatectomy PSA threshold from 0.4 or less to less than 0.1. At around the same time that PSA was introduced, Schuessler and colleagues[3] performed a series of 9 laparoscopic radical prostatectomies (LRPs) with a mean operative time of 9.4 hours, concluding that there were no advantages compared with the gold standard open radical prostatectomy (ORP). However, at the turn of the century, European urologists[4–6] reported shorter operative times and consistently reproducible advantages of the laparoscopic approach, promoting acceptance of this technique.

Introduced in 1999, the da Vinci Surgical System (Intuitive Surgical Inc, CA, USA) was initially intended for cardiac surgery; however, Abbou and colleagues[7] reported the use of the robotic platform for radical prostatectomy in a single case report with an operative time of 420 minutes. The feasibility of this new approach was also shown by Binder and Kramer[8] in a series of 10 robotic-assisted laparoscopic radical prostatectomies (RALPs) with a 30% positive margin rate and 1 case requiring open conversion. The robotic surgical system allows for technical advantages such as three-dimensional magnified vision, enhanced ergonomics, tremor filtration, motion scaling, and improved manual dexterity,[9] from wristed capabilities that allow for 6° of freedom of movement that overcomes some of the limited motion of pure laparoscopy.[9–11] Less than a decade after its introduction, RALP was used in 75% to 85% of radical prostatectomies performed in the United States in 2008.[12,13]

Although enthusiasm for this approach may be driven by good outcomes from studies from high-volume centers, 70% of all radical prostatectomies in the United States are performed by low-volume surgeons,[14] whose findings may go unpublished. A population-based analysis of Surveillance Epidemiology and End Results (SEER)-Medicare linked data demonstrated that those undergoing LRP and RALP versus radical retropubic prostatectomy (RRP) experienced

[1] Both authors contributed equally.

Division of Urology, Brigham & Women's Hospital, 45 Francis Street ASB II-3, Boston, MA 02115, USA
* Corresponding author.
E-mail address: jhu2@partners.org (J.C. Hu).

Urol Clin N Am 37 (2010) 37–47
doi:10.1016/j.ucl.2009.11.005
0094-0143/10/$ – see front matter

shorter hospitalizations (2 vs 3 days) and fewer heterologous transfusions (2.7% vs 20.8%) and strictures (5.8% vs 14%). These advantageous outcomes were likely driven by intrinsic qualities of the minimally invasive approach, such as small incisions with less tension on the abdominal wall, pneumoperitoneum, and superior visualization of the anastomosis. However, LRP and RALP compared with RRP were associated with more genitourinary complications (4.7% vs 2.1%) and diagnoses of incontinence (15.9% vs 12.2%) and erectile dysfunction (26.8% vs 19.2%). Subanalyses demonstrated that cystograms were obtained with 3 times greater frequency with RALP and LRP versus RRP (31.4% vs 9.9%),[15] which may explain the higher rates of anastomotic leak diagnoses. This finding coupled with the greater risk for urinary retention from earlier attempts at catheter removal may contribute to the greater frequency of genitourinary complications observed with RALP and LRP versus RRP.

This article describes the learning curve associated with RALP, reviews in detail the challenging steps of the operation, describes the authors' RALP technique, and concludes with tips to overcome the learning curve.

LEARNING CURVE: THE CHALLENGE OF RADICAL PROSTATECTOMY

In 1936, Wright[16] introduced the concept of a learning curve by proposing a mathematical model for the aircraft industry. Since then, it has been used to characterize the diminishing amount of time required to perform a specific repeated task.[17] However, in the surgical field, no standard definition has been accepted,[18] and the surgical learning curve is typically defined as the number of cases a surgeon needs to perform a particular procedure to achieve acceptable operative times and reasonable outcomes[19]; alternatively, it is a self-declared point at which a surgeon reaches a comfort zone when performing a procedure.[18]

Part of the difficulty in establishing an exact definition is that individuals have different goals when performing a new procedure. Highly experienced surgeons tend to focus on different outcomes than novice surgeons, which could prolong their perception of their learning curve.[18] Moreover, the learning curve also depends on subjective measures such as surgeon confidence, attitude, and previous experience with crossover applicability.[19]

Population-based studies of RRP have shown that greater surgeon experience is associated with fewer perioperative complications, anastomotic strictures, and shorter lengths of stay.[20,21] Hu and colleagues[22] demonstrated that greater LRP and RALP surgeon volume was associated with fewer anastomotic strictures and better cancer control. A study of more than 7000 RRPs at 4 US centers[23] revealed that the learning curve for biochemical recurrence plateaus at 250 cases, and the 5-year probability of recurrence was 10.7% for those treated by surgeons with 250 RRPs, but 17.9% for surgeons with fewer than 10 prior RRPs. Using a similar study design for establishing an LRP cancer control learning curve, Vickers and colleagues[24] demonstrated that the 5-year biochemical recurrence rate for surgeons who performed 10, 250, and 750 prior LRPs were 17%, 16%, and 9%, respectively.

The learning curve for RALP is less challenging than LRP.[10] Patel and colleagues[10] estimated that 20 to 25 cases are required to achieve proficiency with RALP. Conversely, Herrell and Smith[18] defined a learning curve of 150 RALPs for an experienced open surgeon to achieve similar outcomes compared with RRP and 250 RALPs to obtain surgeon comfort and confidence. For laparoscopic surgeons transitioning to RALP, Jaffe and colleagues[25] found that the positive-margin rate for an experienced laparoscopic surgeon was 58% in the first 12 cases, decreasing to 9% after 180 cases.

At the Brigham and Women's Hospital, a single surgeon (JCH) performed more than 700 RALPs after logging 76 RRPs during residency and 397 RALPs during fellowship training. In contrast to the studies mentioned earlier, it was found that the RALP learning curve extends beyond 250 cases, as significant improvements in estimated blood loss (EBL), operative time, and overall complications were observed throughout the first 700 cases. The EBL and operative times were 270.1 mL and 225.8 minutes, respectively during the first 100 cases, and decreased to 197.2 mL and 126.8 minutes during cases 600 to 700. The positive margin rate decreased from 17% for the first 100 cases to 12% after 400 cases, and remained constant up to 700 cases.

The rapid, widespread diffusion of the robotic technique, in conjunction with the RALP learning curve, may help explain why RRP had better outcomes in genitourinary complications, incontinence, and erectile dysfunction in a recent population-based observational cohort study using SEER-Medicare claims.[15] Although learning curves are unavoidable for new techniques, surgeons have the responsibility to portray realistic expectations of outcomes to patients, based on their own data. A recent review of hospital Web sites showed that significant misinformation regarding RALP outcomes has been disseminated: more than 50% of the RALP Web sites had no information regarding erectile function recovery, and of those that did, 50% stated that RALP had better erectile function outcomes than RRP.[26] Such misinformation relays unrealistic expectations, and patients striving to maintain a high level of continence and erectile function may self-select for RALP based on misleading marketing. Consequently, patients treated with RALP may have higher levels of treatment regret than those undergoing RRP.[27] In addition, this potential selection bias may also explain the findings of increased risk of erectile dysfunction and incontinence in RALP patients.

TECHNICAL CHALLENGES OF RALP

Accessing the Space of Retzius: Extraperitoneal Versus Transperitoneal Approach

RALP may be performed via an extraperitoneal or transperitoneal approach. The extraperitoneal approach was first described by Raboy and colleagues in 1997.[28] In retrospective comparative studies, Ruiz and colleagues[29] observed greater operative times in the transperitoneal group with similar early oncologic results for both techniques, whereas Brown and colleagues[30] reported a slightly increased risk of ileus after the transperitoneal approach. No other significant differences between the 2 techniques have been reported.[31,32]

The potential advantages of the extraperitoneal technique include: (1) confinement of potential postoperative bleeding or anastomotic leaks to the closed extraperitoneal space; (2) simulation of the RRP anatomy; (3) absence of bowel in the surgical field; (4) less need for an extreme Trendelenburg position, which improves ventilation, especially in obese patients; and (5) less risk of intra-abdominal complications such as bowel injuries.[11,33]

The potential disadvantages are: (1) limited working space; (2) additional time and equipment required to create the extraperitoneal space; and (3) contraindications in patients with previous extended suprapubic laparotomy, or bilateral hernia repairs.[11]

Bladder Neck Dissection: Standard Technique Versus Bladder Neck Preservation

Bladder neck dissection is one of the most difficult steps for newcomers to LRP and RALP.[34] The absence of tactile sensation and unfamiliar laparoscopic anatomy may prove challenging for those inexperienced with minimally invasive approaches to radical prostatectomy, as shown by the wide variation in techniques to facilitate this step.[35,36]

The standard dissection technique makes no attempt to preserve the muscle fibers of the bladder neck, which results in a larger bladder neck requiring a reconstruction before the urethrovesical anastomosis. Bladder neck preservation has been associated with several advantages, including a lower risk of bladder neck contracture,[37] lower rates of ureteral injury,[35] and earlier return of continence.[38–41] However, others have suggested that preservation of the bladder neck compromises cancer control by increasing the risk of positive margins at the prostate base with no effect on continence.[42–45]

The authors retrospectively evaluated outcomes in a series of 619 men, with 271 submitted to the standard technique and 349 submitted to bladder neck preservation. Bladder neck preservation was associated with earlier return of continence (0 pads per day) and better mean urinary function scores after 24 months of follow-up, using a self-reported validated quality-of-life instrument, the Expanded Prostate Cancer Index (EPIC) short form.[46] Moreover, no differences were observed regarding positive margins at the prostate base.[47]

Nerve-sparing Technique

Nerve preservation during RALP is a challenging and critical step, as it affects postoperative sexual function and cancer control. Several techniques for the release of the NVBs have been described. In an attempt to decrease the rate of positive margins, Villers and colleagues[48] introduced the concept of the extrafascial dissection for ORP. With the improved visualization from laparoscopic approaches, new techniques of interfascial and intrafascial dissection of the NVBs have been proposed.[49] Savera and colleagues[50] first described the intrafascial approach, suggesting that the lateral aspect of the fascia also contains bundles of sensitive parasympathetic nerves, which are not preserved by the traditional technique. With this technique, Menon and colleagues[51] reported a 13% positive margin rate and 100% intercourse rate in patients undergoing bilateral nerve-sparing surgery at 48 months of follow-up (with or without oral medication). Others[52] replicated the feasibility of this technique but with less noteworthy sexual function results and a higher positive margin rate, especially for patients with pT3 disease. Curto and colleagues[53] presented their experience with the intrafascial approach with an overall positive margin rate of 30.7% in more than 2800 procedures. Moreover, the precise role of these nerve fibers spared in the intrafascial approach but sacrificed in the interfascial approach remains unknown[54] and warrants further study.

Regardless of the intra- versus interfascial technique used for nerve sparing, the type and amount of energy used during dissection of the neurovascular bundles is of vital importance for preservation and early recovery of sexual function. In a canine experimental model, Ong and colleagues[55] described that the use of hemostatic energy sources such as monopolar, bipolar, or ultrasound in proximity to the NVBs is associated with the loss of erectile response to cavernous nerve stimulation acutely and after 2 weeks of follow-up.

Other sources of energy have been used in an attempt to control bleeding near the NVBs. Recently, Gianduzzo and colleagues[56] studied the use of potassium titanyl phosphate (KTP) laser energy during nerve-sparing RRP in a canine model. They compared KTP laser with ultrasonic and athermal cold scissor dissection, and found the KTP laser provided effective hemostasis with minimum injury to the adjacent tissues, similar to the amount imparted by the athermal technique. Haber and colleagues[57] proposed an energy-free technique with the use of a bulldog clamp and delicate sutures to control the NVBs. In this technique, a Doppler ultrasound is also used to identify the NVBs, avoiding damage to these structures. Although thermal injuries are significant, Ahlering and colleagues[58] described the eventual recovery of sexual function after 24 months in patients submitted to use of thermal energy during NVB dissection, suggesting these injuries are reversible in the long-term.

The authors' approach to nerve sparing has been described in detail elsewhere.[59] In short, the authors perform a sharp athermal technique with Weck clips and cold scissors after identification of the posteromedial and anterolateral prostatic contours.

Apical Dissection

The apical dissection is one of the most crucial steps in RALP. The surgeon aims to maximize preservation of the urinary sphincter with total resection of the prostate apical tissue, targeting an optimal balance between continence and cancer control.

Different techniques have been described to minimize incontinence after radical prostatectomy. Klein[60] refined the apical dissection technique by describing the mobilization of the distal third of the prostate with minimal damage to the external sphincter. Recently, Porpiglia and colleagues[61] described a selective suture of the DVC for LRP. In this technique, the DVC is sectioned and a selective suture of the plexus is performed with 1 or 2 stitches, avoiding the incorporation of surrounding tissue. At 3 months, 80% of the patients who underwent selective suture ligation of the DVC were continent, compared with 53% of the patients who had surgery without selective suture ligation. Menon and colleagues[62] described their technique of apical dissection, using an adaptation of the same technique previously described for RRP. The DVC is controlled with a single figure-of-eight stitch before it is divided down to the urethra. In their retrospective study, 96% of patients were socially dry (use of 1 pad or less per day) after 3 months of follow-up. Other intraoperative attempts to improve early continence have included the placement of the puboperiurethral stitch after the ligation of the DVC. Patel and colleagues[63] described a suspension technique that resulted in higher continence rates at 3 months after the procedure.

The prostatic apex is generally regarded as the most common site of iatrogenic positive margins.[62,64] Walsh[65] proposed that positive apical margins commonly occur during the release of the DVC and the striated sphincter. Ahlering and colleagues[66] showed that the use of an endovascular stapler to control the DVC decreased the positive margin rates from 27% to 5%, compared with a suture ligation technique. Guru and colleagues[67] proposed that using cold incision of the DVC without previous suture ligation also resulted in lower apical margin rates during RALP. Men who underwent prostatectomy with cold incision apical dissection showed a positive margin rate of 2%, whereas patients with suture ligation had a positive margin rate of 8%.

Vesicourethral Anastomosis

For those early in the learning curve, the vesicourethral anastomosis may be one of the most challenging and time-consuming steps of RALP.[68] Several techniques have been described. A single-knot continuous vesicourethral anastomosis for LRP was proposed by van Velthoven and colleagues.[69] This technique was rapidly adopted for LRP and has been transferred to RALP.[70] This continuous suture is fast and easy to perform, requiring just 1 knot.[71] In a porcine model of vesicourethral anastomosis, continuous suturing was compared with an interrupted suture technique. Both techniques had similar rates of anastomotic leaks. However, histopathologic examination revealed more muscle-layer fibrosis in the group with interrupted sutures,[72] suggesting a higher risk of anastomotic stricture.

On the other hand, the lack of haptic feedback and the potential for suboptimal suture tension after knot tying may increase the risk of anastomotic leakage. Several techniques have been described to mitigate this risk, such as the use of a Lowsley tractor[73] and the use of an absorbable Lapra-Ty (Ethicon Inc, San Angelo, TX, USA) to keep tension and ensure an optimal posterior approximation.[74] The authors' technique of vesicourethral anastomosis combines the more reliable posterior approximation of the interrupted suture with the advantages of the faster running suture.[68]

THE BRIGHAM & WOMEN'S HOSPITAL TECHNIQUE

Positioning/Setup

The patient is initially placed in the supine position with legs extended on flat split leg boards. The split leg boards are spread to allow the robot to dock, and the hips are extended 20°. The patient's arms are tucked and secured with the aid of arm sleds. All pressure points are well padded. After the patient is prepared and draped, a 16-Fr urethral catheter is placed. A Veress needle or Hassan technique is used to achieve pneumoperitoneum to an intra-abdominal pressure of 15 mm Hg. The patient is then reclined in a full Trendelenburg position to approximately 30° for a transperitoneal approach (**Fig. 1**), a standard 6-port template is used (**Fig. 2**), and a 4-arm da Vinci robot is docked. A zero-degree camera is used exclusively throughout the operation, obviating scope changes. The authors start with a curved monopolar scissor in the right da Vinci arm and a bipolar Maryland dissector in the left arm, with a ProGrasp in the fourth arm, docked at the left anterior superior iliac spine. The assistant uses a suction irrigator through a 5-mm assistant trocar positioned cephalad to the umbilicus at the right rectus margin and a nontraumatic grasper through a 12-mm assistant trocar placed just medial to the right anterior superior iliac spine. The monopolar and bipolar currents are set to 25 W.

Accessing the Retropubic Space of Retzius

The operation commences with the high transection of the median umbilical ligament and urachus using generous monopolar cauterization to avoid potential bleeding from a patent umbilical vessel. The peritoneal incision is carried just lateral to the umbilical ligaments, as they course posteriorly to their origin from the hypogastric artery, until the vas deferens is reached. The retropubic space of Retzius is then entered by separating the bladder from the anterior abdominal wall until the pubis is identified. The ProGrasp (fourth arm) applies cephalad traction to the bladder, while overlying fat is cleared from the proximal prostate, the prostatovesical junction, and the endopelvic fascia. The superficial dorsal vein is cauterized with bipolar energy before transaction.

Anterior Bladder Neck Sparing Division

Midprostatic and anterior vesical hemostatic sutures are placed with a 2-0 Vicryl (Ethicon Inc, San Angelo, TX, USA) on a CT-1 needle. Three-dimensionalized anterior-cephalad tension to the bladder is applied by retracting the bladder dome with the fourth arm ProGrasp. This motion tents the anterior bladder to form a ridge that ends distally at the detrusor apron. In addition, this motion allows for visualization of the urethral catheter balloon, as the empty bladder caves in around

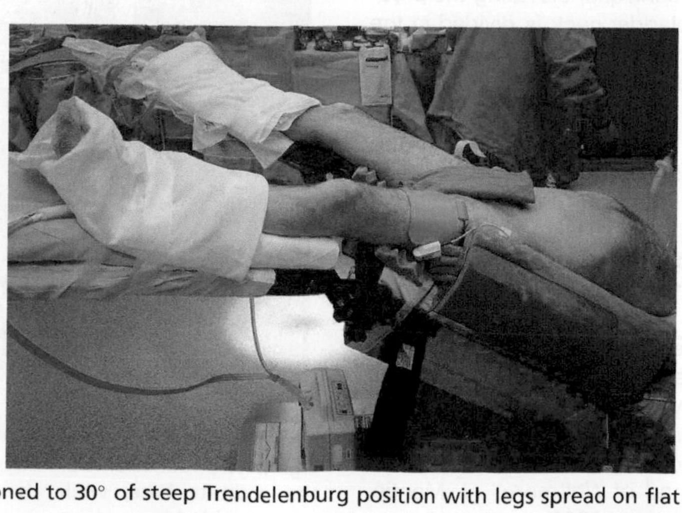

Fig. 1. Patient positioned to 30° of steep Trendelenburg position with legs spread on flat split boards and hips extended about 20°.

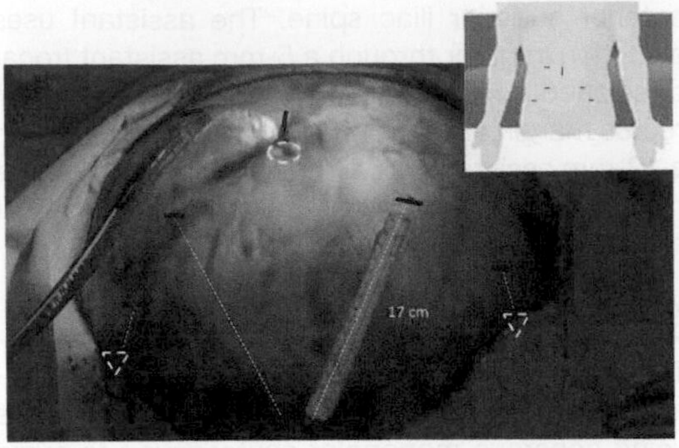

Fig. 2. Standard 6-port template: 12-mm camera trocar just cephalad to the umbilicus, two 8-mm ports placed 17 cm from base of penis and 8 cm from midline on right and left, 8-mm fourth-arm port placed 1 fingerbreadth superior-lateral to the left anterior iliac spine, 12-mm assistant port placed 2 fingerbreadths superior-lateral to right anterior iliac spine, and a 5-mm assistant port placed cephalad, and just medial, to the right-arm 8-mm port.

the balloon. At the proximal detrusor apron, the bladder neck is sharply dissected with the cold scissors while bipolar current is used for hemostasis. The use of bipolar current minimizes the amount of tissue charring, allowing for easier identification of the natural tissue planes. The linear fibers of the bladder neck transitioning to the prostatic urethra are identified in the midline, and the remaining bladder muscle fibers are teased away from the prostate base, preserving a funneled bladder neck. After 270° anterior circumferential dissection of the bladder neck as it transitions to the prostatic urethra, the urethral catheter balloon is deflated, and the bladder neck is incised as distally as possible.[47] The assistant grasps the tip of the urethral catheter using a 1-handed intra- and extracorporeal technique, elevating the prostate. The posterior bladder neck is divided in the midline (**Fig. 3**) until the posterior longitudinal fascia of the detrusor muscle is encountered (**Fig. 4**). For optimal three-dimensionalized traction, the fourth arm ProGrasp retracts the posterior prostate anteriorly, while the assistant grasps the posterior bladder neck for countertraction. Subsequent incision of the posterior longitudinal fascia reveals the seminal vesicles and vas deferens. With the aid of bipolar current for hemostasis, the dissection is continued sharply in a posterior-lateral plane, with care to avoid a posterior cystotomy, entry into the prostate base capsule, or early transection of the lateral pedicle, which can result in bleeding. The dissection is continued until adipose tissue is encountered lateral to the bladder neck, a landmark known as the "fat pad of Whitmore" (J. Montie, personal communication, 2009), which defines

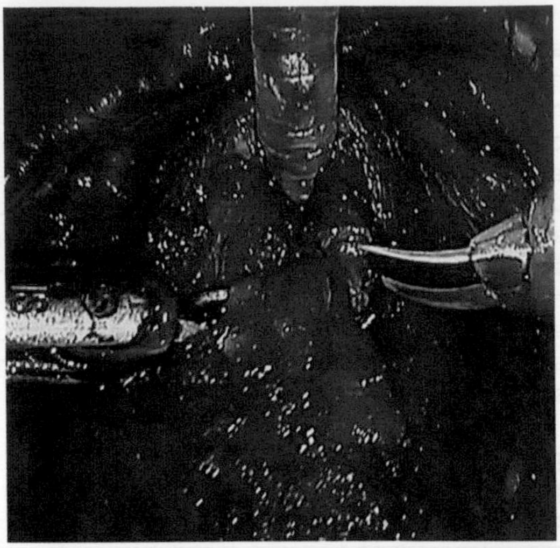

Fig. 3. Isolation of the posterior bladder neck while the assistant elevates the prostate by applying tension to the Foley catheter.

the posterior-lateral limit of the bladder neck dissection, as the NVB lies in close proximity. This complete unhinging of the bladder from the prostate allows for better access to the vasa deferentia.

Isolating the Seminal Vesicles/Posterior Dissection

The fourth arm ProGrasp is readjusted to grab the ampulla of vas and place it on anterior traction. The vas deferens is dissected free from its investing sheath and cut after the assistant places a 10-mm Weck clip on the proximal end. The assistant grasps the proximal cut vas, and the artery to

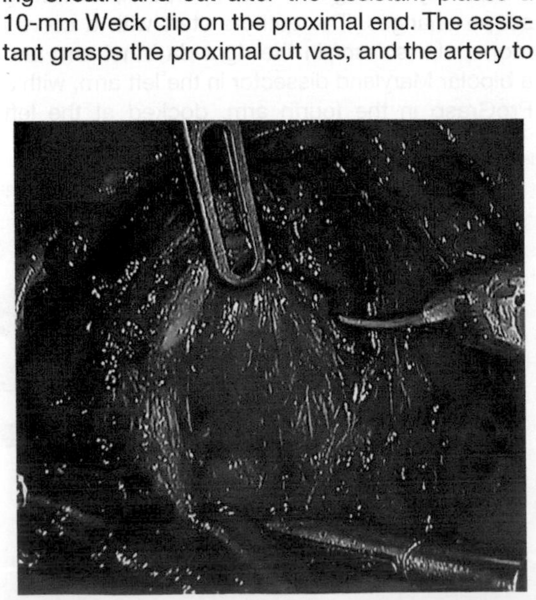

Fig. 4. The fourth arm provides anterior traction on the prostate base, while the assistant grasps the posterior bladder neck.

the vas deferens is identified and secured with small clips or selective use of bipolar current. Frequent readjustment of the fourth arm ProGrasp on the seminal vesicle is helpful in providing the appropriate traction needed to dissect the seminal vesicle free sharply. Thermal energy is avoided to prevent injury to the nearby NVB. Instead, small pedicle windows are created at the tip of the seminal vesicle and small titanium or Weck clips are applied. The contralateral seminal vesicle is dissected in the same manner.

Next, the fourth arm ProGrasp elevates both seminal vesicles, and a sharp incision is made in the midline until the glistening posterior Denonvilliers sheath is identified. With the assistant placing downward traction on the rectum, the posterior dissection is continued between the prostatic and Denonvilliers fascia if a nerve-sparing approach is being used. For higher-risk patients, such as those with high-volume, high-grade disease or those with a palpable nodule, the dissection is performed leaving the entire Denonvilliers fascia with the specimen. A triangle is created with the rectum as the base, the lateral pedicle as the sides, and the middle of the posterior prostate as the apex. The assistant provides countertraction by retracting the corners of the triangle base in a posterior-lateral fashion. Dissection is continued laterally and distally until the medial border of the NVB is appreciated.[59] This maneuver thins out the vascular pedicle, which facilitates subsequent clip placement, and defines the posterior medial prostate contour.

Athermal Lateral Pedicles

A sweeping motion of the monopolar scissors is used to bluntly identify a natural cleavage plane to reflect the levator fascia away from the prostatic fascia until tiny nerve plexus components are identified coursing lateral to the prostate. This technique clearly defines the anterior lateral prostate contour. With the lateral pedicle placed on traction, a series of large Weck clips are used to ligate and divide the lateral pedicle vessels in an athermal fashion. Next, the NVB is gently teased off the prostate to the apex in an antegrade manner using a combination of sharp and blunt dissection (**Fig. 5**). Tumor characteristics determine the amount of periprostatic tissue that is left with the prostate. The contralateral lateral pedicle and NVB are dissected in a similar manner.[59]

Apical Dissection

The prostate is placed on cephalad traction by the fourth arm ProGrasp. The puboprostatic ligaments are transected sharply and the prostate apex is further dissected from the levator fascia. The detrusor apron, the arteries and veins within, are sharply divided, and selective bipolar cautery is used to stop arterial bleeders while allowing pneumoperitoneum to minimize venous bleeding (**Fig. 6**). The distal NVB is swept laterally from the urethra at the apex, and the lateral pillars of the urethra are sharply transected, completely freeing up the prostate and urethra from its surrounding structures. The anterior 270° of urethra are incised until the urethral catheter is identified.

Next, the only instrument changes are made, inserting large needle drivers into both right and left Da Vinci arms. A 3-0 Vicryl on a CT-3 needle is used to re-approximate the cut edges of DVC with a horizontal mattress suture. We believe this precise selective suturing of the DVC provides excellent visualization of the prostatic apex and reduces the risk of positive apical margins and

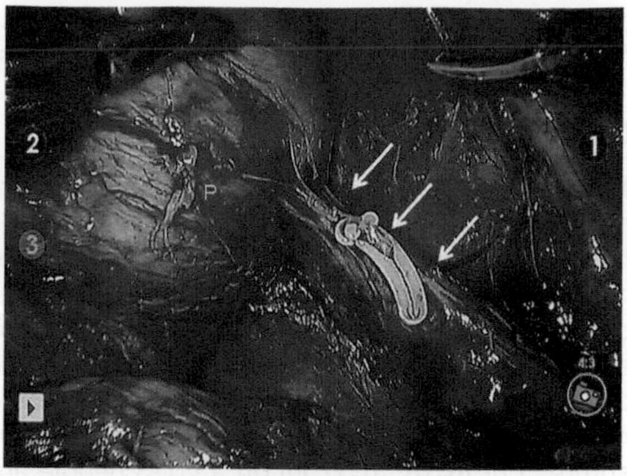

Fig. 5. After the posterior medial and anterior lateral prostatic contours have been defined, the NVB is gently teased off the prostate. P, prostate; arrows, right NVB.

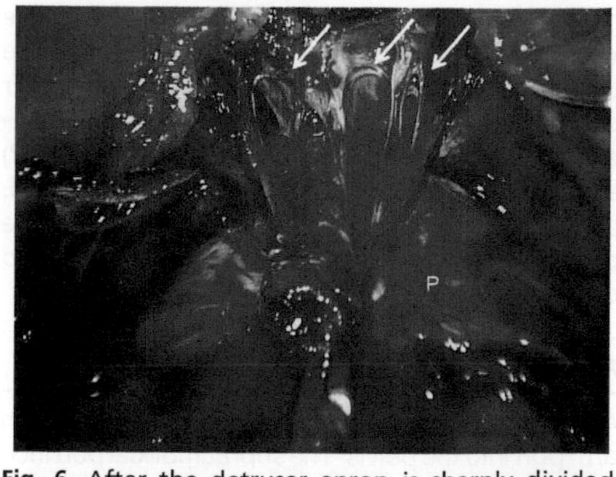

Fig. 6. After the detrusor apron is sharply divided, pneumoperitoneum controls the large dorsal venous complex sinuses, which are easily visible for selective suturing. P, prostate; arrows, dorsal vein complex sinuses.

damage to the rabdosphincter continence mechanism compared with preplaced sutures or staples.

Urethral Anastomosis

The authors prefer a combined running and interrupted suture technique for urethrovesical anastamosis. The posterior stability of this technique is provided by 3 interrupted sutures placed under direct visualization of the knots placed inside the anastamosis on the mucosa, while the remainder of the anastamosis is performed in an efficient running fashion. Two absorbable 3-0 polygalactin sutures cut to 18 cm (7 in) on a CT-3 needle are used.

The urethral catheter is retracted and a 6 o'clock posterior urethral suture is placed inside out before division of the posterior urethra, preventing urethral retraction. The posterior urethra is transected, and the specimen is placed in a laparoscopic bag. Pneumoperitoneum pressure is then brought down to 5 mm Hg, and meticulous hemostasis is obtained with clips or selective suture ligation. The initial suture is then placed on the corresponding posterior bladder neck incorporating mucosa. A surgeon's knot is tied on the bladder neck side to allow for knot tension without tearing the urethral stump. Next 2 lateral posterior sutures are placed on each side of the 6 o'clock suture, with the knot tied on the bladder mucosa. The contralateral needle driver is then used to place full-thickness single bites outside in through the bladder and inside out through the urethra. These sutures are then run in this continuous fashion until both needles are brought out through the urethra at 12 o'clock. Typically 2 or 3 throws of each needle are required. One of the needles is brought inside out on the bladder side so the running sutures are tied down across the anastomosis. The bladder is filled with 120 mL of sterile water to check for anastomotic leak, and the urethral catheter is exchanged for a new 20-Fr catheter. A cystogram is performed before catheter removal if (1) intraoperative leak is noted, (2) extensive bladder neck reconstruction is required, or (3) postoperative urine leak is confirmed by the presence of an increased Jackson-Pratt fluid creatinine concentration.[68]

Retrieval of Specimen/Closure

A Jackson-Pratt drain is placed through the fourth arm port into the pelvis. The supraumbilical port incision is lengthened to allow for specimen removal. The fascia is closed with 0 Vicryl on a UR-6 needle with 3 to 4 figure-of-eight sutures. The skin is reapproximated with a subcuticular suture.

TIPS FOR THE BEGINNER

Although the learning curve for RALP is significant, several measures may shorten the process. A dedicated robotics team must be formed. Initially, this requires significant hospital support, but pays dividends in the long-term. A dedicated surgical assistant is arguably the most helpful. The assistant's role in providing adequate exposure and visualization through retraction and suction, and in applying clips accurately and expeditiously, cannot be overstated. Furthermore, an experienced assistant is able to troubleshoot many of the robotic issues that may arise at the bedside, allowing the surgeon to focus on surgical technique. Moreover, an anesthesiologist familiar with the operation is better able to handle the physiologic effects of prolonged insufflation in the steep Trendelenburg position. An inexperienced anesthesiologist may base fluid management on expectations of blood loss from RRP, leading to overhydration and possible pulmonary edema and congestive heart failure in men with significant cardiovascular disease.

The surgeon unfamiliar with laparoscopy must also learn to depend on visual cues as opposed to tactile feedback. Visual cues are especially important in identifying tissue characteristics and anatomic planes. Rethinking the steps of the operation compared with RRP will also decrease blood loss at critical steps of RALP, leading to better visualization and efficient dissection rather than repeated attempts at hemostasis and guessing the location of the correct anatomic planes. For instance, the authors perform an antegrade RALP in contrast to RRP, which is performed in a retrograde fashion and requires ligation of the DVC initially. Instead, the authors perform the bladder neck dissection first, leaving the apical dissection and the DVC for later. There are several advantages to reversing this sequence. First, the venous anatomy is highly variable at the apex, and incurring blood loss early can obscure anatomic planes for subsequent steps such as nerve-sparing and bladder neck dissection. Moreover, bladder neck dissection and ligation of the lateral pedicles early in RALP leads to an absence of venous back-bleeding when dividing the DVC as one of the final steps. However, because the DVC has not been ligated early, back-bleeder clips must be applied before dividing the lateral pedicle to ensure hemostasis and adequate visualization.

The authors have switched from the posterior approach to seminal vesicle dissection to the anterior approach through the bladder neck because of improved exposure. Dissecting out the vasa deferentia through a peritoneal incision in the cul-de-sac leads to operating in a hole. The fourth arm is occupied with retracting the sigmoid colon cephalad and an assistant instrument is occupied with holding the upper cut edge of the peritoneum to provide exposure. This technique results in poor exposure if bleeding is encountered, often leading to more liberal use of energy for hemostasis.

Another critical component to overcome the learning curve is the continued assessment of technique. This assessment is best done by recording all procedures and reviewing them shortly after. Without the stress of performing an operation, viewing recorded video can provide valuable information about details that facilitate an operation, such as what the fourth arm is doing, and how the assistant is providing exposure. In addition, the neophyte surgeon should review video of more experienced robotic surgeons. A prospectively collected database of perioperative, pathologic, and quality-of-life outcomes should be kept and reviewed for self-assessment, in particular, as modifications of surgical technique may take 18 to 24 months (the interim required for recovery of urinary and sexual function to plateau) to manifest in improved functional outcomes.

The authors believe many of the basic tenets of open surgery must be applied to RALP. A detailed understanding of pelvic anatomy is critical. Meticulous attention to detail and a dedication to performing the same surgical steps in a repetitive fashion are necessary to overcome the prolonged learning curve. Maintaining exposure is necessary for safe and reproducible RALP. The surgical assistant's grasper and fourth arm of the robotic system must always be positioned to provide traction and countertraction, allowing for easier visualization of surgical planes. The surgeon should also avoid working in a hole, which results in poor visualization and difficulty controlling bleeding.

REFERENCES

1. Boxer RJ, Kaufman JJ, Goodwin WE. Radical prostatectomy for carcinoma of the prostate: 1951–1976. A review of 329 patients. J Urol 1977;117:208.
2. Walsh PC. Anatomic radical prostatectomy: evolution of the surgical technique. J Urol 1998;160:2418.
3. Schuessler WW, Schulam PG, Clayman RV, et al. Laparoscopic radical prostatectomy: initial short-term experience. Urology 1997;50:854.
4. Guillonneau B, Vallancien G. Laparoscopic radical prostatectomy: the Montsouris technique. J Urol 2000;163:1643.
5. Guillonneau B, Cathelineau X, Barret E, et al. Laparoscopic radical prostatectomy: technical and early oncological assessment of 40 operations. Eur Urol 1999;36:14.
6. Guillonneau B, Vallancien G. Laparoscopic radical prostatectomy: the Montsouris experience. J Urol 2000;163:418.
7. Abbou CC, Hoznek A, Salomon L, et al. Laparoscopic radical prostatectomy with a remote controlled robot. J Urol 1964;165:2001.
8. Binder J, Kramer W. Robotically-assisted laparoscopic radical prostatectomy. BJU Int 2001;87:408.
9. Chin JL, Luke PP, Pautler SE. Initial experience with robotic-assisted laparoscopic radical prostatectomy in the Canadian health care system. Can Urol Assoc J 2007;1:97.
10. Menon M, Tewari A, Peabody JO, et al. Vattikuti Institute prostatectomy, a technique of robotic radical prostatectomy for management of localized carcinoma of the prostate: experience of over 1100 cases. Urol Clin North Am 2004;31:701.
11. Patel VR, Tully AS, Holmes R, et al. Robotic radical prostatectomy in the community setting–the learning curve and beyond: initial 200 cases. J Urol 2005;174:269.
12. Lepor H. Status of radical prostatectomy in 2009: is there medical evidence to justify the robotic approach? Rev Urol 2009;11:61.
13. Zorn KC, Gautam G, Shalhav AL, et al. Training, credentialing, proctoring and medicolegal risks of robotic urological surgery: recommendations of the society of urologic robotic surgeons. J Urol 2009;182:1126.
14. Wilt TJ, Shamliyan TA, Taylor BC, et al. Association between hospital and surgeon radical prostatectomy volume and patient outcomes: a systematic review. J Urol 2008;180:820.
15. Hu JC, Gu X, Lipsitz SR, et al. Comparative effectiveness of minimally invasive vs open radical prostatectomy. JAMA 2009;302:1557.
16. Wright TP. Factors affecting the cost of airplanes. J Aeronaut Sci 1936;3:122.
17. Steinberg PL, Merguerian PA, Bihrle W 3rd, et al. The cost of learning robotic-assisted prostatectomy. Urology 2008;72:1068.
18. Herrell SD, Smith JA Jr. Robotic-assisted laparoscopic prostatectomy: what is the learning curve? Urology 2005;66:105.
19. Artibani W, Novara G. Cancer-related outcome and learning curve in retropubic radical prostatectomy: "if you need an operation, the most important step is to choose the right surgeon". Eur Urol 2008;53:874.
20. Hu JC, Gold KF, Pashos CL, et al. Role of surgeon volume in radical prostatectomy outcomes. J Clin Oncol 2003;21:401.
21. Begg CB, Riedel ER, Bach PB, et al. Variations in morbidity after radical prostatectomy. N Engl J Med 2002;346:1138.
22. Hu JC, Wang Q, Pashos CL, et al. Utilization and outcomes of minimally invasive radical prostatectomy. J Clin Oncol 2008;26:2278.

23. Vickers AJ, Bianco FJ, Serio AM, et al. The surgical learning curve for prostate cancer control after radical prostatectomy. J Natl Cancer Inst 2007;99:1171.
24. Vickers AJ, Savage CJ, Hruza M, et al. The surgical learning curve for laparoscopic radical prostatectomy: a retrospective cohort study. Lancet Oncol 2009;10:475.
25. Jaffe J, Castellucci S, Cathelineau X, et al. Robot-assisted laparoscopic prostatectomy: a single-institutions learning curve. Urology 2009;73:127.
26. Mulhall JP, Rojaz-Cruz C, Muller A. An analysis of sexual health information on radical prostatectomy websites. BJU Int 2009. [Epub ahead of print]. PMID: 19627282.
27. Schroeck FR, Krupski TL, Sun L, et al. Satisfaction and regret after open retropubic or robot-assisted laparoscopic radical prostatectomy. Eur Urol 2008; 54:785.
28. Raboy A, Ferzli G, Albert P. Initial experience with extraperitoneal endoscopic radical retropubic prostatectomy. Urology 1997;50:849.
29. Ruiz L, Salomon L, Hoznek A, et al. Comparison of early oncologic results of laparoscopic radical prostatectomy by extraperitoneal versus transperitoneal approach. Eur Urol 2004;46:50.
30. Brown JA, Rodin D, Lee B, et al. Transperitoneal versus extraperitoneal approach to laparoscopic radical prostatectomy: an assessment of 156 cases. Urology 2005;65:320.
31. Atug F, Castle EP, Srivastav SK, et al. Positive surgical margins in robotic-assisted radical prostatectomy: impact of learning curve on oncologic outcomes. Eur Urol 2006;49:866.
32. Erdogru T, Teber D, Frede T, et al. Comparison of transperitoneal and extraperitoneal laparoscopic radical prostatectomy using match-pair analysis. Eur Urol 2004;46:312.
33. Atug F, Castle EP, Woods M, et al. Transperitoneal versus extraperitoneal robotic-assisted radical prostatectomy: is one better than the other? Urology 2006;68:1077.
34. Ahlering TE, Skarecky D, Lee D, et al. Successful transfer of open surgical skills to a laparoscopic environment using a robotic interface: initial experience with laparoscopic radical prostatectomy. J Urol 2003;170:1738.
35. Jenkins LC, Nogueira M, Wilding GE, et al. Median lobe in robot-assisted radical prostatectomy: evaluation and management. Urology 2008;71:810.
36. Tewari AK, Rao SR. Anatomical foundations and surgical manoeuvres for precise identification of the prostatovesical junction during robotic radical prostatectomy. BJU Int 2006;98:833.
37. Licht MR, Klein EA, Tuason L, et al. Impact of bladder neck preservation during radical prostatectomy on continence and cancer control. Urology 1994;44:883.
38. Gomez CA, Soloway MS, Civantos F, et al. Bladder neck preservation and its impact on positive surgical margins during radical prostatectomy. Urology 1993;42:689.
39. Soloway MS, Neulander E. Bladder-neck preservation during radical retropubic prostatectomy. Semin Urol Oncol 2000;18:51.
40. Selli C, De Antoni P, Moro U, et al. Role of bladder neck preservation in urinary continence following radical retropubic prostatectomy. Scand J Urol Nephrol 2004;38:32.
41. Lowe BA. Comparison of bladder neck preservation to bladder neck resection in maintaining postprostatectomy urinary continence. Urology 1996;48:889.
42. Marcovich R, Wojno KJ, Wei JT, et al. Bladder neck-sparing modification of radical prostatectomy adversely affects surgical margins in pathologic T3a prostate cancer. Urology 2000;55:904.
43. Katz R, Salomon L, Hoznek A, et al. Positive surgical margins in laparoscopic radical prostatectomy: the impact of apical dissection, bladder neck remodeling and nerve preservation. J Urol 2003;169:2049.
44. Srougi M, Nesrallah LJ, Kauffmann JR, et al. Urinary continence and pathological outcome after bladder neck preservation during radical retropubic prostatectomy: a randomized prospective trial. J Urol 2001;165:815.
45. Aydin H, Tsuzuki T, Hernandez D, et al. Positive proximal (bladder neck) margin at radical prostatectomy confers greater risk of biochemical progression. Urology 2004;64:551.
46. Wei JT, Dunn RL, Litwin MS, et al. Development and validation of the expanded prostate cancer index composite (EPIC) for comprehensive assessment of health-related quality of life in men with prostate cancer. Urology 2000;56:899.
47. Freire MP, Weinberg AC, Lei Y, et al. Anatomic bladder neck preservation during robotic-assisted laparoscopic radical prostatectomy: description of technique and outcomes. Eur Urol 2009;56(6): 972–80.
48. Villers A, Stamey TA, Yemoto C, et al. Modified extrafascial radical retropubic prostatectomy technique decreases frequency of positive surgical margins in T2 cancers <2 cm (3). Eur Urol 2000;38:64.
49. Menon M, Kaul S, Bhandari A, et al. Potency following robotic radical prostatectomy: a questionnaire based analysis of outcomes after conventional nerve sparing and prostatic fascia sparing techniques. J Urol 2005;174:2291.
50. Savera AT, Kaul S, Badani K, et al. Robotic radical prostatectomy with the "Veil of Aphrodite" technique: histologic evidence of enhanced nerve sparing. Eur Urol 2006;49:1065.
51. Menon M, Shrivastava A, Kaul S, et al. Vattikuti Institute prostatectomy: contemporary technique and analysis of results. Eur Urol 2007;51:648.

52. Potdevin L, Ercolani M, Jeong J, et al. Functional and oncologic outcomes comparing interfascial and intrafascial nerve sparing in robot-assisted laparoscopic radical prostatectomies. J Endourol 2009;23(9):1479.
53. Curto F, Benijts J, Pansadoro A, et al. Nerve sparing laparoscopic radical prostatectomy: our technique. Eur Urol 2006;49:344.
54. Rassweiler J. Intrafascial nerve-sparing laproscopic radical prostatectomy: do we really preserve relevant nerve-fibres? Eur Urol 2006;49:955.
55. Ong AM, Su LM, Varkarakis I, et al. Nerve sparing radical prostatectomy: effects of hemostatic energy sources on the recovery of cavernous nerve function in a canine model. J Urol 2004;172:1318.
56. Gianduzzo TR, Colombo JR Jr, Haber GP, et al. KTP laser nerve sparing radical prostatectomy: comparison of ultrasonic and cold scissor dissection on cavernous nerve function. J Urol 2009;181:2760.
57. Haber GP, Aron M, Ukimura O, et al. Energy-free nerve-sparing laparoscopic radical prostatectomy: the bulldog technique. BJU Int 2008;102:1766.
58. Ahlering TE, Eichel L, Skarecky D. Evaluation of long-term thermal injury using cautery during nerve sparing robotic prostatectomy. Urology 2008;72:1371.
59. Berry A, Korkes F, Hu JC. Landmarks for consistent nerve sparing during robotic-assisted laparoscopic radical prostatectomy. J Endourol 2008; 22:1565.
60. Klein EA. Modified apical dissection for early continence after radical prostatectomy. Prostate 1993; 22:217.
61. Porpiglia F, Fiori C, Grande S, et al. Selective versus standard ligature of the deep venous complex during laparoscopic radical prostatectomy: effects on continence, blood loss, and margin status. Eur Urol 2009;55:1377.
62. Menon M, Hemal AK, Tewari A, et al. The technique of apical dissection of the prostate and urethrovesical anastomosis in robotic radical prostatectomy. BJU Int 2004;93:715.
63. Patel VR, Coelho RF, Palmer KJ, et al. Periurethral suspension stitch during robot-assisted laparoscopic radical prostatectomy: description of the technique and continence outcomes. Eur Urol 2009;56(3):472.
64. Sofer M, Hamilton-Nelson KL, Civantos F, et al. Positive surgical margins after radical retropubic prostatectomy: the influence of site and number on progression. J Urol 2002;167:2453.
65. Walsh PC. Re: radical prostatectomy: the value of preoperative, individually labeled apical biopsies. J Urol 2001;165:915.
66. Ahlering TE, Eichel L, Edwards RA, et al. Robotic radical prostatectomy: a technique to reduce pT2 positive margins. Urology 2004;64:1224.
67. Guru KA, Perlmutter AE, Sheldon MJ, et al. Apical margins after robot-assisted radical prostatectomy: does technique matter? J Endourol 2009;23:123.
68. Berry AM, Korkes F, Ferreira M, et al. Robotic urethrovesical anastomosis: combining running and interrupted sutures. J Endourol 2008;22:2127.
69. Van Velthoven RF, Ahlering TE, Peltier A, et al. Technique for laparoscopic running urethrovesical anastomosis: the single knot method. Urology 2003;61: 699.
70. Kaul S, Menon M. Robotic radical prostatectomy: evolution from conventional to VIP. World J Urol 2006;24:152.
71. Emiliozzi P, Martini M, d'Elia G, et al. A new technique for laparoscopic vesicourethral anastomosis: preliminary report. Urology 2008;72:1341.
72. Lieber D, Tran V, Belani J, et al. Comparison of running and interrupted vesicourethral anastomoses in a porcine model. J Endourol 2005;19:1109.
73. Garrett JE, LaGrange CA, Chenven E, et al. Use of Lowsley tractor during laparoscopic prostatectomy to reduce urethrovesical anastomotic tension. J Endourol 2006;20:220.
74. Zorn KC. Robotic radical prostatectomy: assurance of water-tight vesicourethral anastomotic closure with the Lapra-Ty clip. J Endourol 2008;22:863.

The Case for Open Radical Prostatectomy

Edward M. Schaeffer, MD, PhD*,
Stacy Loeb, MD, Patrick C. Walsh, MD

KEYWORDS

- Prostate cancer • Radical retropubic prostatectomy
- Laparoscopic prostatectomy • Outcome

Radical prostatectomy was first performed at Johns Hopkins Hospital in 1904, and today it remains the surgical standard of care for clinically localized prostate cancer. Hugh Hampton Young initially approached the prostate from the perineum. Thereafter, perineal prostatectomy became the primary surgical approach to prostate cancer treatment; nevertheless, only approximately 7% of prostate cancer patients underwent surgery in the early 1980s.[1]

The first radical retropubic prostatectomy (RRP) was performed in 1947 by Millin. However, the procedure was uncommonly used for several decades due to the considerable associated morbidity. Finally, in the 1980s, improved delineation of the surgical anatomy (including the dorsal venous complex and neurovascular bundles) enabled several important modifications in RRP technique, and the first modern nerve-sparing RRP was performed by the senior author (P.C.W.) in 1982.[2]

In the 1990s, laparoscopic prostatectomy techniques were developed[3]; however, due to the technical difficulty of the procedure, it failed to attain widespread use until the advent of the da Vinci robotic interface by Intuitive Surgical.[4] Since that time, the use of robotic prostatectomy (RALRP) has steadily increased.[5] RALRP is rapidly becoming the predominant form of surgical management for prostate cancer in the United States.

Continued refinements to both techniques have built on each other to trigger an overall improvement in surgical outcomes.[1] This article reviews the fundamentals of radical prostatectomy including oncologic outcomes, functional outcomes, complications, convalescence, and cost. A critical assessment of surgical outcomes is necessary as clinicians strive to attain the "holy grail" of prostate cancer by providing the best cancer control with minimal morbidity.

TECHNIQUE

Although the steps of the radical prostatectomy itself are anatomically similar, there are many differences between the robotic and open techniques from start to finish. Beginning with patient positioning, open RRP is traditionally performed with the table flat or slightly flexed at the midline. By contrast, RALRP typically uses steep Trendelenburg (head-down) positioning to shift the abdominal contents for optimal exposure. Prolonged Trendelenburg positioning has been associated with head edema,[6] increased intraocular pressure,[7] and cardiopulmonary alterations, particularly in obese patients. In addition, insufflation with carbon dioxide during RALRP may lead to problematic hypercarbia and acidosis, particularly when the intra-abdominal insufflation pressure is increased in the event of troublesome bleeding.[6] Overall, judicious monitoring of end-tidal carbon dioxide levels and controlled ventilation are important to avoid respiratory compromise during RALRP.

Other anesthetic issues also may differ between the procedures. For example, open RRP may be performed under general, epidural, or spinal anesthesia. Indeed, the senior author exclusively uses spinal anesthesia in the majority of patients. By contrast, general anesthesia is necessary for

Johns Hopkins Medical Institution, Brady Urological Institute, 600 North Wolfe Street, Marburg 145, Baltimore, MD 21287, USA
* Corresponding author.
E-mail address: eschaeffer@jhmi.edu (E.M. Schaeffer).

Urol Clin N Am 37 (2010) 49–55
doi:10.1016/j.ucl.2009.11.008

RALRP, potentially increasing the overall "invasiveness" of the procedure.

Another readily apparent difference is the skin incision. Open RRP can be performed through a midline or Pfannenstiel 8-cm incision, as has been used by the senior author since August 2007 with improved cosmetic results. By contrast, RALRP involves 5 to 6 smaller incisions to accommodate trocars ranging from 5 to 12 mm in diameter. Because prostatic morcellation is not performed, one of these incisions must be extended sufficiently at the end of the prostatectomy to permit intact specimen removal. The relative cosmetic appeal of multiple smaller incisions higher on the abdomen, compared with a single somewhat larger incision lower on the abdomen, is a matter of personal preference.

The extent and yield of pelvic lymphadenectomy (PLND) may also differ between open RRP and RALRP. Among 1278 consecutive patients treated at University of California—San Francisco, Cooperberg and colleagues[8] reported that PLND was less frequently performed during RALRP compared with open RRP (31.8% vs 47.8%, respectively, *P*<.01). Moreover, after controlling for year of surgery and CAPRA risk score (Cancer for Prostate Risk Assessment), RALRP remained significantly associated with a lower odds of PLND (odds ratio [OR] 0.18, 95% confidence interval [CI] 0.11–0.32). In addition, the mean lymph node yield was 9.3 in RALRP versus 14.4 in open RRP (*P*<.01). Due to stage migration and the declining rate of lymph node metastases at diagnosis, the impact of these differences in nodal yield may be of lesser magnitude than in the past. Nevertheless, the risk of occult nodal metastases remains substantial for patients in the high-risk group, necessitating adherence to the same high surgical standards. Of note, a technique for more extended PLND during RALRP was recently described in 99 patients, involving more cephalad trocar placement.[9] Using this method, Feicke and colleagues reported a mean lymph node yield of 19, although it required an additional 51 minutes of operative time to complete.

Another important difference between RRP and RALRP is the timing of PLND during the operation. In the classic open RRP, PLND is done at the beginning of the case, providing the opportunity to examine the lymph nodes (by palpation or, less commonly, with frozen sections) prior to prostatectomy. By contrast, PLND is typically reserved until after prostatic removal during RALRP. At that point, the excised lymph nodes may be removed either through the assistant port, in the same Endocatch bag with the prostate, or by using separate specimen bags. This action precludes the ability to examine the lymph nodes grossly or histologically before prostatectomy.

Another difference between RRP and RALRP is the technique used for the vesicourethral anastomosis. During open RRP, the anastomosis uses approximately 4 to 8 interrupted sutures. By contrast, the vesicourethral anastomosis during RALRP is typically performed in a running fashion with a single knot, as described by Van Velthoven and colleagues.[10] The long-term impact of this technical modification on continence requires further study.

A final major difference is that open RRP is entirely an extraperitoneal procedure, whereas RALRP can be performed through a transperitoneal or extraperitoneal approach. However, the limited working space makes extraperitoneal RALRP more technically challenging. In consequence, in contrast to open RRP, most RALRP are currently performed transperitoneally.[11] Despite its designation as "minimally invasive surgery," one could argue that violating the peritoneal cavity makes transperitoneal RALRP considerably more invasive than open RRP.

The issue of relative "invasiveness" was studied from a unique perspective by Jurczok and colleagues[12] by comparing levels of acute phase reactants (as a marker for the systemic response) before, during, and after laparoscopic versus open RRP. Overall, they found no difference in C-reactive protein (CRP), serum amyloid A, interleukin (IL)-6, and IL-10 between the 2 groups at any time point. The investigators concluded that "the so-far assumed less invasiveness of laparoscopic radical prostatectomy is not objectively supported by the data from this study." By contrast, Fracalanza and colleagues[13] reported significantly higher blood levels of CRP, IL-6, and lactate after open RRP than RALRP, although still within the normal range. Based on these findings, the investigators concluded that "RALRP induces lower tissue trauma than RRP." Although the clinical significance of these minor variations in acute phase reactants is unclear, additional study is warranted into the physiologic response to open radical prostatectomy and RALRP at both the systemic and tissue level.

There are several major intraoperative advantages of RALRP, including 3-dimensional magnified visualization and the computer-assisted elimination of intention tremor. RALRP is also less physically and technically demanding than pure laparoscopic radical prostatectomy. Another well-documented advantage of RALRP is lower average intraoperative blood loss than open RRP, which has been verified in numerous studies. In one series, the average estimated blood loss (EBL) was 200 mL in RALRP compared with 550 mL in open RRP.[12] In a matched analysis by Rocco and colleagues,[14] EBL was 200 mL in RALRP versus 800 mL in RRP ($P<.0001$). Farnham and colleagues[15] similarly reported an average EBL of 191 and 664 mL in RALRP and RRP, respectively. Nevertheless, there was no difference in the transfusion rate in their series. Thus, the long-term clinical significance of such differences in intraoperative blood loss is unclear.

COST

The cost of a surgical intervention is a complex issue to study. Not only is it affected by the cost of the surgical equipment but also by surgeon-related factors, operative time, length of hospital stay, hospital volume and charges, lost work time, rates of hospital readmission and complications, marketing costs, and many other factors.

To start, the initiation of a robotic prostatectomy program involves considerable expense, including the cost to purchase the robotic system (approximately \$1.5 million), as well as annual maintenance fees of \$100,000 to \$200,000, and at least \$1000 for disposable instruments per case.[16] Furthermore, the initial learning curve has been associated with substantial expense. Using a theoretical model with different rates of surgeon improvement, Steinberg and colleagues[17] estimated this cost to range from \$95,000 with a learning curve of 24 cases, to \$1,365,000 for a learning curve of 360 cases. A major contributory factor to this increased cost clearly is the significantly longer operative times during the early learning curve, which have been well documented in numerous studies.[14]

In a recent cost-benefit analysis, Steinberg and colleagues[18] estimated that at least 78 cases are needed per year to maintain profits following the purchase of a robotic system. The investigators concluded accordingly that surgical volume at a particular center and patient demand may represent important determinants for the profitability of implementing a RALRP program. To minimize the costs associated with RALRP would involve a high-volume center with an experienced surgeon, short length of stay, and the absence of complications, readmissions, or secondary therapy.

A few studies have demonstrated significantly shorter length of hospital stay with RALRP than RRP, which would help to balance the aforementioned costs.[5] Nevertheless, many other studies reporting similar clinical care pathways and length of hospitalization for RALRP versus RRP would negate this advantage.[19]

In the words of Emanuel, "novelty cannot be equated with benefit."[20] Particularly in light of the current economic crisis and discussions regarding health care reform, a critical assessment of new technology is warranted, including RALRP.

PERIOPERATIVE OUTCOMES

With respect to the perioperative period, there is conflicting evidence regarding differences in length of hospital stay (LOS) and convalescence between RRP and RALRP. Among Medicare beneficiaries treated from 2003 to 2005, Hu and colleagues[5] reported a significantly longer LOS following open RRP than laparoscopic approaches (4.4 vs 1.4 days, $P<.0001$). However, the LOS in this study may not reflect other contemporary RRP series.

At the authors' institution, the same clinical care pathway is used for open RRP and RALRP. Following an uncomplicated open or robotic procedure, patients are given a clear liquid diet and patient-controlled anesthesia (PCA) on the night of surgery. On the first postoperative day, the diet is gradually advanced, the PCA is discontinued, and frequent ambulation is encouraged. The timing of discharge (ie, postoperative day 1 or 2) is then determined based on patient-specific factors (eg, tolerating a regular diet, pain control, ambulating) and physician preference, but not by surgical approach. Nelson and colleagues[19] similarly reported a common clinical care pathway and LOS for RRP and RALRP patients treated at Vanderbilt. Prior studies have also shown similar postoperative pain after RRP and RALRP. For example, Jurczok and colleagues[12] reported no difference in morphine equivalents between patients treated by the 2 approaches.

After discharge, patients at the authors' institution treated by RRP and RALRP are provided with the same instructions regarding the return to work and resumption of physical activity. The duration of catheterization is determined based on patient-specific factors and physician discretion, rather than surgical approach.

With regard to complication rates, published studies have varying results when comparing RRP to RALRP. In the study by Hu and colleagues,[5] RALRP was associated with a significantly lower odds of short-term perioperative complications (OR 0.7, 95% CI 0.6–0.9), but a significantly higher frequency of strictures (OR 1.4, 95% CI 1.04–1.9). As expected, in both open RRP and RALRP, the risk of perioperative complications and strictures has been shown to decrease with surgeon experience.[21,22]

ONCOLOGICAL OUTCOMES

Surgical Margins

There is no better way to cure a cancer that is localized to the prostate than total surgical excision. Multiple factors impact the long-term oncologic outcomes after radical prostatectomy, including stage, Gleason grade, and the use of adjuvant or salvage therapies.[23,24] One imperative of optimal cancer control is complete removal of the tumor, hence a critical examination of surgical margin status must be considered when determining the optimal surgical approach.

Of the 10,446 open radical prostatectomies performed at Johns Hopkins Hospital from 1993 to 2004, the positive surgical margin rate for organ-confined prostate cancer was 1.3%.[25] However, other reports of open radical prostatectomy have reported positive margin rates up to 24% for organ-confined disease, using different pathologic processing techniques.[26] Other large series of open prostatectomy report overall positive surgical margin rates between 8.0% and 35%, depending on clinical and pathologic features.[26]

Relative to RRP, robotic-assisted radical prostatectomy is a much newer procedure, and initial reports of margin rates were high. For example, in the first 100 cases, Atug and colleagues[27] reported positive surgical margin rates of 45.4%, 21.2%, and 11.7%, with a significant decrease over time ($P = .0053$).

Furthermore, more recent reports from large robotic series have reported margin rates that are comparable to large open series. In a contemporary report by Ahlering and colleagues,[28] margin status in the last 500 cases was 3.1% for organ-confined cancer. For men with organ-confined disease, Tewari and colleagues[29] and Patel and colleagues[30] similarly reported positive margin rates of 4.7%, and 2.5%, respectively. The largest series published to date by Menon and colleagues[31] including 2766 men reported positive margin rates of 13.0% and 35% for pathologic stage T2 and T3 disease, respectively. Thus, with increasing volume and surgeon experience there has been an improvement in published surgical margin rates in RALRP.

Of interest is that evidence from several institutions suggests that the location and degree (length) of positive surgical margin may differ between RRP and RALRP. The most common site of a positive margin in RRP is at the apex, whereas in RALRP it is typically posterior-lateral. At this time, it is unclear whether the location of positive margins affects the biochemical progression-free survival. Further, van der Kwast and colleagues[32] reported a similar response to adjuvant radiation therapy among men with positive margins at the apex and other locations. In contrast, emerging evidence does suggest that the length of positive margin may affect oncological outcomes. For example, Chuang and colleagues[25] reported a significantly lower 5-year progression-free survival rate with capsular incision of 3 mm or more.

In conclusion, recent studies suggest comparable positive surgical margin rates between RRP and RALRP performed by expert surgeons. A cautionary note is that "expert" surgeons with the highest lifetime number of procedures comprise the minority of many published series.[33,34] Further, the reduction in intraoperative blood loss with RALRP, coupled with heavy direct-to-consumer advertising,[11] have led to its widespread adoption in the community. In consequence, published margin rates for open or robotic prostatectomy from high-volume academic centers may not be generalizable to other settings.

Biochemical Progression and Secondary Therapy

Long-term follow-up is not yet available for RALRP. Some studies have reported comparable 5-year biochemical progression-free survival rates comparing open RRP with RALRP. For example, Drouin and colleagues[35] reported 5-year progression-free survival rates of 87.8%, 88.1%, and 89.6% for patients treated at by open, laparoscopic, and robotic prostatectomy at their institution from 2000 to 2004 ($P = .93$).

Another metric that has been used to compare oncologic outcomes between the techniques is the rate of secondary therapy. Hu and colleagues[5] reported that salvage treatment was greater than 3 times more likely within 6 months after RALRP than RRP. Data on clinical and pathologic features were not available in this population, precluding an assessment of the reasons for such high rates of early salvage treatment among RALRP patients. In addition, whether these high early failure rates will translate into worse long-term outcomes is unknown.

On the whole, the current literature comparing oncologic outcomes between approaches is substantially limited by the short follow-up for RALRP. Given the long natural history of prostate cancer,[36] this issue requires further study after the accrual of additional follow-up. In particular, future studies are necessary to determine whether more meaningful long-term clinical end points (ie, metastasis and cancer-specific survival) are comparable using RALRP.

FUNCTIONAL OUTCOMES

Urinary Control

Urinary incontinence is a major side effect of radical prostatectomy, which may limit its widespread acceptance by both patients and urologists. Although incontinence was once a common problem, today in experienced hands the rate of long-term incontinence after RRP is only 2% to 7%.[22] Nevertheless, rates of incontinence after open RRP vary across different practice settings in the community. In the Prostate Cancer Outcomes Study, Stanford and colleagues[37] reported 3 or more pads per day in 3.3% and moderate to severe urinary disturbance in 8.7% of men at 24 months after radical prostatectomy. Of note, high continence rates of 95% have also been reported after RALRP.[38]

Despite the generally favorable long-term continence results in contemporary series, experienced open surgeons have continued to modify the technique to hasten the early return of urinary control. For example, based on the premise that passive urinary control is dependent on both the striated urethral sphincter and the preprostatic sphincter/bladder neck, in 2002 the senior author implemented buttressing sutures to prevent passive opening of the bladder neck with filling.[39] This technique of bladder neck "intussusception" was associated with earlier return of urinary control. Patient-reported continence specifically was 82% at 3 months, compared with 54% using a conventional bladder neck reconstruction. Others have tried to recapitulate the normal anatomic support of the urethra and bladder neck after radical prostatectomy. For example, Rocco and colleagues[40] described a modification that involves suturing the posterior striated sphincter to the Denonvilliers fascia posterior to the bladder wall. Although this "Rocco stitch" was initially described in men undergoing open RRP, it is widely used during RALRP prior to the running vesicourethral anastomosis (described earlier). Using this modification, the investigators reported earlier recovery of continence than a group of historical controls.

Similar efforts have been made to improve continence after RALRP using anatomic approaches. For example, Tewari and colleagues[41] recently described a "total restoration technique" with improvements in the early recovery of urinary control. Menon and colleagues[42] performed a randomized trial to determine whether a 2-layered anatomic reconstruction improved urinary control after RALRP, and did not find an improvement compared with the conventional method.

Sexual Function

Sexual function is an important quality of life measure after radical prostatectomy. The description of the location and surgical techniques to preserve the cavernous nerves has allowed surgeons to preserve potency during RRP.[2] In the senior author's series, 68% of men overall are potent and 93% of men with normal sexual function preoperatively are potent after surgery. Nonetheless, variable rates for potency after nerve-sparing radical prostatectomy have been reported, with some reported rates as low as 56%.[37]

Recent anatomic studies have suggested that branches of the pelvic plexus may travel more anteriorly. Building on these observations, Kaul and colleagues[43] first described a technique to preserve prostatic fascial tissue more anteriorly. Using this technique of a high, intrafascial nerve release along the length of the prostate, 96% of men achieved intercourse at least once in 4 weeks and 71% returned to baseline erectile function at 1 year. One concern with this technique is the proximity of the dissection to the prostate, and potentially, cancer. This concern has stemmed from the description of the technique and accompanying histologic images, wherein the dissection approaches as close as 0.3 mm from the cancer.[43]

Building on this principle of a high release of the neurovascular bundle, Nielsen and colleagues[44] reported a technique for a high anterior release (HAR) of the levator fascia in RRP. This technique differs from that of Kaul and colleagues in that the high release is performed more toward the apex of the prostate and in a plane between the levator fascia and the prostatic fascia, rather than between the prostatic fascia and the capsule of the prostate. With this approach, patients reported earlier potency (93% vs 77% at 12 months) and improved return to baseline function (70% vs 54%) compared with a matched cohort of men with standard nerve-sparing. Of note, men who had either unilateral or bilateral HAR had similar rates of recovery, suggesting that preservation of the anterior nerve fibers, noted in anatomic dissections, likely does not contribute to better recovery. Rather, the authors have speculated that the HAR dissection allows for a precise apical dissection with more complete nerve release with less traction.

Satisfaction

A recent study from Duke assessed satisfaction and regret among 400 men treated by either open or robotic prostatectomy.[45] Patients treated by RALRP had a 3-fold increased odds of regret, which the investigators attributed potentially to a "higher expectation of an innovative procedure." In general, direct-to-consumer advertising may engender unrealistic patient expectations regarding the outcomes of what remains a major surgical operation.[11] Overall, continued technical advances in both open RRP and RALRP will likely result in further improvements in both outcomes and patient satisfaction.

SUMMARY

Both open and robotic surgeons continue to search for the "holy grail" of oncological control with optimal functional outcomes. Analogous to the progress in RRP with the advent of modern external beam radiation therapy,[1] the introduction of robotics has identified new areas for improvement in the surgical management of prostate cancer and has accelerated progress in the technique of open RRP. The accrual of additional follow-up of contemporary RALRP will enable comparisons of essential long-term outcomes between the 2 techniques. Whatever approach surgeons use, they must continue to try to perfect their technique. In doing so, if the complications of radical prostatectomy can be reduced to a minimum, eventually there will no longer be a controversy about the best way to treat localized disease.

REFERENCES

1. Walsh PC. 2008 Whitmore lecture: radical prostatectomy—where we were and where we are going. Urol Oncol 2009;27(3):246–50.
2. Walsh PC, Lepor H, Eggleston JC. Radical prostatectomy with preservation of sexual function: anatomical and pathological considerations. Prostate 1983;4(5):473–85.
3. Guillonneau B, Vallancien G. Laparoscopic radical prostatectomy: initial experience and preliminary assessment after 65 operations. Prostate 1999; 39(1):71–5.
4. Menon M, Shrivastava A, Tewari A, et al. Laparoscopic and robot assisted radical prostatectomy: establishment of a structured program and preliminary analysis of outcomes. J Urol 2002;168(3):945–9.
5. Hu JC, Wang Q, Pashos CL, et al. Utilization and outcomes of minimally invasive radical prostatectomy. J Clin Oncol 2008;26(14):2278–84.
6. Stolzenburg JU, Aedtner B, Olthoff D, et al. Anaesthetic considerations for endoscopic extraperitoneal and laparoscopic transperitoneal radical prostatectomy. BJU Int 2006;98(3):508–13.
7. Awad H, Santilli S, Ohr M, et al. The effects of steep Trendelenburg positioning on intraocular pressure during robotic radical prostatectomy. Anesth Analg 2009;109(2):473–8.
8. Cooperberg MR, Kane CJ, Cowan JE, et al. Adequacy of lymphadenectomy among men undergoing robot-assisted laparoscopic radical prostatectomy. BJU Int 2009. [Epub ahead of print].
9. Feicke A, Baumgartner M, Talimi S, et al. Robotic-assisted laparoscopic extended pelvic lymph node dissection for prostate cancer: surgical technique and experience with the first 99 cases. Eur Urol 2009;55(4):876–83.
10. Van Velthoven RF, Ahlering TE, Peltier A, et al. Technique for laparoscopic running urethrovesical anastomosis: the single knot method. Urology 2003; 61(4):699–702.
11. Ghavamian R. The urologic oncologist, robotic, and open radical prostatectomy: the need to look through the hype and propaganda and serve our patients. Urol Oncol 2009;27(3):233–5.
12. Jurczok A, Zacharias M, Wagner S, et al. Prospective non-randomized evaluation of four mediators of the systemic response after extraperitoneal laparoscopic and open retropubic radical prostatectomy. BJU Int 2007;99(6):1461–6.
13. Fracalanza S, Ficarra V, Cavalleri S, et al. Is robotically assisted laparoscopic radical prostatectomy less invasive than retropubic radical prostatectomy? Results from a prospective, unrandomized, comparative study. BJU Int 2008;101(9):1145–9.
14. Rocco B, Matei DV, Melegari S, et al. Robotic vs open prostatectomy in a laparoscopically naive centre: a matched-pair analysis. BJU Int 2009. [Epub ahead of print].
15. Farnham SB, Webster TM, Herrell SD, et al. Intraoperative blood loss and transfusion requirements for robotic-assisted radical prostatectomy versus radical retropubic prostatectomy. Urology 2006; 67(2):360–3.
16. Gianino MM, Galzerano M, Tizzani A, et al. Critical issues in current comparative and cost analyses between retropubic and robotic radical prostatectomy. BJU Int 2008;101(1):2–3.
17. Steinberg PL, Merguerian PA, Bihrle W 3rd, et al. The cost of learning robotic-assisted prostatectomy. Urology 2008;72(5):1068–72.
18. Steinberg PL, Merguerian PA, Bihrle W 3rd, et al. A da Vinci robot system can make sense for a mature laparoscopic prostatectomy program. JSLS 2008; 12(1):9–12.
19. Nelson B, Kaufman M, Broughton G, et al. Comparison of length of hospital stay between radical retropubic prostatectomy and robotic assisted laparoscopic prostatectomy. J Urol 2007;177(3): 929–31.
20. Emanuel EJ, Fuchs VR, Garber AM. Essential elements of a technology and outcomes assessment initiative. JAMA 2007;298(11):1323–5.

21. Erickson BA, Meeks JJ, Roehl KA, et al. Bladder neck contracture after retropubic radical prostatectomy: incidence and risk factors from a large single-surgeon experience. BJU Int 2009. [Epub ahead of print].
22. Kundu SD, Roehl KA, Egginer SE, et al. Potency, continence and complications in 3,477 consecutive radical retropubic prostatectomies. J Urol 2004; 172(6 Pt 1):2227–31.
23. Stephenson AJ, Kattan MW, Eastham JA, et al. Prostate cancer-specific mortality after radical prostatectomy for patients treated in the prostate-specific antigen era. J Clin Oncol 2009;27(26):4300–5.
24. Thompson IM, Tangen CM, Paradelo J, et al. Adjuvant radiotherapy for pathological T3N0M0 prostate cancer significantly reduces risk of metastases and improves survival: long-term followup of a randomized clinical trial. J Urol 2009;181(3):956–62.
25. Chuang AY, Nielsen ME, Hernandez DJ, et al. The significance of positive surgical margin in areas of capsular incision in otherwise organ confined disease at radical prostatectomy. J Urol 2007; 178(4 Pt 1):1306–10.
26. Smith JA Jr, Chan RC, Chang SS, et al. A comparison of the incidence and location of positive surgical margins in robotic assisted laparoscopic radical prostatectomy and open retropubic radical prostatectomy. J Urol 2007;178(6):2385–9 [discussion: 2389–90].
27. Atug F, Castle EP, Srivastav SK, et al. Positive surgical margins in robotic-assisted radical prostatectomy: impact of learning curve on oncologic outcomes. Eur Urol 2006;49(5):866–71 [discussion: 871–2].
28. Yee DS, Narula N, Amin MB, et al. Robot-assisted radical prostatectomy: current evaluation of surgical margins in clinically low-, intermediate-, and high-risk prostate cancer. J Endourol 2009;23(9):1461–5.
29. Tewari A, Rao S, Martinez-Salamanca JI, et al. Cancer control and the preservation of neurovascular tissue: how to meet competing goals during robotic radical prostatectomy. BJU Int 2008;101(8): 1013–8.
30. Patel VR, Shah S, Arend D. Histopathologic outcomes of robotic radical prostatectomy. Scientific World Journal 2006;6:2566–72.
31. Badani KK, Kaul S, Menon M. Evolution of robotic radical prostatectomy: assessment after 2766 procedures. Cancer 2007;110(9):1951–8.
32. Van der Kwast TH, Bolla M, Van Poppel H, et al. Identification of patients with prostate cancer who benefit from immediate postoperative radiotherapy: EORTC 22911. J Clin Oncol 2007;25(27):4178–86.
33. Vickers AJ, Bianco FJ, Serio AM, et al. The surgical learning curve for prostate cancer control after radical prostatectomy. J Natl Cancer Inst 2007; 99(15):1171–7.
34. Vickers AJ, Savage CJ, Hruza M, et al. The surgical learning curve for laparoscopic radical prostatectomy: a retrospective cohort study. Lancet Oncol 2009;10(5):475–80.
35. Drouin SJ, Vaessen C, Hupertan V, et al. Comparison of mid-term carcinologic control obtained after open, laparoscopic, and robot-assisted radical prostatectomy for localized prostate cancer. World J Urol 2009;27(5):599–605.
36. Pound CR, Partin AW, Eisenberger MA, et al. Natural history of progression after PSA elevation following radical prostatectomy. JAMA 1999;281(17):1591–7.
37. Stanford JL, Feng Z, Hamilton AS, et al. Urinary and sexual function after radical prostatectomy for clinically localized prostate cancer: the prostate cancer outcomes study. JAMA 2000;283(3):354–60.
38. Raman JD, Dong S, Levinson A, et al. Robotic radical prostatectomy: operative technique, outcomes, and learning curve. JSLS 2007;11(1):1–7.
39. Walsh PC, Marschke PL. Intussusception of the reconstructed bladder neck leads to earlier continence after radical prostatectomy. Urology 2002; 59(6):934–8.
40. Rocco F, Carmignani L, Acquati P, et al. Restoration of posterior aspect of rhabdosphincter shortens continence time after radical retropubic prostatectomy. J Urol 2006;175(6):2201–6.
41. Tewari A, Bigelow K, Rao S, et al. Anatomic restoration technique of continence mechanism and preservation of puboprostatic collar: a novel modification to achieve early urinary continence in men undergoing robotic prostatectomy. Urology 2007;69(4):726–31.
42. Menon M, Muhletaler F, Campos M, et al. Assessment of early continence after reconstruction of the periprostatic tissues in patients undergoing computer assisted (robotic) prostatectomy: results of a 2 group parallel randomized controlled trial. J Urol 2008;180(3):1018–23.
43. Kaul S, Savera A, Badani K, et al. Functional outcomes and oncological efficacy of Vattikuti Institute prostatectomy with veil of Aphrodite nerve-sparing: an analysis of 154 consecutive patients. BJU Int 2006;97(3):467–72.
44. Nielsen ME, Schaeffer EM, Marschke P, et al. High anterior release of the levator fascia improves sexual function following open radical retropubic prostatectomy. J Urol 2008;180(6):2557–64 [discussion: 2564].
45. Schroeck FR, Krupski TL, Sun L, et al. Satisfaction and regret after open retropubic or robot-assisted laparoscopic radical prostatectomy. Eur Urol 2008;54(4):785–93.

Controversies Surrounding Lymph Node Dissection for Prostate Cancer

Ganesh S. Palapattu, MD, FACS[a,*], Eric A. Singer, MD, MA[b],
Edward M. Messing, MD, FACS[c]

KEYWORDS

• Lymph node dissection • Lymph node
• Prostate cancer • Lymphadenectomy
• Radical prostatectomy • Review

Almost 35 years after the revolution in the technique of radical prostatectomy was introduced by Walsh and Donker,[1] controversy remains regarding the utility of performing a concomitant pelvic lymph node dissection. High-level scientific evidence, in the form of randomized controlled trials, examining the efficacy of lymphadenectomy in this setting is lacking. Hence, we must make do with a trove of retrospective data to assist us in determining the best course of action. In this article, the authors discuss the appropriate candidate, the influence of imaging, the anatomic boundaries, the surgical approach, the prognostic and therapeutic implications, and complications that surround the role of pelvic lymph node dissection in the management of prostate cancer.

DETERMINING IN WHOM TO PERFORM PELVIC LYMPHADENECTOMY

The preoperative parameters conventionally used to assess the need for pelvic lymph node dissection at the time of radical prostatectomy focus on determining the probability of finding positive lymph nodes. The greater the predicted likelihood of lymph node involvement, the stronger the recommendation to perform lymphadenectomy. However, current predictive tools do not consider possible therapeutic benefit. The predominant variables used by all preoperative prediction algorithms for lymph node disease are prostate-specific antigen (PSA) at diagnosis, clinical stage, and Gleason score on biopsy.[2] In the past few years, several investigators have combined these 3, in varying ways, and have been able to achieve predictive accuracies ranging from 75% to 88%.[3–5] When these factors are augmented by other variables, such as the number of positive biopsy cores or an endorectal magnetic resonance imaging (MRI) of the pelvis, accuracy can be further improved to approximately 90%.[6,7] Interestingly, Karam and colleagues[8] showed close to 98% predictive accuracy of lymph node involvement by adding preoperative serum endoglin level, a cell surface protein highly expressed in endothelial cells, to the 3 traditional variables (**Table 1**).

Each statistical model, whether a nomogram, a table, or something else, is limited by the data used to create it. Predicative accuracy can only be determined by final pathology, which, in this situation, is largely a function of surgical template. Almost all predictive models are formulated from

Funding support to acknowledge: Z01 BC 011023 Clinical Fellowship Training Program.
[a] Department of Urology, The Methodist Hospital, 6560 Fannin, Suite 2100, Houston, TX 77030, USA
[b] Urologic Oncology Branch, National Cancer Institute, 10 Center Drive, Building 10, Room 1-5940, Bethesda, MD 20814, USA
[c] Department of Urology, University of Rochester Medical Center, 601 Elmwood Avenue, Box 656, Rochester, NY 14642, USA
* Corresponding author.
E-mail address: gpalapattu@tmhs.org (G.S. Palapattu).

Urol Clin N Am 37 (2010) 57–65
doi:10.1016/j.ucl.2009.11.002
0094-0143/10/$ – see front matter

Table 1
Preoperative predictors of lymph node involvement for prostate cancer

Authors	Year	Subjects	Variables	Lymph Node Involvement (%)	Accuracy (%)
Briganti et al[4]	2006	602	PSA, clinical stage, Gleason score on biopsy	11	76
Wang et al[7]	2006	411	PSA, Gleason score on biopsy, endorectal MRI	5	89.2
Briganti et al[6]	2007	278	PSA, clinical stage, Gleason score on biopsy, percentage of positive cores	10.4	83
Makarov et al[3]	2007	5730	PSA, clinical stage, Gleason score on biopsy	1	88
Karam et al[8]	2008	425	PSA, clinical stage, Gleason score on biopsy, preoperative plasma endoglin level	3.3	97.8
Bhojani et al[5]	2009	839 235	PSA, clinical stage, Gleason score on biopsy in 2 cohorts	2 5	82 75

data obtained by a standard or more limited pelvic lymph dissection (see later discussion). One might surmise then that the models derived from an extended pelvic lymph node dissection would possess higher predictive accuracy. Briganti and colleagues[4] were unable to show a clinically significant benefit in predictive accuracy for detecting lymph node positive disease from the data garnered from pelvic lymph nodes removed within an extended template.

Although it seems clear that PSA, clinical stage, and Gleason score on biopsy are vital to the prediction model, an improvement in the ability to predict the presence of lymph node disease would require the addition of other informative variables (eg, radiography, biomarkers) to the equation.

The 2009 National Comprehensive Cancer Network guidelines state that "a pelvic lymph node dissection can be excluded in patients with <7% predicted probability of nodal metastasis by nomograms, although some patients with lymph node metastases will be missed."[9] Depending on the definition used, the probability of lymph node disease in men deemed to possess low preoperative risk of lymph node metastasis is anywhere between less than 1% and 8%. Data from clinical practice since 2001 obtained from Cancer of the Prostate Strategic Urologic Research Endeavor database seem to reveal acceptance of this recommendation by practitioners; more than 90% of men deemed high risk received a pelvic lymph node dissection, whereas less than 75% of those at low risk did so.[10] If the goal is to improve the detection rate of men with lymph node positive disease, confining pelvic lymph node dissection to higher-risk men will yield better results. Whether this logic is true when the aim is therapeutic, however, is open to question and is discussed later.

EVALUATING THE ROLE OF IMAGING IN IDENTIFYING LYMPH NODE INVASION

If a radiological technique that was able to detect lymph node metastases with high sensitivity and specificity existed, the need for pelvic lymph node dissection for staging purposes would be obviated. Current computed tomography (CT) and MRI modalities only have a sensitivity of approximately 35% for detecting lymph node involvement.[11–13] This is because of the poor performance of these modalities in detecting subcentimeter lesions and the high prevalence of micrometastases in the PSA era.[11] Several innovations in imaging technology have dramatically improved the ability to identify lymph node disease preoperatively. The addition of lymphotropic contrast agents, such as paramagnetic iron oxide nanoparticles and ferumoxtran-10, can increase the sensitivity and specificity to 80% to 90% and 96% to 98%, respectively.[14–16] Imaging based on a lymphotropic agent relies on the tendency of these compounds to concentrate and flow within the lymphatic system. The absence of lymphotropic contrast agent in a visualized lymphatic chain may occur if the lymph node in question is infiltrated with cancer, or less commonly, if a benign process is at work (eg, fibrosis or lipomatosis).[2] Thoeny and colleagues[17] reported an exciting development in lymph node imaging using ultrasmall superparamagnetic particles of iron oxide coupled with diffusion-weighted MRI. These authors found that this technique was capable of identifying lymph node invasion with 92% accuracy in patients with bladder and prostate cancer.[17]

Positron emission tomography/CT, although useful in advanced testicular cancer, has demonstrated marginal utility for detecting lymph node disease in men with prostate cancer.[18] Advancements using modifications of MRI technology or perhaps delivery of agents such as indocyanine green, a lymphotropic contrast agent, into the lymphatic system hold promise for improved lymph node staging in the future.[19]

EXAMINING THE IMPORTANCE OF THE ANATOMIC TEMPLATE

One of the fundamental issues that has fueled the controversy on pelvic lymphadenectomy in prostate cancer has been the matter of which nodes need to be removed. Anatomic studies in men without known cancer done with labeling agents injected directly into the prostate have demonstrated that the draining lymphatics typically involve 3 main areas: (1) along the pelvic side wall comprising the internal and external iliac lymphatics up to their junction with the common iliac lymphatic chain, (2) inferior to the prostate to the perineal floor to the lymphatics at and below the level of the internal iliac artery, and (3) the presacral area.[20] The extent of pelvic lymph node dissection can be termed either standard or extended (**Fig. 1**, **Table 2**). Most investigators agree that the standard template is limited to the bladder (medially), the pelvic side wall (laterally), the femoral canal (distally), the bifurcation of the common iliac vessels (proximally), the external iliac vein (superiorly), and the obturator nerve (inferiorly).[21–23] Definitions of an extended dissection differ but invariably include the area bounded by the standard template with the addition of removal of the fibrofatty tissue in the hypogastric region,

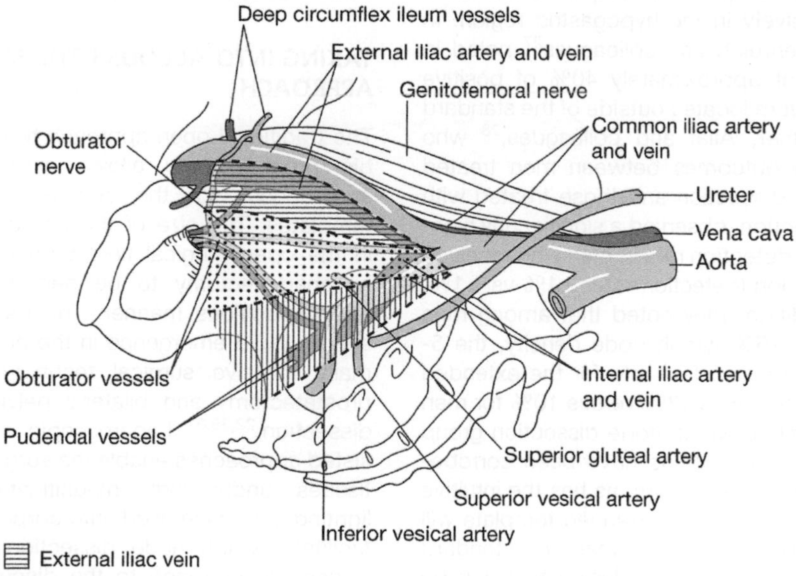

Fig. 1. Anatomic boundaries of lymphadenectomy. Standard lymphadenectomy includes the nodal tissue from the external iliac vein and obturator fossa, whereas an extended lymphadenectomy also includes the tissue overlying the internal iliac (hypogastric) and common iliac vessels as well as the presacral area. (*Reprinted from* Burkhard FC, Schumacher M, Studer UE. The role of lymphadenectomy in prostate cancer. Nat Clin Pract Urol 2005;2:336–42; with permission.)

Table 2
Lymphatic tissue removed during pelvic lymphadenectomy

	Standard Template	Extended Template
Medial to external iliac vein	✓	✓
Obturator	✓	✓
Hypogastric	×	✓
Presacral	×	✓
Common iliac	×	✓
Lateral to external iliac vein	×	✓

with possible inclusion of the presacral, common iliac, and nodal tissue lateral to the external iliac vein.[21] Golimbu and colleagues[24] observed in their series in the pre-PSA era that among men with lymph node positive disease, the presacral and presciatic regions were involved as commonly as the external iliac and obturator nodes. From the same time period, Fujioka and colleagues[25] found that lymph node disease was always present in the hypogastric region.

With regard to prostate cancer lymph node detection, numerous investigators have shown that an extended template is much more likely to find cancer than a more limited one. For example, Bader and colleagues[26] noted in their cohort that close to 20% of positive lymph nodes were located exclusively in the hypogastric region. In addition, Heidenreich and colleagues[27] noted in their series that approximately 40% of positive lymph nodes were located outside of the standard template. Further, Allaf and colleagues,[28] who compared the outcomes between men treated with extended dissection and those treated with standard dissection, observed a significantly higher lymph node detection rate in men who received a wider dissection (detection rate, 3.1% vs 1.1%; $P<.01$). In addition, they noted that among men with less than 15% lymph node density, the 5-year PSA progression-free rate for the extended lymph node group was 43% versus 10% for men in the more limited lymph node dissection group ($P = .01$).[28] These findings have been corroborated by several investigators, as has the intuitive notion that, in general, an extended template will yield more lymph nodes than a standard one.[24,29–31] The obvious conclusion that can be drawn from these data is that the wider the template, the more the lymph nodes will be removed and the more likely lymph node metastases will be detected.

Some investigators have emphasized the number of lymph nodes retrieved, irrespective of the template used. Surgeons who routinely obtain a higher lymph node yield typically perform a more extended dissection. The total lymph node count may have diagnostic and potentially therapeutic implications, as discussed later. Nevertheless, the surgeon can only control the template, and the ultimate lymph node count is, to some degree, dependent on the pathologist performing the analysis. In radical cystectomy for bladder cancer, for example, investigators have shown that submitting individual packets of fibrofatty tissue for analysis increases the number of lymph nodes identified by the pathologist versus en bloc submission.[32–34] Other factors, such as the technique of surgical specimen processing and examination, and the skill of the histopathologist can also influence the total lymph node count.[35]

TAKING INTO ACCOUNT THE SURGICAL APPROACH

The traditional open approach to radical retropubic prostatectomy allows excellent exposure and access for the standard and extended templates. The size of the operative workspace in the open surgical field permits a meticulous lymphadenectomy to be performed in a safe and expeditious manner. The past decade has seen a rapid emergence in the adoption of minimally invasive surgical techniques for radical prostatectomy and bilateral pelvic lymph node dissection.[22,36,37] Laparoscopic and robotic-assisted approaches enable the surgeon to visualize tissues under high magnification; enhanced lighting and increased intracorporeal pressures facilitate lymph node dissection. Two specific issues are germane to the discussion vis-à-vis minimally invasive pelvic lymphadenectomy. The first is port placement. Placing the midline port for the laparoscope too inferiorly to enhance visualization of the prostatic apex and vesicourethral anastomosis may hinder access to the more proximal lymphatic tissues in the extended template.[23,38,39] The second is the peritoneal approach. The extraperitoneal robotic-assisted technique, by virtue of its anatomic position, makes visualization and access beyond the standard template challenging.[38] In contrast, the transperitoneal robotic-assisted approach has no such encumbrances.[38]

ASSESSING THE RATIONALE FOR PELVIC LYMPH NODE DISSECTION

As discussed earlier, there are essentially 2 reasons to perform a pelvic lymphadenectomy at the time of radical prostatectomy: (1) for staging and prognostic purposes and (2) for possible therapeutic benefit. No one can argue that performing a pelvic lymph node dissection (standard or extended) gives greater information for pathologic staging than not doing one at all. Improved pathologic staging translates into better prognostic information that can aid the decision-making process regarding adjuvant therapies (eg, the survival benefit seen with the use of early androgen deprivation therapy for men with lymph node positive disease[40,41]). Confounding issues are (1) the current low prevalence of lymph node positive disease in men undergoing radical prostatectomy and (2) the lack of uniformity in prognosis among men with lymph node metastases.

In large contemporary series from Johns Hopkins (n = 5744) and a multiinstitutional group led by Memorial Sloan-Kettering (n = 7014), the overall lymph node positive incidence rate was found to be 5% and 3.7%, respectively.[42,43] As discussed earlier, preoperative prediction tools can be used to increase this proportion by identifying men at higher risk.

What of the outcomes of men with lymph node positive prostate cancer detected at radical prostatectomy? In a large cohort of men spanning the period from 1972 to 1999, Daneshmand and colleagues[44] observed that the overall recurrence-free probability at 10 years for men with nodal disease was 65%, with those with a lymph node density of more than 20% at greatest risk of recurrence. Close to one-third of the men in this study received adjuvant treatment. Masterson and colleagues[45] reported the 5-year and 10-year biochemical recurrence-free probability for men with positive lymph nodes to be approximately 23% and 19%, respectively. These results were found to be unaffected by approximately 15% of men in this study who received neoadjuvant hormone therapy. Among men with N0 disease, there was a trend toward better recurrence-free survival for those with a greater number of lymph nodes removed (*P* = .01). In a study from Bern, Switzerland, Bader and colleagues[46] observed a biochemical recurrence-free probability at 5 and 10 years of 25% and 10%, respectively, for all men in their study (no adjuvant therapy) with lymph node invasion, with those men with more than 2 nodes positive having the poorest outcome (5- and 10-year PSA recurrence-free probability of 21% and 7%, respectively). Boorjian and colleagues[47] from the Mayo Clinic reported on a cohort of 507 men with lymph node positive disease treated between 1988 and 2001, of whom close to 90% received adjuvant therapy. They also found that at 5 and 10 years, 69% and 56%, respectively, were free of biochemical recurrence. Two or more lymph nodes positive as well as a pathologic Gleason score of 8 to 10, positive surgical margins, and tumor aneuploid status conferred an increased risk of disease progression.[47] Cheng and colleagues[48] from the Mayo Clinic, also reported on men with lymph node involvement encompassing a slightly earlier timeframe and found that in the 322 men studied, the 5- and 10-year PSA progression-free probability rates were 74% and 64%, respectively.[48] Approximately 90% of these men also received adjuvant therapy and once again men with 1 lymph node positive fared better than those with 2 or more lymph nodes positive. Similar results were reported by Briganti and colleagues[49] in a 2-institution study wherein all men received adjuvant hormone therapy. In a report from Johns Hopkins where no man received adjuvant hormone therapy (n = 143), the authors noted the 5-year PSA-free progression rate to be 27% among all men with lymph node positive disease with a lymph node density of more than 15% distinguishing men with the poorest prognosis (5-year recurrence-free survival of 10%).[50]

In total, these data show that not all men with lymph node positive disease share the same prognosis. The number of lymph nodes that are positive (>2 or lymph node density of >15%–20%) is directly proportional to the risk of recurrence. In addition, there are some men with N1 disease who are free of disease at 10 years follow-up.[40,51] Among node-negative patients, higher lymph node yield has been associated with improved outcomes in bladder,[52] breast,[53] colon,[54] and lung cancer.[55] Masterson and colleagues[45] observed a similar finding in prostate cancer as mentioned earlier. Moreover, in an analysis of the SEER-Medicare database focusing on men with N0 disease, Joslyn and Konety[56] detected a 15% lower risk of cancer-specific death among men who had more than10 lymph nodes removed compared with those who had fewer nodes sampled. These findings have not been universally corroborated. DiMarco and colleagues[57] from the Mayo Clinic (n = 7036) found no difference in progression or survival outcomes in pN0 men treated during the PSA era, regardless of the number of lymph nodes removed. Similarly, Bhatta-Dhar and colleagues[58] noted no difference in recurrence-free survival in men (pN0, n = 806) with low-risk disease based on the presence or absence of a pelvic lymph node dissection. If a therapeutic benefit does exist for pelvic lymph node dissection in men with N0 disease, it is most likely because of the removal of micrometastases/histologically occult disease.

At the outset of this article, we pointed out that the field is devoid of randomized clinical trials, and hence, the interpretation of the retrospective data should be done with some caution. One particular item that should be kept in mind when reviewing the literature, as is the case for pelvic lymph node dissection, is the Will Rogers phenomenon.[59] This statistical effect occurs when an element from one dataset (set A) is moved to another dataset (set B), and consequently the averages of both datasets increase. For this to occur, the element in question must have a value (eg, outcome) lower than its original dataset (set A) and higher than its new dataset (set B). This phenomenon becomes relevant in oncology when data from 2 distinct groups (eg, pN0 vs pN1 or extended vs standard dissection) are compared. Consider a comparison in outcomes among men treated with an extended lymph node dissection: an extended lymph node dissection can improve the outcomes of men with both N0 and N1 disease by enriching the N0 cohort for true node-negative patients and by adding men with smaller nodal tumor volume (micrometastases) to the N1 group. In this scenario, the N1 group also benefits, as the prognosis of men with minimal burden of disease is better than those with more substantial N1 disease. Men who are pN0 as determined by an extended dissection are more likely to be truly node negative than men who are deemed pN0 via a standard dissection. Hence, men thought to be pN0 treated with a standard lymph node dissection may actually be pN1 and bring down the outcomes of node-negative men treated with a more limited lymph node dissection. Randomized controlled trials eliminate this effect because the probability of the Will Rogers phenomenon occurring is equal in all cohorts. Although Clark and colleagues[60] performed a randomized controlled trial of pelvic lymphadenectomy in men with localized prostate cancer, the study had some methodological issues (ie, underpowered, n = 123; each man received an extended dissection on one side and a standard dissection on the other) that precluded a final conclusion to be drawn from this report.

CONTEMPLATING THE RISKS OF PELVIC LYMPH NODE DISSECTION

The most common complications relating to pelvic lymphadenectomy for prostate cancer include symptomatic lymphocele, lower extremity edema, deep vein thrombosis, infected lymphocele (pelvic abscess), vascular injury, and ureteral injury. All can occur with either the standard or extended dissection but may be more common with an extended dissection, particularly lymphocele. The overall complication rate has been reported to be between 2% and 51%.[2] Recently, Briganti and colleagues[61] examined the complication rate in 963 men who underwent either an extended (n = 767) or a standard (n = 196) lymph node dissection. They noted an overall complication rate of 20% for the extended and 8% for the standard group (*P*<.01). This was largely because of an increased rate of lymphocele formation in the extended group (10% vs 5%, *P* = .01). In contrast, Heidenreich and colleagues[27] observed no differences in complications between the extended (n = 103) and standard (n = 100) templates of dissection. In a series of 365 men treated with extended lymphadenectomy, Bader and colleagues[26] reported a 2% lymphocele rate, whereas Pepper and colleagues[62] observed a symptomatic lymphocele formation rate of approximately 4% among 260 men who underwent a standard lymph node dissection.

Using a laparoscopic approach, Stone and colleagues[63] (n = 189) reported an overall complication rate of 36% for men who received an extended dissection and 2% for those who were treated with a standard template (*P*<.01). Among men treated with a robotic approach, Zorn and colleagues[22] found that those receiving a standard pelvic lymph node dissection (n = 296) had no increased complication rate compared with those who received none at all (n = 859). Interestingly, in a study investigating laparoscopic instruments, Box and colleagues[64] studied the lymphatic sealing properties of monopolar scissors, Harmonic ACE scalpel (Ethicon, Inc, Cincinnati, OH, USA), LigaSure V (Valleylab, Inc, Boulder, CO, USA), EnSeal (Ethicon, Inc, Cincinnati, OH, USA), and Trissector (Gyrus/ACMI, Southborough, MA, USA) and found that only the monopolar scissors was unable to generate an effective lymphatic seal.

In general, lymphadenectomy is associated with some risk of complications, the most common of which is symptomatic lymphocele, and the risk increases with increase in the extent of dissection.

SUMMARY

In the PSA era, lymph node metastasis is relatively uncommon. Various prediction tools can be used to identify men at greatest risk of harboring nodal disease. Current imaging modalities are unable to visualize lymph node involvement with acceptable fidelity and precision, although several emerging techniques show promise. Dissection in the extended template, versus the standard, yields more nodes and is associated with a higher positive lymph node detection rate. Given the high rate of involvement noted by most investigators, the removal of lymphatic tissue in the hypogastric region is suggested to optimize lymph node staging. Lymph node dissection performed by open, laparoscopic, or robotic techniques are largely equivalent, although extraperitoneal minimally invasive techniques pose some unique challenges. Not all men with pN1 disease share the same prognosis; higher number of positive lymph nodes (ie, >2) and lymph node density (ie, >15%–20%) portend a poorer outcome. There may be some therapeutic benefit to the removal of lymph nodes in men with node-negative disease, although this is currently speculative. Level I evidence supporting the use of early androgen deprivation therapy in men with nodal disease diagnosed during pelvic lymphadenectomy has been reported and is reviewed in greater detail elsewhere in this issue. Complications from pelvic lymph node dissection, although generally not prohibitive, increase proportionally in relation to the size of the template.

It is therefore reasonable for urologic surgeons to recommend pelvic lymphadenectomy to men with high-risk and selected intermediate-risk prostate cancer.[9,65,66] The diagnostic and therapeutic role of a pelvic lymph node dissection, and its optimal extent, can and should be addressed with a properly powered, prospective, randomized, multicenter clinical trial.

ACKNOWLEDGMENTS

This research was supported by the Intramural Research Program of the NIH, National Cancer Institute, Center for Cancer Research.

REFERENCES

1. Walsh PC, Donker PJ. Impotence following radical prostatectomy: insight into etiology and prevention. J Urol 1982;128(3):492–7.
2. Briganti A, Blute ML, Eastham JH, et al. Pelvic lymph node dissection in prostate cancer. Eur Urol 2009; 55(6):1251–65.
3. Makarov DV, Trock BJ, Humphreys EB, et al. Updated nomogram to predict pathologic stage of prostate cancer given prostate-specific antigen level, clinical stage, and biopsy Gleason score (Partin tables) based on cases from 2000 to 2005. Urology 2007;69(6):1095–101.
4. Briganti A, Chun FK, Salonia A, et al. Validation of a nomogram predicting the probability of lymph node invasion based on the extent of pelvic lymphadenectomy in patients with clinically localized prostate cancer. BJU Int 2006;98(4):788–93.
5. Bhojani N, Salomon L, Capitanio U, et al. External validation of the updated partin tables in a cohort of French and Italian men. Int J Radiat Oncol Biol Phys 2009;73(2):347–52.
6. Briganti A, Karakiewicz PI, Chun FK, et al. Percentage of positive biopsy cores can improve the ability to predict lymph node invasion in patients undergoing radical prostatectomy and extended pelvic lymph node dissection. Eur Urol 2007;51(6): 1573–81.
7. Wang L, Hricak H, Kattan MW, et al. Combined endorectal and phased-array MRI in the prediction of pelvic lymph node metastasis in prostate cancer. AJR Am J Roentgenol 2006;186(3):743–8.
8. Karam JA, Svatek RS, Karakiewicz PI, et al. Use of preoperative plasma endoglin for prediction of lymph node metastasis in patients with clinically localized prostate cancer. Clin Cancer Res 2008; 14(5):1418–22.
9. NCCN.NCCN clinical practice guidelines in oncology: prostate cancer. Available at: http://www.nccn.org/professionals/physicians_gls/pdf/prostate.pdf. Accessed September 5, 2009.
10. Kawakami J, Meng MV, Sadetsky N, et al. Changing patterns of pelvic lymphadenectomy for prostate cancer: results from CaPSURE. J Urol 2006; 176(4 Pt 1):1382–6.
11. Wolf JS Jr, Cher M, Dall'era M, et al. The use and accuracy of cross-sectional imaging and fine needle aspiration cytology for detection of pelvic lymph node metastases before radical prostatectomy. J Urol 1995;153(3 Pt 2):993–9.
12. Katz S, Rosen M. MR imaging and MR spectroscopy in prostate cancer management. Radiol Clin North Am 2006;44(5):723–34, viii.
13. Tempany CM, McNeil BJ. Advances in biomedical imaging. JAMA 2001;285(5):562–7.
14. Harisinghani MG, Barentsz J, Hahn PF, et al. Noninvasive detection of clinically occult lymph-node metastases in prostate cancer. N Engl J Med 2003;348(25):2491–9.
15. Bellin MF, Roy C, Kinkel K, et al. Lymph node metastases: safety and effectiveness of MR imaging

with ultrasmall superparamagnetic iron oxide particles–initial clinical experience. Radiology 1998;207(3):799–808.
16. Heesakkers RA, Hovels AM, Jager GJ, et al. MRI with a lymph-node-specific contrast agent as an alternative to CT scan and lymph-node dissection in patients with prostate cancer: a prospective multicohort study. Lancet Oncol 2008;9(9):850–6.
17. Thoeny HC, Triantafyllou M, Birkhaeuser FD, et al. Combined ultrasmall superparamagnetic particles of iron oxide-enhanced and diffusion-weighted magnetic resonance imaging reliably detect pelvic lymph node metastases in normal-sized nodes of bladder and prostate cancer patients. Eur Urol 2009;55(4):761–9.
18. Schiavina R, Scattoni V, Castellucci P, et al. 11C-choline positron emission tomography/computerized tomography for preoperative lymph-node staging in intermediate-risk and high-risk prostate cancer: comparison with clinical staging nomograms. Eur Urol 2008;54(2):392–401.
19. Marshall J, Cardin A, Singer E, et al. Laparoscopic pelvic lymphadenectomy with real time lymphatic imaging using near infrared fluorescence (NIRF) cameras. J Urol 2009;181(Suppl 4):274.
20. Brossner C, Ringhofer H, Hernady T, et al. Lymphatic drainage of prostatic transition and peripheral zones visualized on a three-dimensional workstation. Urology 2001;57(2):389–93.
21. Burkhard FC, Schumacher M, Studer UE. The role of lymphadenectomy in prostate cancer. Nat Clin Pract Urol 2005;2(7):336–42.
22. Zorn KC, Katz MH, Bernstein A, et al. Pelvic lymphadenectomy during robot-assisted radical prostatectomy: assessing nodal yield, perioperative outcomes, and complications. Urology 2009;74(2): 296–302.
23. Van Appledorn S, Bouchier-Hayes D, Agarwal D, et al. Robotic laparoscopic radical prostatectomy: setup and procedural techniques after 150 cases. Urology 2006;67(2):364–7.
24. Golimbu M, Morales P, Al-Askari S, et al. Extended pelvic lymphadenectomy for prostatic cancer. J Urol 1979;121(5):617–20.
25. Fujioka T, Koike H, Aoki H, et al. Significance of staging pelvic lymphadenectomy for prostatic cancer. Urol Int 1987;42(5):380–4.
26. Bader P, Burkhard FC, Markwalder R, et al. Is a limited lymph node dissection an adequate staging procedure for prostate cancer? J Urol 2002;168(2):514–8 [discussion: 518].
27. Heidenreich A, Varga Z, Von Knobloch R. Extended pelvic lymphadenectomy in patients undergoing radical prostatectomy: high incidence of lymph node metastasis. J Urol 2002;167(4):1681–6.
28. Allaf ME, Palapattu GS, Trock BJ, et al. Anatomical extent of lymph node dissection: impact on men with clinically localized prostate cancer. J Urol 2004;172(5 Pt 1):1840–4.
29. Mattei A, Fuechsel FG, Bhatta Dhar N, et al. The template of the primary lymphatic landing sites of the prostate should be revisited: results of a multimodality mapping study. Eur Urol 2008;53(1):118–25.
30. McLaughlin AP, Saltzstein SL, McCullough DL, et al. Prostatic carcinoma: incidence and location of unsuspected lymphatic metastases. J Urol 1976; 115(1):89–94.
31. Briganti A, Chun FK, Salonia A, et al. A nomogram for staging of exclusive nonobturator lymph node metastases in men with localized prostate cancer. Eur Urol 2007;51(1):112–9 [discussion: 119–20].
32. Bochner BH, Herr HW, Reuter VE. Impact of separate versus en bloc pelvic lymph node dissection on the number of lymph nodes retrieved in cystectomy specimens. J Urol 2001;166(6):2295–6.
33. Stein JP, Penson DF, Cai J, et al. Radical cystectomy with extended lymphadenectomy: evaluating separate package versus en bloc submission for node positive bladder cancer. J Urol 2007;177(3):876–81 [discussion: 881–2].
34. Barth PJ, Gerharz EW, Ramaswamy A, et al. The influence of lymph node counts on the detection of pelvic lymph node metastasis in prostate cancer. Pathol Res Pract 1999;195(9):633–6.
35. Thorn CC, Woodcock NP, Scott N, et al. What factors affect lymph node yield in surgery for rectal cancer? Colorectal Dis 2004;6(5):356–61.
36. Sivalingam S, Oxley J, Probert JL, et al. Role of pelvic lymphadenectomy in prostate cancer management. Urology 2007;69(2):203–9.
37. Finelli A, Moinzadeh A, Singh D, et al. Critique of laparoscopic lymphadenectomy in genitourinary oncology. Urol Oncol 2004;22(3):246–54 [discussion: 254–5].
38. Menon M, Tewari A, Peabody JO, et al. Vattikuti Institute prostatectomy, a technique of robotic radical prostatectomy for management of localized carcinoma of the prostate: experience of over 1100 cases. Urol Clin North Am 2004;31(4):701–17.
39. Gonzalgo ML, Patil N, Su LM, et al. Minimally invasive surgical approaches and management of prostate cancer. Urol Clin North Am 2008;35(3):489–504, ix.
40. Messing EM, Manola J, Yao J, et al. Immediate versus deferred androgen deprivation treatment in patients with node-positive prostate cancer after radical prostatectomy and pelvic lymphadenectomy. Lancet Oncol 2006;7(6):472–9.
41. Messing EM, Manola J, Sarosdy M, et al. Immediate hormonal therapy compared with observation after radical prostatectomy and pelvic lymphadenectomy in men with node-positive prostate cancer. N Engl J Med 1999;341(24):1781–8.
42. Cagiannos I, Karakiewicz P, Eastham JA, et al. A preoperative nomogram identifying decreased risk

of positive pelvic lymph nodes in patients with prostate cancer. J Urol 2003;170(5):1798–803.
43. Han M, Snow PB, Brandt JM, et al. Evaluation of artificial neural networks for the prediction of pathologic stage in prostate carcinoma. Cancer 2001;91(Suppl 8):1661–6.
44. Daneshmand S, Quek ML, Stein JP, et al. Prognosis of patients with lymph node positive prostate cancer following radical prostatectomy: long-term results. J Urol 2004;172(6 Pt 1):2252–5.
45. Masterson TA, Bianco FJ Jr, Vickers AJ, et al. The association between total and positive lymph node counts, and disease progression in clinically localized prostate cancer. J Urol 2006;175(4):1320–4 [discussion: 1324–5].
46. Bader P, Burkhard FC, Markwalder R, et al. Disease progression and survival of patients with positive lymph nodes after radical prostatectomy. Is there a chance of cure? J Urol 2003;169(3):849–54.
47. Boorjian SA, Thompson RH, Siddiqui S, et al. Long-term outcome after radical prostatectomy for patients with lymph node positive prostate cancer in the prostate specific antigen era. J Urol 2007; 178(3 Pt 1):864–70 [discussion: 870–1].
48. Cheng L, Zincke H, Blute ML, et al. Risk of prostate carcinoma death in patients with lymph node metastasis. Cancer 2001;91(1):66–73.
49. Briganti A, Karnes JR, Da Pozzo LF, et al. Two positive nodes represent a significant cut-off value for cancer specific survival in patients with node positive prostate cancer. A new proposal based on a two-institution experience on 703 consecutive N+ patients treated with radical prostatectomy, extended pelvic lymph node dissection and adjuvant therapy. Eur Urol 2009;55(2):261–70.
50. Palapattu GS, Allaf ME, Trock BJ, et al. Prostate specific antigen progression in men with lymph node metastases following radical prostatectomy: results of long-term followup. J Urol 2004;172(5 Pt 1):1860–4.
51. Schumacher MC, Burkhard FC, Thalmann GN, et al. Good outcome for patients with few lymph node metastases after radical retropubic prostatectomy. Eur Urol 2008;54(2):344–52.
52. Herr HW, Bochner BH, Dalbagni G, et al. Impact of the number of lymph nodes retrieved on outcome in patients with muscle invasive bladder cancer. J Urol 2002;167(3):1295–8.
53. Axelsson CK, During M, Christiansen PM, et al. Impact on regional recurrence and survival of axillary surgery in women with node-negative primary breast cancer. Br J Surg 2009;96(1):40–6.
54. Joseph NE, Sigurdson ER, Hanlon AL, et al. Accuracy of determining nodal negativity in colorectal cancer on the basis of the number of nodes retrieved on resection. Ann Surg Oncol 2003;10(3): 213–8.
55. Gajra A, Newman N, Gamble GP, et al. Effect of number of lymph nodes sampled on outcome in patients with stage I non-small-cell lung cancer. J Clin Oncol 2003;21(6):1029–34.
56. Joslyn SA, Konety BR. Impact of extent of lymphadenectomy on survival after radical prostatectomy for prostate cancer. Urology 2006;68(1):121–5.
57. DiMarco DS, Zincke H, Sebo TJ, et al. The extent of lymphadenectomy for pTXNO prostate cancer does not affect prostate cancer outcome in the prostate specific antigen era. J Urol 2005;173(4):1121–5.
58. Bhatta-Dhar N, Reuther AM, Zippe C, et al. No difference in six-year biochemical failure rates with or without pelvic lymph node dissection during radical prostatectomy in low-risk patients with localized prostate cancer. Urology 2004;63(3):528–31.
59. Gofrit ON, Zorn KC, Steinberg GD, et al. The Will Rogers phenomenon in urological oncology. J Urol 2008;179(1):28–33.
60. Clark T, Parekh DJ, Cookson MS, et al. Randomized prospective evaluation of extended versus limited lymph node dissection in patients with clinically localized prostate cancer. J Urol 2003;169(1):145–7 [discussion: 147–8].
61. Briganti A, Chun FK, Salonia A, et al. Complications and other surgical outcomes associated with extended pelvic lymphadenectomy in men with localized prostate cancer. Eur Urol 2006;50(5): 1006–13.
62. Pepper RJ, Pati J, Kaisary AV. The incidence and treatment of lymphoceles after radical retropubic prostatectomy. BJU Int 2005;95(6):772–5.
63. Stone NN, Stock RG, Unger P. Laparoscopic pelvic lymph node dissection for prostate cancer: comparison of the extended and modified techniques. J Urol 1997;158(5):1891–4.
64. Box GN, Lee HJ, Abraham JB, et al. Comparative study of in vivo lymphatic sealing capability of the porcine thoracic duct using laparoscopic dissection devices. J Urol 2009;181(1):387–91.
65. Heidenreich A, Aus G, Bolla M, et al. EAU guidelines on prostate cancer. Eur Urol 2008;53(1):68–80.
66. Thompson I, Thrasher JB, Aus G, et al. Guideline for the management of clinically localized prostate cancer: 2007 update. J Urol 2007;177(6): 2106–31.

Primary and Salvage Cryotherapy for Prostate Cancer

David S. Finley, MD[a,*], Frederic Pouliot, MD, PhD[a], David C. Miller, MD, MPH[b,c], Arie S. Belldegrun, MD, FACS[a]

KEYWORDS

- Cryotherapy • Cryoablation • Prostate
- Prostate cancer • Focal therapy • Focal ablation

Cryotherapy is a technique to ablate tissue by local induction of extremely cold temperatures. This technology was pioneered in the 1960s by Cooper and Lee.[1] Several years later, Gonder and colleagues[2] performed transurethral cryoablation of the prostate with digital rectal guidance of the ice ball for benign prostatic hypertrophy. Initial forays were hampered by difficulty in accurate placement of cryoprobes and by imprecise monitoring of the ice ball, which resulted in incomplete treatment and high complication rates. During the past 40 years, however, considerable inroads have been made in cryotechnology and imaging, allowing for precision, safety, and efficacy. In 2005, approximately 6600 procedures were performed in the United States.[3] Indeed, it has now been more than a decade since the American Urological Association (AUA) recognized cryotherapy as a therapeutic option for prostate cancer, removing the label of "investigational." In 2008, an AUA Best Practice Statement recognized cryoablation of the prostate as an established treatment option for men with newly diagnosed or radiorecurrent organ-confined prostate cancer. In their analysis of the current state of the art, the panel identified a constellation of key advancements such as improved cryotechnology, advanced ultrathin cryoprobes with precise isotherm delineation, real-time ultrasonographic ice-ball monitoring, active urethral warming, and, in particular, the use of multipoint thermal sensors to protect nontarget tissues (eg, rectum, external urethral sphincter).[4] Improved patient outcomes have been seen commensurate with refinement of surgical technique and evolution of technology.[5–7]

CRYOINJURY

The principles of cryotherapy, including the mechanisms of cell injury and cell death, have been well described.[8–10] Cryotherapy induces cell damage by a variety of direct and indirect mechanisms, some immediate and others delayed. The end result is the induction of coagulative necrosis in the targeted tissue. The direct and immediate effects of injury occur because of the destructive effects of freezing and warming tissue. The indirect and delayed effects occur due to microcirculatory damage/ischemia, inflammation, and apoptosis.[9–13] A full discussion of the mechanism of cryoinjury is beyond the scope of this article.

FACTORS AFFECTING TISSUE DESTRUCTION DURING CRYOTHERAPY

The key variables that affect cellular destruction include the rates of cooling and warming and the nadir temperature achieved in the tissue.[4,9,10,12,13]

Disclosure: Chairman of Galil, Medical Advisory Board, Consultant, Galil Medical (Arie S. Belldegrun).
[a] Department of Urology, Institute of Urologic Oncology, David Geffen School of Medicine at UCLA, 924 Westwood Boulevard, Suite 1050, Box 957207, Los Angeles, CA 90095-7207, USA
[b] Department of Urology, University of Michigan School of Medicine, University of Michigan, 1031 Michigan House 2301, Commonwealth, Ann Arbor, MI 48106, USA
[c] VA Center for Clinical Management Research, University of Michigan School of Medicine, University of Michigan, 1031 Michigan House 2301, Commonwealth, Ann Arbor, MI 48106, USA
* Corresponding author.
E-mail address: dfinley@mednet.ucla.edu (D.S. Finley).

Urol Clin N Am 37 (2010) 67–82
doi:10.1016/j.ucl.2009.11.007
0094-0143/10/$ – see front matter

urologic.theclinics.com

Tatsutani and colleagues[14] studied thermal parameters associated with prostate cancer destruction in an ND-1 cell line; they demonstrated that temperatures less than −40°C were required for complete cell death. In addition, the investigators noted a faster freezing rate (ie, 2°C/min vs 1°C/min or 5°C/min) resulted in optimal cellular destruction, a finding reported by other groups.[15–17] In practice, however, the cooling rate proximal to the probe is much higher than that of peripheral tissue, resulting in differential rates of cooling. Others have suggested that the cooling rate is not the most important factor determining cell death.[17] However, there is evidence to suggest that the subsequent thaw cycle is more destructive at slower rates.[9,18,19] In addition, numerous investigators have reported that a double freeze/thaw cycle significantly increased cell destruction.[20,21] A second cycle has been found to increase the extent of necrosis up to 80% of the previously frozen volume.[9,10,12,13,22] A second cycle also results in a lower lethal isotherm of approximately −20°C, permitting a closer approach to the margins of the prostate without endangering the rectum. Clinically, double freeze-thaw cycles have been associated with lower posttreatment positive biopsy rates and improved prostate-specific antigen (PSA) results, compared with a single freeze-thaw cycle.[4,21,23–25] For patients who had undergone focal cryoablation before radical prostatectomy (RP) with 2 consecutive 10-minute freeze cycles, pathologic examination revealed a larger area of coagulative necrosis than with a single 20-minute freeze.[22] **Fig. 1** shows an example of a 1.47-mm ablation needle (IceRod, Galil Medical) and the corresponding isotherm map. **Fig. 2** depicts a typical needle insertion template.

Key variables associated with maximum cell death

1. Nadir temperature: minimum of −20°C, preferably −40°C
2. Freezing rate: as rapid as possible (ie, 25°C/min)
3. Thawing rate: slow, passive thawing
4. Freeze/thaw cycles: a double freeze-thaw cycle (ie, 10 min freeze/5 min thaw)

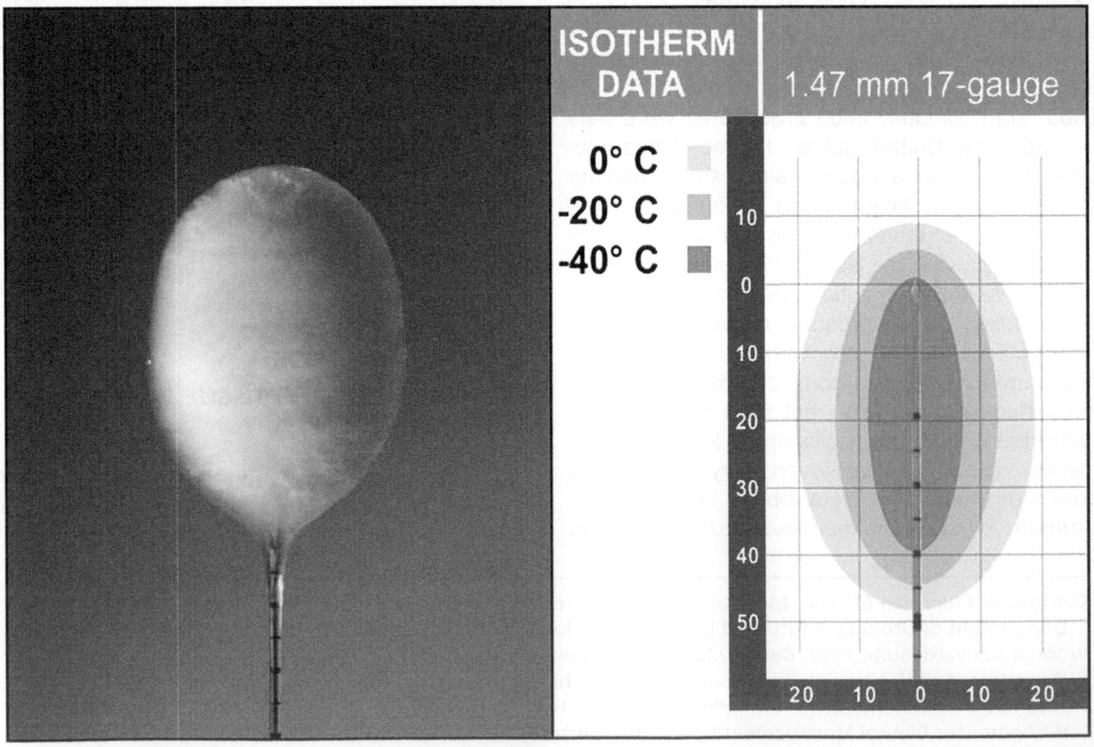

Fig. 1. A 1.47-mm ablation needle (IceRod, Galil Medical) and the corresponding isotherm map. (*Courtesy of* Galil Medical, Inc., Plymouth Meeting, PA; with permission.)

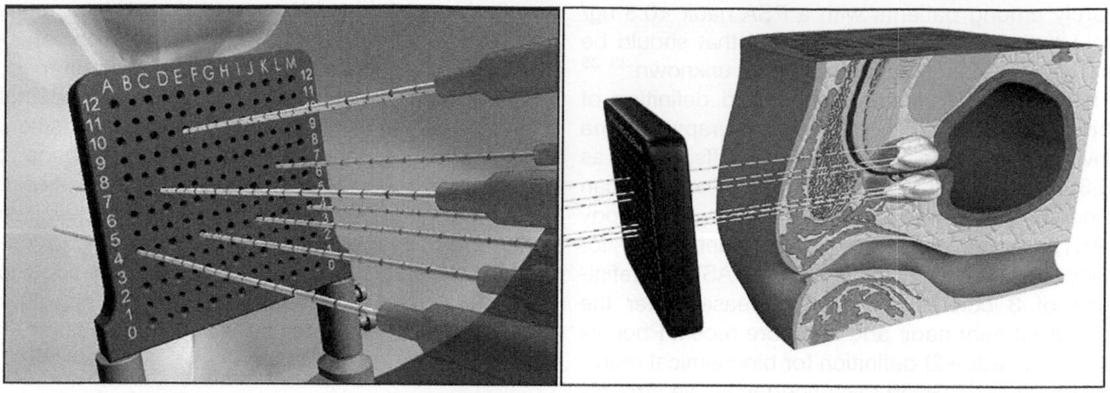

Courtesy of Galil Medical

Fig. 2. Depicts a typical needle insertion template. (*Courtesy of* Galil Medical, Inc., Plymouth Meeting, PA; with permission.)

Primary Cryotherapy

In general, patients with clinical stage T1c-T2 disease, who have no evidence of metastatic disease, greater than 10-year life expectancy, and who are not concerned with potency are candidates for whole-gland primary cryotherapy. The AUA Best Practice Policy Statement of cryosurgery proposed that the role of cryosurgery remains undetermined for patients with clinical stage T3 disease.[4] Cryotherapy represents a good option for many patients who do not wish to undergo RP or radiation therapy (RT). Many patients who are candidates for external beam radiotherapy (EBRT) may consider primary cryotherapy because treatment can be conveniently administered as an outpatient procedure as opposed to 1 to 2 months of treatment. High-risk patients may require multimodal therapy.[4] Patients with gross extracapsular extension or seminal vesicle invasion are treated with neoadjuvant hormone therapy to reduce the tumor volume and allow for easier inclusion within the ice ball. Due to limitations in isotherm coverage based on currently available probes, prostates larger than 50 cm^3 may be incompletely enveloped by the ice ball; neoadjuvant hormone therapy is indicated in these cases to reduce the target volume to allow for complete coverage.[4,21,23,26–29] To date, there are no data to suggest that neoadjuvant or concurrent androgen deprivation therapy (ADT) improves postcryosurgery cancer control outcomes.[4]

Cryotherapy may offer certain advantages to patients with comorbidities that may preclude them from candidacy for RP or RT (eg, men with Crohn disease, ulcerative colitis, prior pelvic irradiation or pelvic surgery, cardiac disease, morbid obesity, or body habitus unfavorable for RP or RT). Finally, cryosurgery can also be considered in a salvage setting (ie, radiation failure) in patients who have negative metastatic workup.

Contraindications to cryosurgery

Absolute

- Metastatic disease
- Anorectal fistula

Relative

- Gland size >50 cm^3
- Prior transurethral resection of prostate (TURP) (particularly for salvage cryotherapy)
- PSA >20 ng/mL
- cT3 disease
- Prior pelvic surgery/trauma with distorted anatomy

Data from Miller DC, Pisters LL, Belldegrun AS. Cryotherapy for Prostate Cancer, Chapter 101. In: Wein AJ, Kavoussi LR, Novick AC, et al, editors. Campbell-Walsh Urology, 9th edition. Saunders, 2007.

SURVEILLANCE AFTER CRYOTHERAPY

Generally, we follow patients with clinical examinations and serial PSA measurements every 3 months for the first year and then biannually thereafter along with routine biopsies. Initially following the procedure, serum PSA levels spike due to release of intracellular PSA from cellular necrosis.[30] The PSA nadir is generally reached in 3 months.[31] However, serum PSA levels after cryotherapy may not decrease to an undetectable level because of the necessary preservation of a thin rim of periurethral tissue for whole-gland ablation or from a more substantial spared portion of the gland with subtotal treatment.[4] Although data have shown that a lower PSA nadir is associated with an increased chance of a stable PSA and negative biopsy (eg, residual cancer is found rarely among patients with a PSA nadir <0.5 ng/mL),[32] the actual PSA nadir level that should be achieved after cryotherapy is unknown.[33–35] There is no universally established definition of biochemical failure after cryotherapy. Some investigators use static PSA cutoffs, such as 0.3, 0.4, 0.5, and 1.0 ng/mL.[32,36–44] The American Society for Therapeutic Radiology and Oncology (ASTRO) has put forth various definitions for biochemical failure: the traditional ASTRO definition of 3 consecutive PSA increases after the posttreatment nadir and the more recent Phoenix (ie, PSA nadir+2) definition for biochemical recurrence.[5,37,44,45] Given this uncertainty, we strongly advocate performing routine prostate biopsy after cryotherapy to assess local control. If biopsies are considered, however, we recommend waiting approximately 6 months to allow for resolution of inflammation.

PRIMARY CRYOTHERAPY

Following primary cryotherapy prostate biopsy has been routinely performed as part of a standard protocol 6 to 12 months after cryotherapy in a few studies; the positive biopsy rate ranges from 2% to 25%.[21,23,24,39,44,46–48] Cohen and colleagues[5] reported a 10-year positive biopsy rate of 23%. The investigators noted that higher baseline PSA levels and clinical T stage were independent risk factors for positive postcryosurgery biopsies. In a series of 168 men who underwent primary cryoablation with third-generation cryosurgical technology, Ellis and colleagues[48] found that 10.1% of men had a positive biopsy at an average of 10 months postablation. Among a subset of 336 patients from the Cryo On-Line Data (COLD) Registry who underwent posttreatment biopsy, a positive biopsy rate of 38% (49/129) was observed for patients with evidence of biochemical recurrence, compared with only 14.5% (30/207) among patients with no clinical evidence for biochemical recurrence.[6] These data underscore the important observation that rates of local control can vary significantly depending on whether biopsies are performed as part of a standard surveillance protocol (ie, independent of postcryotherapy PSA levels) compared with biopsy only in patients with a rising PSA after the procedure. In most series that have advocated routine postcryotherapy biopsies, positive biopsy rates are usually reported in less than 10% of patients treated with third-generation systems and a double freeze-thaw cycle.[44] The areas of the prostate or seminal vesicles that have been reported to have the highest recurrence rates are at the apex and the seminal vesicles compared with the midgland and base because of their peripheral location.[34,49]

Pathologists should be experienced in interpretation of prostate tissue that has undergone cryoablation. Pathologic findings include stromal fibrosis, hyalinization, basal cell hyperplasia with ductal and acinar regeneration, hemosiderin deposition, squamous metaplasia, and stromal hemorrhage[50]; coagulative necrosis is seen up to 30 weeks following treatment. Although there is no definitive method to evaluate tumor viability following cryoablation, keratin 34βE12, p63 (basal cell–specific markers), and racemase expression persist after cryoablation which may be of adjunctive value.[50]

Biochemical Recurrence-Free Survival

In 2008, collaborators of the COLD Registry reported on pooled multicenter PSA outcomes for 2558 patients treated with primary whole-gland cryosurgical ablation.[51] Among this large group of men, the 5-year actuarial biochemical recurrence-free survival was 83.7 (ASTRO definition) and 82.7% (Phoenix definition). When stratified according to D'Amico risk categories, 5-year biochemical recurrence-free survival rates (by ASTRO) were 89.2% for patients in the low-risk group, 83.7% for moderate-risk patients, and 80.2% for patients in the high-risk group. According to the Phoenix (nadir+2) definition, the corresponding rates were 84.3%, 79.0%, and 69.6% for low-, intermediate-, and high-risk groups, respectively.[44,51] Cohen and colleagues[5] reported long-term outcomes of approximately 200 men treated with cryoablation of the prostate from 1991 to 1996. Their reported 10-year PSA recurrence-free survival rates (Phoenix) were 80.6%, 74.2%, and 45.5% for low-, intermediate-, and high-risk groups, respectively. Variables that were significantly associated with postcryosurgery biochemical recurrence by multivariate analysis included patient age, pretreatment PSA, and the posttreatment PSA nadir.[5] Similarly, Shinohara correlated the rate of biochemical and biopsy failure with the PSA nadir after cryotherapy in 132 patients.[34] Biochemical failure was lowest in patients who achieved a PSA nadir of less than 0.1 ng/mL (21%). In addition, biopsy failure was rare in patients with a PSA nadir of less than 0.1 ng/mL (1.5%). Yet, among patients with a PSA nadir greater than 0.5 ng/mL, 55% had a positive follow-up prostate biopsy. The investigators observed that biochemical and biopsy failure usually occurred within the first 12 months after treatment (96% and 88% of biochemical and biopsy failures, respectively).[34,44]

As noted in the AUA Best Practice Policy Statement of cryosurgery, to date, there are no long-term data for disease-specific or metastasis-free survival. Given this dearth of information, oncologic comparison between cryosurgery and other treatment modalities are limited.

FOCAL CRYOTHERAPY

Definition

The 2008 report from the Consensus Conference on Focal Treatment of Prostatic Carcinoma defined focal cryotherapy as "an individualized treatment that selectively ablates known disease and preserves existing functions, with the overall objective of minimizing lifetime morbidity without compromising life expectancy."[52] Focal therapy can involve the local application of treatment to a specific focus, and the term, "image-guided focal therapy," is used when it is done under real-time imaging.[53,54] Focal therapy has been further subdivided into hemiablation when treatment involves a complete lobe, and subtotal ablation when both lobes are targeted with the exception of a rim of parenchyma close to the neurovascular bundle(s) (**Fig. 3**).[25,55–60]

Patient Selection

Conceptually, prostate-sparing focal therapy has the advantages of treating the index lesion while minimizing morbidity that occurs with more radical treatments. Although this strategy is attractive to men with minimal disease who are concerned about potential over-treatment with RP or under-treatment as with active surveillance, at the present time it should be limited to patients who meet rigorous selection criteria. Although no universally accepted selection criteria currently exist, the 2008 Consensus Panel proposed several specific selection factors. Eggener and colleagues[55] also suggested a comprehensive set of selection factors for focal therapy.

It has been shown in several studies that low-risk prostate cancers are unifocal in about 20% of cases at RP, a finding that provides a biologic basis for such a therapy. However, a major concern is our ability to accurately identify preoperatively the patients that harbor unilateral prostate cancer. Several studies have attempted to determine whether the prevalence of unifocal prostate cancer on RP specimens can be predicted by unilateral or unifocal prostate cancer at biopsy. Iczkowski and colleagues[58] analyzed a series of 393 perineal RP specimens with preoperative biopsy (average of 11 cores) and observed that prostate cancers were unilateral in approximately 71% to 76% at prostatectomy when they were unilateral at biopsy. In addition, the ability of preoperative biopsy to assess unilaterality at prostatectomy correlated with the number of biopsy cores. Yoon and colleagues[59] reviewed the prostatectomy specimens for which the preoperative biopsy predicted limited disease (Gleason score ≤6, <3 positive cores, <50% of cancer in any core). The investigators found 13% had a significant tumor (>0.5 cm^3) contralateral to the index tumor, half of which were located in the transition zone. At RP, 20% of the patients had an adverse pathologic feature on the contralateral side of the biopsy, described as tumor volume

Proposed patient selection criteria for focal ablation according to the 2008 report of the Consensus Panel[4]

- ≥5-year life expectancy
- The primary consideration for focal therapy is the location of the cancer
- Stage T1 to T3 disease: ablation of all known cancer is possible in a minimally morbid fashion
- PSA <15 ng/mL
- M1 disease is considered a contraindication
- Nodal involvement is a relative contraindication

Data from Babaian RJ, Donnelly B, Bahn D, et al. Best practice statement on cryosurgery for the treatment of localized prostate cancer. J Urol 2008;180:1993–2004.

Proposed clinical, biopsy and imaging criteria for focal therapy patient selection[55]

Clinical

- Clinical stage T1 or T2a
- PSA <10 ng/mL
- PSA density <0.15 ng/mL/cm^3
- PSA velocity <2 ng/mL yearly in the year before diagnosis

Biopsy

- Minimum of 12 cores
- No Gleason grade 4 or 5
- Maximum percentage of cancer in each core (eg, 20%)
- Maximum length of cancer in each core (eg, 7 mm)
- Maximum percentage of total cores with cancer (eg, 33%)

Imaging

- Single lesion with a maximum size (eg, 12 mm)
- Maximum length of capsular contact (eg, 10 mm)
- No evidence of extraprostatic extension or seminal vesicle invasion

Data from Eggener SE, Scardino PT, Carroll PR, et al. Focal therapy for localized prostate cancer: A critical appraisal of rationale and modalities. J Urol 2007;178:2260–7.

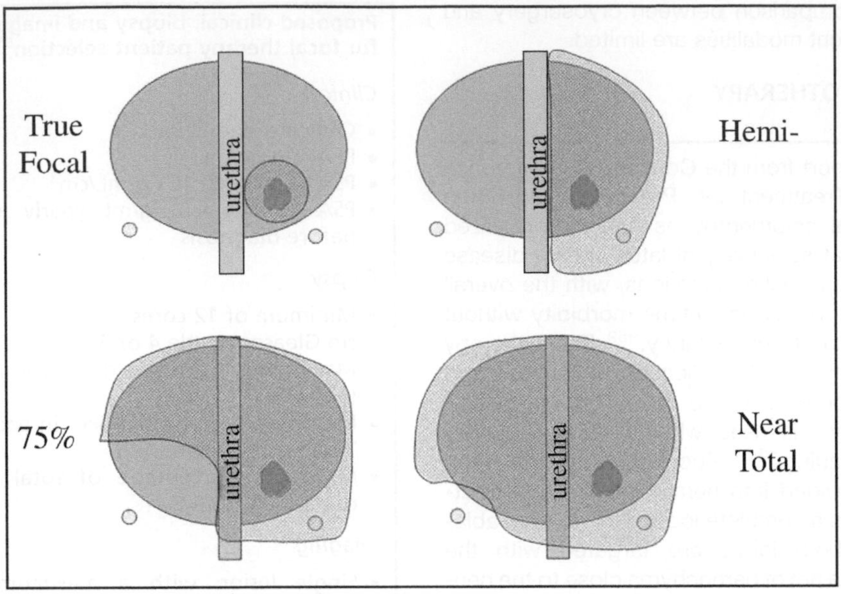

Fig. 3. Ablation templates. (*Courtesy of* Dr Katz.)

greater than 0.5 cm^3, positive margin, extraprostatic extension, or Gleason score greater than 6. However, one limitation of that study was the lack of detail regarding the number of biopsy cores obtained preoperatively. The importance of accurately sampling the prostate has led some investigators to suggest a second biopsy or even saturation biopsies to reduce the risk of contralateral cancer at follow-up.[61]

Outcomes of Focal Ablation

Table 1 summarizes the first pilot clinical trials of focal hemiablation for unilateral lesions and targeted cryoablation of a presumed unifocal lesion. In 2002, Onik and colleagues[60] reported an initial pilot study of 9 men treated with focal, unilateral, nerve-sparing cryotherapy. Using this technique, they attempted to exploit the ability of cryotherapy to treat extracapsular extension while minimizing the sexual function morbidity associated with whole-gland ablation. At a mean follow-up of 36 months, all 9 men had stable PSA levels; the 6 patients who had posttreatment biopsies had no evidence of residual cancer. The same group reported more mature follow-up on a larger cohort of patients treated with focal ablation between June 1995 and December 2005.[61,63] Before treatment, patients underwent three-dimensional mapping saturation rebiopsy. Approximately 50% of patients who were initially believed to have unilateral disease were found to have bilateral lesions and were excluded from the study. Although follow-up was short (mean 3.6 years), 95% had a stable PSA at last follow-up. The investigators determined that the postcryosurgery PSA stabilization level was at some fraction of the preoperative PSA level, depending on the extent of gland ablation; the mean preoperative PSA level for this cohort was 8.3 ng/mL, whereas the mean postoperative PSA was 2.4 ng/mL. Among the 4 patients noted to have an unstable PSA level in the first posttreatment year, prostate biopsy determined that each patient harbored cancer in an untreated portion of the gland. A subset of patients underwent routine biopsy at 1 year, all of which were negative. Although standardized questionnaires were not used, potency was reportedly maintained in 85% of patients. No patients developed de novo urinary incontinence.[61]

Lambert and colleagues[62] reported on subtotal cryoablation (hemiablation) of the prostate among 25 patients with unilateral prostate cancer. In this study, each patient had unilateral, histologically proven prostate cancer meeting the following criteria: (1) Gleason score 6 or Gleason score 7 (3+4) prostate cancer that involved only a single lobe of the gland; (2) involvement of only 1 or 2 contiguous biopsy cores; and (3) tumor volume of less than 10% in a 12-core biopsy. The neurovascular bundle on the treated side was ablated, whereas the contralateral neurovascular bundle was spared. The investigators provided variable definitions of biochemical disease-free survival

Table 1
Cancer control and potency rates after focal and unilateral cryoablation

References	N	No. of bx Cores	Median FU (mo)	Cryounit	bDFS (%)	PSA Cutoff	Bx-proven Recurrence	Potency Preserved
Lambert et al[62]	25	12	28	SeedNet[b]	84	<50% nadir, nadir+2	12% (8% untreated lobe, 4% treated lobe)	71%
Bahn et al[39,a]	31	6–12	70	Cryocare[c]	93	ASTRO	4% untreated lobe	88.9% total (48.1% full recovery, 40.8% medically assisted)
Onik et al[63]	21	7–8	50	Cryocare	95	ASTRO	0 (1 case of CaP was found on MRIS in untreated lobe)	80%
Ellis et al[64]	60	ND	12	Cryocare	80.5	ASTRO	23%[d]	70.6%

Bx, biopsy; bDFS, biochemical disease-free survival; CaP, cancer of the prostate; PSA, prostate-specific antigen; MRIS, MRI spectroscopy.
[a] Results from a 2-center trial.
[b] SeedNet, Galil Medical, Plymouth, PA, USA.
[c] Cryocare Endocare, Irvine, CA, USA.
[d] Twenty-three percent for the entire series of 60 patients, but biopsies were only taken from 35 patients. Forty percent (14/35) of those from whom a biopsy was taken had a positive biopsy, 13/14 on the contralateral side of cryotherapy.

rates; for example, using a PSA nadir of less than 1 ng/mL as the definition of biochemical failure, the investigators reported 36% biochemical disease-free survival (median follow-up 28 months). Using a PSA less than 2 ng/mL or less than 3 ng/mL as the definitions for biochemical control, the PSA recurrence-free survival rates were higher at 48% and 72%, respectively. Among 7 patients who underwent posttreatment biopsy, 3 had recurrent cancer, including 1 patient with tumor in the previously ablated lobe. In terms of morbidity, 71% of patients maintained potency and none developed postoperative urinary incontinence.

Ellis and colleagues[65] reported on results of data extracted from the COLD registry comprising 341 patients treated with focal cryoablation. Biochemical disease-free survival according to ASTRO and Phoenix criteria for low-, intermediate-, and high-risk groups were 762.2%, 87.2%, 75% and 62.3%, 68.1%, 62.5%, respectively. Rectal fistula and incontinence rates at 12 months were 0.3% and 1.6%, respectively. Among men who were potent before the procedure, posttreatment potency rates were greater than 74% at 36 months.[44]

Despite the promising data that continue to emerge for subtotal (including focal) cryoablation, overall clinical experience is limited and long-term results are largely unavailable.[4] Moreover, there are still no precise means to definitively identify histologically and/or biologically unifocal tumors.[55] In select cases for whom focal therapy may be appropriate, we recommend performing repeat biopsies with a saturation template on the disease-free side to confirm the absence of disease before treatment. We strongly agree with the recommendations from the AUA Best Practices Consensus Panel and the International Task Force on Prostate Cancer and the Focal Lesion Paradigm, that the potential application of subtotal or focal cryotherapy must be carefully investigated in prospective clinical trials.[4,54]

At present, current imaging modalities are insufficient to localize small lesions. In the future, there will be improved imaging resolution with techniques such as 7 Tesla magnetic resonance imaging (MRI), MRI spectroscopy (MRSI), functional MRI, [^{11}C]choline positron emission tomography (PET)/computed tomography (CT), molecular imaging and contrast-enhanced ultrasound (CEUS). Early experience with CEUS imaging shows significant advantages over standard ultrasound gray-scale imaging. Improved imaging may help select patients with true unifocal disease, allow more precise probe placement for true focal ablation (vs hemiablation), enhance protection of the neurovascular bundles (NVBs), and aid in posttreatment monitoring given the inherent difficulties of using PSA in the setting of subtotal treatment.

SALVAGE CRYOTHERAPY

Radiation Failures

Approximately one-third of men with newly diagnosed prostate cancer undergo primary treatment with EBRT and/or brachytherapy annually.[65,66] It estimated that between 20% and 60% of men who undergo primary RT for prostate cancer may develop a postradiotherapy PSA recurrence.[44,67,68] Among this group, local-only failure rates range from 25% to 32%.[69] Radioresistant or radiorecurrent prostate cancer is typically an aggressive form of localized prostate cancer; in many cases radiorecurrent disease involves high-volume and/or poorly differentiated tumors at the time of diagnosis,[67,68] rendering salvage therapies less likely to fully eradicate the cancer. Following primary RT, the identification of residual cancer by early PSA detection and positive biopsies increases the likelihood of successful salvage therapy.[44,67,68] Salvage cryotherapy can be undertaken in patients following EBRT and brachytherapy. Salvage therapy can provide a curative treatment option that improves local control and possibly increases long-term survival.[4]

In our practice, candidacy for salvage cryotherapy is reserved for patients who meet the following criteria: an increasing PSA value after radiation, a positive postradiation biopsy, and a negative metastatic workup.[4,44,70] Although the AUA Best Practice Consensus Statement acknowledges that there are no clear guidelines in patient section for salvage cryotherapy, they note that patients should ideally have a life expectancy of greater than 10 years, PSA 4 ng/mL or less, absence of seminal vesicle invasion, and a long PSA doubling time.[4] We prefer to wait at least 18 to 24 months after RT and to perform a biopsy of the prostate if the PSA value increases above the nadir level and there are 3 consecutive increases. When performing a biopsy, multiple cores should be obtained. Because seminal vesicle invasion is common in patients undergoing salvage RP, it is recommended to also perform concurrent seminal vesicle biopsies.[4] The pathologist should have experience interpreting postradiation prostate biopsies as nuclear and cytoplasmic alterations can confound the diagnosis of residual cancer.[71] Although the incidence of positive biopsy after RT varies widely in the literature, it seems that the rates are higher after EBRT compared with brachytherapy.[72] In addition, patients with a postradiation PSA greater than 10 ng/mL or a PSA doubling time of 16 months or less are more likely to fail salvage cryotherapy.[4,44,73,74]

Once it has been established that primary therapy has failed, it is key to differentiate a local recurrence from a distant recurrence. Local failure requires a histologically proven active adenocarcinoma on prostate biopsy in the absence of radiographic evidence of metastatic disease.[44] A major problem with radiographic evaluation for metastases in biochemically recurrent prostate cancer, however, is the relative lack of sensitivity and specificity of CT, PET-CT, MRI, bone scan, and, more recently, monoclonal antibody-labeled nuclear scans.[44,75,76] Emerging techniques under investigation, such as high-resolution MRI with lymphotropic superparamagnetic nanoparticle imaging, may offer increased sensitivity for the detection of lymph node metastases.[67,77] Although these technologies have limitations, if recurrence is suspected, they are mandatory to exclude the presence of overt metastatic disease, which may potentially save the patient from unnecessary invasive treatment. There may be a limited role for laparoscopic/robotic or open lymph node sampling in select patients.[4]

Focal ablation has been applied to localized radiorecurrent disease. Eisenberg and Shinohara[78] reported their preliminary results with partial salvage cryoablation of the prostate among men with radiorecurrent prostate cancer. In this series, 19 patients with a unilateral focus of radiorecurrent prostate cancer were treated with hemigland ablation in the salvage setting. The investigators reported biochemical recurrence-free survival rates (ASTRO definition) of 89%, 67%, and 50% at 1, 2, and 3 years respectively. Using the Phoenix criteria, biochemical control rates were 89%, 79%, and 79% at 1, 2, and 3 years, respectively.[44] At 1 year, 1/10 (10%) patients undergoing posttreatment biopsy harbored residual cancer. Reported complications in this series were rare. The investigators concluded that, in selected patients with a unilateral focus of radiorecurrent prostate cancer, acceptable oncologic results may be achieved with partial cryoablation of the prostate, while at the same time minimizing postcryotherapy morbidity. It is our opinion that focal salvage cryoablation of the prostate is highly experimental because the interpretation of PSA recurrence after primary and salvage procedures might be difficult to interpret without systematic rebiopsy.

Local Recurrence Following RP

For patients with biopsy-proven or radiographically identified local recurrence after RP, cryoablation may provide an alternative to radiotherapy. To our knowledge, there is only 1 report in this select patient population. Siddiqui and colleagues[79] offered salvage cryotherapy to men with isolated, radiographically identified, biopsy-proven local recurrence after radical retropubic prostatectomy. Forty percent of patients showed a sustained decline in PSA, whereas 60% suffered from disease progression. Factors that correlated with success were Gleason score of 6 and an MRI lesion of 1 cm or less. Despite a PSA response, the ability and safety of salvage cryoablation to eradicate prostate cancer completely in the prostate bed after prostatectomy is unknown. For instance, recurrence close to the rectum or sphincter would not be treated safely by salvage cryoablation. This limitation of the technology adds to the inaccuracy of current clinical predictors to determine whether a local recurrence is local or systemic.

OUTCOMES

Prognostic Variables

A few clinical variables have been identified that may predict the efficacy of salvage cryoablation. In a seminal article, Pisters and colleagues[80] analyzed 145 men who underwent salvage cryotherapy; the investigators identified that a PSA greater than 10 ng/mL and Gleason score of the recurrent cancer greater than or equal to 9 were associated with salvage failure. In another large series by Izawa and associates,[81] among 131 patients who had received EBRT and then went on to salvage cryotherapy, they found that androgen-independent local recurrences, Gleason score, and preradiation clinical stage were key predictors of disease-specific survival and disease-free survival.[44,81] Several recent studies have demonstrated that a postradiation PSA level greater than 10 ng/mL or a PSA doubling time of 16 months or less was associated with increased salvage failure rates.[4,44,73,74,81]

Although the proportions of patients with positive biopsies after salvage cryoablation for radiorecurrent disease vary widely, they usually range from 15% to 35% in most series.[7,44,74] For example, Ng and colleagues[74] reported a positive biopsy rate of 16.6% among a large series of 187 patients treated with third-generation systems. In addition, among 279 COLD Registry patients who underwent postcryoablation prostate biopsy, 15/46 (32.2%) were found to have residual cancer; of 15 patients with evidence of biochemical recurrence, 8 (53.3%) had a positive biopsy.

Biochemical Control

Ismail and colleagues[82] reported on a cohort of 100 patients treated with salvage cryoablation of the prostate between 2000 and 2005. With a median follow-up of 33.5 months, a biochemical recurrence-free survival (defined as PSA <0.5 ng/mL) of 73%, 45%, and 11% was observed for patients with low-, intermediate-, and high-risk disease, respectively. More favorable outcomes were seen among patients with a postcryoablation PSA nadir of 0.1 ng/mL or less.[44] Ng and colleagues[74] reported biochemical failure results for 187 patients treated with salvage cryotherapy between 1995 and 2004. The investigators found that preablation PSA level was a significant independent predictor of treatment failure; among patients with a presalvage PSA level of 4 ng/mL or less, 5-year and 8-year biochemical recurrence-free survival was 56% and 37%, respectively. By contrast, patients who had a presalvage PSA of 10 ng/mL or more were found to have poor biochemical recurrence-free survival rates of only 14% and 7%, at 5 and 8 years, respectively. The COLD registry investigators reported biochemical outcomes among 279 patients treated with salvage cryosurgical ablation. The investigators observed 5-year biochemical recurrence-free survival rates of 59% and 55%, based on the ASTRO and Phoenix criteria, respectively.[7] These data suggest that salvage cryosurgical ablation of the prostate is associated with biochemical control rates of approximately 50% to 60% at 4 or more years after salvage therapy, with improved outcomes seen with lower presalvage PSA levels and postsalvage PSA nadirs.[44,73,74,82,83]

Recently, cancer control and morbidity outcomes following salvage cryosurgery, salvage prostatectomy, and salvage brachytherapy were reviewed by Nguyen and colleagues[67] and Allen and colleagues.[68] The investigators reported that, in the absence of prospective comparative trials, it is not currently possible to determine whether 1 treatment is superior with respect to biochemical recurrence-free survival or other cancer control outcomes. Five-year biochemical recurrence-free survival rates following salvage RP range from 50% to 60%[67,68]; slightly less favorable PSA control rates have been reported following salvage cryotherapy and brachytherapy. A recent study by Pisters and colleagues[83] reported on findings of a retrospective comparison of cancer control outcomes following salvage cryotherapy and salvage RP among a cohort of patients with presalvage PSA less than 10 ng/mL, post-RT biopsy Gleason score of 8 or less, and no prior ADT. They found that salvage RP yielded improved outcomes compared with salvage cryotherapy based on 2 separate definitions of biochemical failure (PSA >0.4 ng/mL: salvage RP 61% vs salvage cryo 21%, at 5 years; 2 increases above PSA nadir: salvage RP 66% vs salvage cryo 42%) and superior overall survival at 5 years (salvage RP 95% vs salvage cryo 85%). Disease-specific survival at 5 years was similar for both groups (salvage cryo 96% vs salvage RP 98%). The investigators concluded that younger patients with radiorecurrent prostate cancer should consider salvage RP because it can offer superior progression-free survival.[44,83]

The following clinical variables predict a greater likelihood of PSA recurrence-free survival: (1) low-risk tumor (ie, clinical stage T1c or T2a, PSA <10 ng/mL, and Gleason score $\leq$6) at the time of original diagnosis; (2) PSA velocity before initial RT <2 ng/mL per year; (3) time to postradiation PSA failure >3 years; (4) postradiation PSA doubling time >12 months; and (5) negative bone scan and pelvic imaging.[44,67] Although infrequent, serious adverse complications are more common following salvage versus primary therapy for all 3 treatment modalities with respect to erectile dysfunction (ED), urinary incontinence, stricture formation, and rectal injury/fistulae.[4,67,68]

Retreatment After Cryotherapy Failure

Although treatment options for primary cryotherapy failures are incompletely reported in the literature, many surgeons commonly perform repeat cryoablation. Repeat cryotherapy for the prostate is safe and may be effective for select candidates with truly localized disease. Bahn and colleagues[39] performed a second round of cryotherapy on 32 patients with positive biopsies following primary cryotherapy. Reported PSA recurrence-free survival rates at 63 months were 68%, 72%, and 91% using variable definitions of failure of 0.5 ng/mL, 1.0 ng/mL, and the ASTRO criteria, respectively. We eagerly await reports of repeat cryotherapy to elucidate its efficacy.

COMPLICATIONS OF CRYOTHERAPY

Rectourethral Fistula

The most feared complication of cryoablation is rectourethral fistula. However, in contemporary series, rectourethral fistula formation has been reported to occur in only 0% to 3% of patients treated.[4,6,7,37,38,40,81,84] Improved ultrasound imaging combined with real-time temperature monitoring of the anterior rectal wall have reduced the incidence of this devastating complication to almost 0% in modern series.[4,6,7,25] In our practice, we place multitemperature sensing probes in the anterior rectal wall and in the Denovillier space to ensure safe temperatures (**Fig. 4**). In addition, manipulation of the probe upwards along the Y-axis can open up the space between the prostate and rectum significantly, virtually guaranteeing the prevention of this complication.

Fistulae may present early after the procedure or up to several months later. Fecaluria, watery diarrhea, or pneumaturia should raise the suspicion of possible fistula formation. A voiding

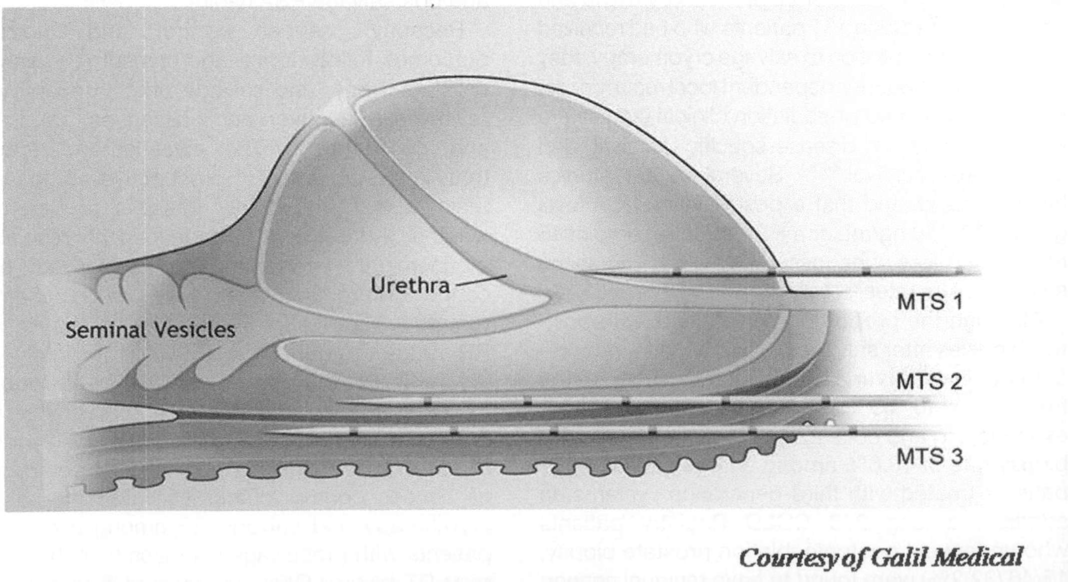

Fig. 4. Sagittal view of the prostate depicting multitemperature sensing probe (MTS) position at the apex of the prostate (MTS 1), Denovillier space (MTS 2), and the anterior rectal wall (MTS 3). (*Courtesy of* Galil Medical, Inc., Plymouth Meeting, PA; with permission.)

cystourethrography (VCUG) or CT scan may help confirm the diagnosis and localize the site of the fistula. Some fistulas may respond to conservative treatment with Foley catheter drainage and a low residue diet. Conservative measures usually fail in patients who develop fistulae following postradiation salvage cryotherapy. In this setting, early fecal and urinary diversion may be required. Formal fistula repair should be postponed until the inflammatory cascade has fully resolved, usually by 6 months. A transperineal, posterior, or anterior approach for closure has been recommended.[81,85]

ED

ED after whole-gland prostate cryotherapy is common. Although some series have reported rates ranging from 40% to 47%,[47] more recent series report rates between 50% and 90%.[6,33,37,39,40,43,44] Potency rates associated with subtotal and focal cryotherapy range from 71% to 85%.[60,62] The high incidence of ED after cryosurgery is undoubtedly due to extension of the ice ball beyond the prostate into the NVBs. Although some investigators have reported that up to 50% of patients regain erectile function 3 to 5 years after cryosurgical ablation,[47,48] we do not routinely perform whole-gland cryotherapy in patients who have a strong interest in maintaining erectile function. With currently available systems, we believe that complete ablation of the NVBs is mandatory to ensure complete cancer kill.

Urinary Retention

A urinary catheter is routinely left after the procedure for a variable amount of time. Transient urinary retention following catheter removal is due to persistent glandular edema. This complication usually resolves after repeat short-term catheterization.

Urinary Incontinence

The incidence of incontinence after cryotherapy varies widely among studies because of differences in definitions and reporting of incontinence (ie, zero pad, security pad, ≤1 pad/d), heterogenous patient populations, and variable use of an effective urethral warming catheter. Long-term mild stress incontinence occurs in approximately 1% to 10% of patients undergoing contemporary (ie, third- or fourth-generation) cryosurgical ablation; the upper end of this range is generally seen in patients undergoing salvage cryosurgery.[4,6,7,25,44,64,82] Severe incontinence occurs in less than 1% to 8% of patients.[48] The potential causes of postcryotherapy urinary incontinence include striated sphincter damage leading to intrinsic sphincter deficiency, urethral sloughing, urethral stricture or bladder neck contracture formation, pudendal nerve injury, and possibly detrusor instability.

Urethral Sloughing and/or Urethral Stricture

The use of an effective urethral warming catheter is critical to minimize the risk of tissue sloughing. Symptomatic sloughing is a minor event occurring in fewer than 5% to 15% of patients.[4,6] Treatment of urethral sloughing consists of antibiotics and adequate urinary drainage. We encourage patients to perform clean intermittent catheterization, which often leads to sloughed tissue dislodgment. Transurethral resection or removal of the necrotic tissue is rarely necessary. Urethral stricture is almost never seen after cryotherapy if a urethral warming device is used properly.[44]

Pelvic and/or Rectal Pain

Transient pelvic, rectal, and/or perineal pain after cryotherapy is common (range 0%–50%).[4,7,21,82,86–88] This complaint was more frequently reported in older series, particularly among patients undergoing salvage treatment.[23,89] Seigne and colleagues[90] reported that 2.7% of patients undergoing salvage cryoablation developed symptomatic osteitis pubis. This complication has been best managed with antiinflammatories once a urinoma or abscess has been ruled out. Han and colleagues[40] reported that transient penile paresthesia occurred in 3% of patients following cryotherapy, probably due to damage of the dorsal nerve.

Quality-of-Life Outcomes

To our knowledge, there is only 1 randomized prospective trial of quality-of-life (QOL) outcomes with whole-gland prostate cryoablation versus EBRT.[91] Two-hundred forty-four men were randomly assigned to cryoablation (third-generation) or EBRT (median dose 68 Gy, range: 68–73.5 Gy); all patients received neoadjuvant ADT for 3 to 6 months. Following local treatment, all patients underwent a 36-month 10-core prostate biopsy. Patients completed the European Organisation for Research and Treatment of Cancer (EORTC) Quality of Life Questionnaire (QLQ) C30 (domains include physical activity, emotional state, social interaction, global health status/QOL, financial impact, and other symptom scales) and the University of California, Los Angeles (UCLA) Patient Classification Index (PCI) (domains include sexual, urinary, bowel; higher score = better function) at baseline and at posttreatment intervals up to 36 months. Approximately 90% to 92% of patients completed the assigned questionnaires at 24 and 36 months. There was no statistically significant difference at 6 weeks or 3 years in EORTC QLQ C30 scores. Differences were detected for the UCLA PCI, however. At 3 months, patients treated with cryoablation had significantly lower urinary function scores (69.4 vs 90.7) and sexual function scores (7.2 vs 32.9); bowel function was similar (83.7 vs 81.4). At 36 months, urinary and bowel domains recovered to baseline in both treatment groups. However, men who were potent before cryoablation treatment reported worse sexual function scores at 36 months (16 vs 36.7, *P*<.001). Among the men who were potent before treatment who underwent cryoablation (n = 34) or EBRT (n = 30) (61.8% and 54.6% of the entire cohort, respectively, were capable of unassisted intercourse at baseline), at 12 months posttreatment, 17.7% and 44.4% were capable of having intercourse (*P*<.01). By 36 months posttreatment, however, this difference lost statistical significance (22% vs 36%, respectively).

A retrospective review of 89 consecutive patients who underwent cryoablation of the prostate was compared with a contemporaneous series of patients undergoing brachytherapy.[92] QOL was measured by percent return to baseline score of the UCLA PCI and American Urological Association Symptom Score (AUAss). Fourteen of 89 patients underwent subtotal cryoablation (focal or nerve sparing). In addition, 28 patients received preoperative ADT. The cryoablation cohort was older and had significant baseline ED; the average age was 72.1 years and the mean baseline sexual function score was 25.9 (on a scale of 0–100). Men with a baseline score of 30 were excluded from analysis (n = 31), leaving only 20 men for analysis (mean baseline = 59.6). Among this group of men, at 12 months posttreatment, only 20% returned to baseline function. For the corresponding brachytherapy cohort, in whom the pretreatment function was higher, 56% regained baseline activity. Trends toward increased urinary and bowel problems was observed among the brachytherapy group. Based on these data, the investigators concluded that, relative to patients treated with brachytherapy, patients undergoing primary cryosurgical ablation experience worse sexual function but fewer irritative and obstructive voiding complaints with their consequent detrimental effects on urinary health-related QOL (HRQOL). Moreover, urinary function among patients treated with cryosurgery may improve up to 24 months after treatment. A problem with such a retrospective case series is the tendency to over-emphasize the value of data extrapolated from poorly matched cohorts. In this series, baseline characteristics between groups differed significantly; the cryoablation group was older (72.1 vs 65.5 years, *P*<.001) and had a higher clinical stage and pretreatment PSA level. In addition, the brachytherapy group had significantly higher baseline sexual and urinary function scores (36.8 vs 25.9, *P* = .04 and 88.7 vs 80.3, *P* = .03). Moreover, only 71% and 51% of patients in the cryotherapy and brachytherapy groups completed a baseline questionnaire and at least 1 posttreatment questionnaire. Despite these limitations, it seems that radiotherapy is associated with improved sexual function compared with whole-gland cryoablation.

Asterling and Green[93] prospectively followed the sexual function of 53 patients undergoing whole-gland cryosurgery according to the patients' perception of their sexual function. Among this group of men with a median age of 66 years, before treatment, 17 of 53 (32%) reported ED, 9 (17%) reported partial erections, and 25 (47%) described full potency. Among men who were potent before cryosurgery, 9 of 23 (39%) regained full erectile function by 24 months.

The concern about loss of sexual function with whole-gland cryoablation has led to increased interest in so-called nerve-sparing cryoablation. Nerve-sparing cryotherapy attempts to protect an NVB during ablation by active warming (using a helium-driven probe) or injection of antifreeze proteins. Alternatively, during focal ablation, the contralateral NVB is unaffected. The feasibility of nerve-sparing cryotherapy by active warming of the NVB was initially evaluated in a canine model.[94] Prostate lobes treated with active warming demonstrated complete or partial NVB preservation. All prostate lobes treated with a double freeze-thaw cycle demonstrated complete and uniform ablation of prostate tissue. In a pilot study of focal nerve-sparing cryosurgery, Onik and colleagues[60] treated 1 lobe in 9 patients, sparing 1 NVB. Potency was maintained in 7 of 9 patients. Interesting studies include the feasibility of injecting antifreeze proteins[95] or saline to protect or separate the NVBs.

SUMMARY

Contemporary prostate cryotherapy is a minimally invasive treatment option for men with organ-confined or locally recurrent prostate cancer. Current data suggest that short-term oncologic results, complication rates, and QOL outcomes are acceptable compared with other treatment options. Long-term oncologic data are forthcoming. Focal ablation at the present time is an experimental technique that should currently be considered only under prospective investigational protocols. Emerging imaging technology will continue to drive focal therapy into mainstream practice.

REFERENCES

1. Cooper IS, Lee AS. Cryostatic congelation: a system for producing a limited, controlled region of cooling or freezing of biologic tissues. J Nerv Ment Dis 1961; 133:259.
2. Gonder MJ, Soanes WA, Shulman S. Cryosurgical treatment of the prostate. Invest Urol 1966;3(4):372–8.
3. Millennium Research Group. US markets for urological devices. Toronto, Ontario, Canada: Millennium Research Group, Inc; 2006.
4. Babaian RJ, Donnelly B, Bahn D, et al. Best practice statement on cryosurgery for the treatment of localized prostate cancer. J Urol 2008;180:1993–2004.
5. Cohen JK, Miller RJ, Ahmed S, et al. Ten-year biochemical disease control for patients with prostate cancer treated with cryosurgery as primary therapy. Urology 2008;71:515–8.
6. Jones JS, Rewcastle JC, Donnelly BJ, et al. Whole gland primary prostate cryoablation: initial results from the cryo on-line data registry. J Urol 2008; 180:554–8.
7. Pisters LL, Rewcastle JC, Donnelly JC, et al. Salvage prostate cryoablation: initial results from the cryo on-line data registry. J Urol 2008;180:559–64.
8. Gonder MJ, Soanes WA, Smith V. Experimental prostate cryosurgery. Invest Urol 1964;14:610–9.
9. Baust JG, Gage AA, Klossner D, et al. Issues critical to the successful application of cryosurgical ablation of the prostate. Technol Cancer Res Treat 2007;6:97–109.
10. Hoffmann NE, Bischof JC. The cryobiology of cryosurgical injury. Urology 2002;60:40–9.
11. Cooper IS, Hirose T. Application of cryogenic surgery to resection of parenchymal organs. N Engl J Med 1966;274:15–8.
12. Gage AA, Baust JG. Cryosurgery for tumors. J Am Coll Surg 2007;205:342–56.
13. Baust JG, Gage AA. The molecular basis of cryosurgery. BJU International 2005;95:1187–91.
14. Tatsutani K, Rubinsky B, Onik G, et al. Effect of thermal variables on frozen human primary prostatic adenocarcinoma cells. Urology 1996;48:441–7.
15. Mazur P. Physical-chemical factors underlying cell injury in cryosurgical freezing. In: Rand R, Rinfret A, von Leden H, editors. "Cryosurgery". Springfield (IL): Thomas; 1968. p. 32–51.
16. Mazur P. Freezing of living cells: mechanisms and implications. Am J Physiol 1984;143:C125–42.
17. Farrant J, Walter CA. The cryobiological basis for cryosurgery. J Dermatol Surg Oncol 1977;3:403–7.
18. Gage AA, Baust J. Mechanisms of tissue injury in cryosurgery. Cryobiology 1998;37:171–86.
19. Whittaker DK. Ice crystals formed in tissue during cryosurgery. II. Electron microscopy. Cryobiology 1974;11:202–17.
20. Onik GM, Lee F, Bahn D. Cryosurgical techniques, caveats, and refinements. In: Onik GM, Rubinsky B, Watson G, Ablin RJ, editors. Percutaneous prostate cryoablation. St. Louis (MO): Quality Medical Publishing; 1994. p. 78–84, chapter 6.
21. Shinohara K, Connolly JA, Presti JC Jr, et al. Cryosurgical treatment of localized prostate cancer (stages T1 to T4): preliminary results. J Urol 1996; 156:115–20 [discussion: 120–1].
22. Larson TR, Robertson DW, Corica A, et al. In vivo interstitial temperature mapping of the human prostate during cryosurgery with correlation to histopathologic outcomes. Urology 2000;55:547–52.
23. Pisters LL, von Eschenbach AC, Scott SM, et al. The efficacy and complications of salvage cryotherapy of the prostate. J Urol 1997;157:921–5.
24. Wong WS, Chinn DO, Chinn M, et al. Cryosurgery as a treatment for prostate carcinoma: results and complications. Cancer 1997;79:963–74.
25. Mouraviev V, Polascik TJ. Update on cryotherapy for prostate cancer in 2006. Curr Opin Urol 2006;16:152–6.
26. Bales GT, Williams MJ, Sinner M, et al. Short-term outcomes after cryosurgical ablation of the prostate in men with recurrent prostate carcinoma following radiation therapy. Urology 1995;46:676–80.
27. Baust J, Gage AA, Ma H, et al. Minimally invasive cryosurgery—technological advances. Cryobiology 1997;34:373–84.
28. Miller RJ Jr, Cohen JK, Shuman B, et al. Percutaneous, transperineal cryosurgery of the prostate as salvage therapy for post radiation recurrence of adenocarcinoma. Cancer 1996;77:1510–4.
29. Cespedes RD, Pisters LL, von Eschenbach AC, et al. Long-term followup of incontinence and obstruction after salvage cryosurgical ablation of the prostate: results in 143 patients. J Urol 1997; 157:237–40.
30. Leibovici D, Zisman A, Lindner A, et al. PSA elevation during prostate cryosurgery and subsequent decline. Urol Oncol 2005;23:8–11.
31. Wieder J, Schmidt JD, Casola G, et al. Transrectal ultrasound-guided transperineal cryoablation in the treatment of prostate carcinoma: preliminary results. J Urol 1995;154:435–41.
32. Greene GF, Pisters LL, Scott SM, et al. Predictive value of prostate specific antigen nadir after salvage cryotherapy. J Urol 1998;160:86–90.
33. Ellis DS. Cryosurgery as primary treatment for localized prostate cancer: a community hospital experience. Urology 2002;60:34–9.
34. Shinohara K, Rhee B, Presti JC Jr, et al. Cryosurgical ablation of prostate cancer: patterns of cancer recurrence. J Urol 1997;158:2206–9 [discussion 2209–10].

35. Benoit RM, Cohen JK, Miller RJ Jr. Cryosurgery for prostate cancer: new technology and indications. Curr Urol Rep 2000;1:41.
36. Koppie TM, Shinohara K, Grossfeld GD, et al. The efficacy of cryosurgical ablation of prostate cancer: the University of California, San Francisco experience. J Urol 1999;162:427–32.
37. Long JP, Bahn D, Lee F, et al. Five-year retrospective, multi-institutional pooled analysis of cancer-related outcomes after cryosurgical ablation of the prostate. Urology 2001;57:518–23.
38. Ghafar MA, Johnson CW, De La Taille A, et al. Salvage cryotherapy using an argon based system for locally recurrent prostate cancer after radiation therapy: the Columbia experience. J Urol 2001; 166:1333–7 [discussion: 1337–8].
39. Bahn DK, Lee F, Badalament R, et al. Targeted cryoablation of the prostate: 7-year outcomes in the primary treatment of prostate cancer. Urology 2002;60:3–11.
40. Han KR, Cohen JK, Miller RJ, et al. Treatment of organ confined prostate cancer with third generation cryosurgery: preliminary multicenter experience. J Urol 2003;170:1126–30.
41. Chinn DO, Wong WW, Chinn M, et al. Temperature monitored prostate cryosurgery: 8 year accrued clinical experience. J Urol 2004;171:219.
42. Donnelly BJ, Saliken JC, Ernst DS, et al. Role of transrectal ultrasound guided salvage cryosurgery for recurrent prostate carcinoma after radiotherapy. Prostate Cancer Prostatic Dis 2005;8: 235–42.
43. Polascik TJ, Nosnik I, Mayes JM, et al. Short-term cancer control after primary cryosurgical ablation for clinically localized prostate cancer using third-generation cryotechnology. Urology 2007;70: 117–21.
44. Miller DC, Pisters LL, Belldegrun AS. Cryotherapy for prostate cancer, Chapter 101. In: Wein AJ, Kavoussi LR, Novick AC, et al, editors. Campbell-Walsh Urology, 9th edition. Saunders, 2007.
45. Prepelica KL, Okeke Z, Murphy A, et al. Cryosurgical ablation of the prostate: high risk patient outcomes. Cancer 2005;103:1625–30.
46. Connolly JA, Shinohara K, Carroll PR. Cryosurgery for locally advanced (T3) prostate cancer. Semin Urol Oncol 1997;15:244–9.
47. Donnelly BJ, Saliken JC, Ernst DS, et al. Prospective trial of cryosurgical ablation of the prostate: five-year results. Urology 2002;60:645–9.
48. Ellis DS, Manny TB Jr, Rewcastle JC. Cryoablation as primary treatment for localized prostate cancer followed by penile rehabilitation. Urology 2007;69: 306–10.
49. Bahn DK, Lee F, Solomon MH, et al. Prostate cancer: US-guided percutaneous cryoablation: work in progress. Radiology 1995;194:551–6.
50. Bostwick DG, Meiers I. Diagnosis of prostatic carcinoma after therapy. Arch Pathol Lab Med 2007;131: 360–71.
51. Katz A, Jones S, Ellis D, et al. Primary prostate cryoablation: updated results from 2558 patients tracked with the COLD registry. Abstract Number: 08-AB-95457-AUA.
52. Bostwick DG, Waters DJ, Farley ER, et al. Group consensus reports from the Consensus Conference on Focal Treatment of Prostatic Carcinoma, Celebration, Florida, February 24, 2006. Urology 2007; 70(Suppl 6):42–4.
53. Barqawi AB, Crawford ED. The current use and future trends of focal surgical therapy in the management of localized prostate cancer. Cancer J 2007;13(5):313–7.
54. Barzell WE, Melamed MR. Appropriate patient selection in the focal treatment of prostate cancer: the role of transperineal 3-dimensional pathologic mapping of the prostate–a 4-year experience. Urology 2007;70(Suppl 6):27–35.
55. Eggener SE, Scardino PT, Carroll PR, et al. Focal therapy for localized prostate cancer: a critical appraisal of rationale and modalities. J Urol 2007; 178:2260–7.
56. Polascik TJ, Mayes JM, Mouraviev V. From whole-gland to targeted cryoablation for the treatment of unilateral or focal prostate cancer. Oncology (Williston Park) 2008;22(8):900–6 [discussion: 906–7, 914].
57. Ahmed HU, Moore C, Emberton M. Minimally-invasive technologies in uro-oncology: the role of cryotherapy, HIFU and photodynamic therapy in whole gland and focal therapy of localised prostate cancer. Surg Oncol 2009;18(3):219–32.
58. Iczkowski KA, Hossain D, Torkko KC, et al. Preoperative prediction of unifocal, unilateral, margin-negative, and small volume prostate cancer. Urology 2008;71(6):1166–71.
59. Yoon GS, Wang W, Osunkoya AO, et al. Residual tumor potentially left behind after local ablation therapy in prostate adenocarcinoma. J Urol 2008; 179(6):2203–6 [discussion: 2206].
60. Onik G, Narayan P, Vaughan D, et al. Focal "nerve-sparing" cryosurgery for treatment of primary prostate cancer: a new approach to preserving potency. Urology 2002;60:109–14.
61. Levine MA, Ittman M, Melamed J. Two consecutive sets of transrectal ultrasound guided sextant biopsies of the prostate for the detection of prostate cancer. J Urol 1998;159(2):471–5.
62. Lambert EH, Bolte K, Masson P, et al. Focal cryosurgery: encouraging health outcomes for unifocal prostate cancer. Urology 2007;69:1117–20.
63. Onik G, Vaughan D, Lotenfoe R, et al. The "male lumpectomy": focal therapy for prostate cancer using cryoablation results in 48 patients with at least

2-year follow up. Seminars and Original Investigations. Urol Oncol 2008;26:500–5.
64. Ellis D, Jones S, Pisters L, et al. Subtotal/partial gland prostate cryoablation: results of 341 patients from multiple centers tracked with the COLD registry. Abstract Number: 08-AB-95484-AUA.
65. Mettlin CJ, Murphy GP, McDonald CJ, et al. The National Cancer Data Base Report on increased use of brachytherapy for the treatment of patients with prostate carcinoma in the U.S. Cancer 1999;86:1877–82.
66. Mettlin CJ, Murphy GP, Rosenthal DS, et al. The National Cancer Data Base report on prostate carcinoma after the peak in incidence rates in the U.S. The American College of Surgeons Commission on Cancer and the American Cancer Society. Cancer 1998;83:1679–84.
67. Nguyen PL, D'Amico AV, Lee AK, et al. Patient selection, cancer control, and complications after salvage local therapy for postradiation prostate-specific antigen failure. Cancer 2007;110:1417–28.
68. Allen GW, Howard AR, Jarrard DF, et al. Management of prostate cancer recurrences after radiation therapy-brachytherapy as a salvage option. Cancer 2007;110:1405–16.
69. Touma NJ, Izawa JI, Chin JL. Current status of local salvage therapies following radiation failure for prostate cancer. J Urol 2005;173:373–9.
70. Mouraviev V, Evans B, Polascik TJ. Salvage prostate cryoablation after primary interstitial brachytherapy failure: a feasible approach. Prostate Cancer Prostatic Dis 2006;9:99–101.
71. Cheng L, Cheville JC, Bostwick DG. Diagnosis of prostate cancer in needle biopsies after radiation therapy. Am J Surg Pathol 1999;23:1173–83.
72. Stone NN, Stock RG, Unger P, et al. Biopsy results after real-time ultrasound-guided transperineal implants for stage T1-T2 prostate cancer. J Endourol 2000;14:375–80.
73. Spiess PE, Lee AK, Leibovici D, et al. Presalvage prostate-specific antigen (PSA) and PSA doubling time as predictors of biochemical failure of salvage cryotherapy in patients with locally recurrent prostate cancer after radiotherapy. Cancer 2006;107:275–80.
74. Ng CK, Moussa M, Downey DB, et al. Salvage cryoablation of the prostate: followup and analysis of predictive factors for outcome. J Urol 2007;178:1253–7.
75. Albertsen PC, Hanley JA, Harlan LC, et al. The positive yield of imaging studies in the evaluation of men with newly diagnosed prostate cancer: a population based analysis. J Urol 2000;163:1138–43.
76. Sodee DB, Malguria N, Faulhaber P, et al. Multicenter ProstaScint imaging findings in 2154 patients with prostate cancer. The ProstaScint Imaging Centers. Urology 2000;56:988–93.
77. Harisinghani MG, Barentsz J, Hahn PF, et al. Noninvasive detection of clinically occult lymph-node metastases in prostate cancer. N Engl J Med 2003;348:2491–9.
78. Eisenberg ML, Shinohara K. Partial salvage cryoablation of the prostate for recurrent prostate cancer after radiotherapy failure. Urology 2008;72:1315–8.
79. Siddiqui SA, Mynderse LA, Zincke H, et al. Treatment of prostate cancer local recurrence after radical retropubic prostatectomy with 17-gauge interstitial transperineal cryoablation: initial experience. Urology 2007;70:80–5.
80. Pisters LL, Perrotte P, Scott SM, et al. Patient selection for salvage cryotherapy for locally recurrent prostate cancer after radiation therapy. J Clin Oncol 1999;17:2514–20.
81. Izawa JI, Ajam K, McGuire E, et al. Major surgery to manage definitively severe complications of salvage cryotherapy for prostate cancer. J Urol 2000;164:1978–81.
82. Ismail M, Ahmed S, Kastner C, et al. Salvage cryotherapy for recurrent prostate cancer after radiation failure: a prospective case series of the first 100 patients. BJU Int 2007;100:760–4.
83. Pisters LL, Leibovici D, Blute M, et al. Locally recurrent prostate cancer after initial radiation therapy: a comparison of salvage radical prostatectomy versus cryotherapy. J Urol 2009;182:517–25.
84. Cox RL, Crawford ED. Complications of cryosurgical ablation of the prostate to treat localized adenocarcinoma of the prostate. Urology 1995;45:932–5.
85. Nyam DC, Pemberton JH. Management of iatrogenic rectourethral fistula. Dis Colon Rectum 1999;42:994–7 [discussion: 997–9].
86. Coogan CL, McKiel CF. Percutaneous cryoablation of the prostate: preliminary results after 95 procedures. J Urol 1995;154:1813–7.
87. Cohen JK, Rooker GM, Miller RJ Jr, et al. Cryosurgical ablation of the prostate: treatment alternative for localized prostate cancer. Cancer Treat Res 1996;88:167–86.
88. Long JP, Fallick ML, LaRock DR, et al. Preliminary outcomes following cryosurgical ablation of the prostate in patients with clinically localized prostate carcinoma. J Urol 1998;159:477–84.
89. De La Taille A, Benson MC, Bagiella E, et al. Cryoablation for clinically localized prostate cancer using an argon-based system: complication rates and biochemical recurrence. BJU Int 2000;85:281–6.
90. Seigne JD, Pisters LL, von Eschenbach AC. Osteitis pubis as a complication of prostate cryotherapy. J Urol 1996;156(1):182.
91. Hubosky SG, Fabrizio MD, Schellhammer PF, et al. Single center experience with third- generation cryosurgery for management of organ-confined prostate cancer: critical evaluation of short-term outcomes,

complications, and patient quality of life. J Endourol 2007;21:1521–31.
92. Robinson JW, Donnelly BJ, Siever JE, et al. A randomized trial of external beam radiotherapy versus cryoablation in patients with localized prostate cancer: quality of life outcomes. Cancer 2009; 115:4695–704.
93. Asterling S, Greene DR. Prospective evaluation of sexual function in patients receiving cryosurgery as a primary radical treatment for localized prostate cancer. BJU Int 2009;103(6):788–92.
94. Janzen NK, Han KR, Perry KT, et al. Feasibility of nerve-sparing prostate cryosurgery: applications and limitations in a canine model. J Endourol 2005; 19:520–5.
95. Jia Z, Davies PL. Antifreeze proteins: an unusual receptor-ligand interaction. Trends Biochem Sci 2002;27:101–6.

Current Topics in the Treatment of Prostate Cancer with Low-Dose-Rate Brachytherapy

Richard G. Stock, MD[a,*], Nelson N. Stone, MD[b]

KEYWORDS

- Prostate cancer • Brachytherapy • Ultrasound
- Treatment

The treatment of prostate cancer with low-dose-rate prostate brachytherapy has grown rapidly over the last 20 years. Outcome analyses performed in this period have enriched understanding of this modality. Many topics can be covered in a review of this subject, but limitations of the current article format prevent a thorough comprehensive review of all of these. Instead, this article focuses on a more limited number of topics that the authors believe are relevant to current understanding of brachytherapy. These topics include the development of a real-time ultrasound-guided implant technique, the importance of radiation dose, trimodality treatment of high-risk disease, long-term treatment outcomes, and treatment-associated morbidity.

THE DEVELOPMENT OF A REAL-TIME ULTRASOUND-GUIDED IMPLANT TECHNIQUE

The advent of transrectal ultrasound-guided brachytherapy was first reported by Holm and Gammelgaard[1] in Denmark in 1981. These investigators described the use of transrectal ultrasound to help guide needle and seed placement in the treatment of localized prostate cancer using iodine 125 (^{125}I) radioactive seeds.[2] In the last 26 years, there have been many significant advances in low-dose-rate brachytherapy techniques, all derived from this initial approach. This article outlines the real-time method of ultrasound-guided implantation developed at Mount Sinai Hospital, New York, in 1990.[3]

The original technique was based on the concept that a preplan of seed placement could never be exactly duplicated in the operating room because of changes in the shape of the prostate and its position relative to the bladder and rectum. Instead, a technique was developed to take into account prostate mobility and use the imaging capabilities of transrectal real-time ultrasound. Using ultrasound, the physician could monitor the position of the prostate during the operation and the seeds could be placed based on the live image of the gland. To further simplify the planning aspect, a lookup table was developed. The amount of radioactivity to implant was derived from the original Memorial Sloan Kettering Cancer Center (MSKCC) nomogram for ^{125}I volume implants. This nomogram allowed calculation of the amount of radioactivity to implant based on the volume measured to deliver a matched peripheral dose of 160 Gy.[4]

The basic concept behind the technique is simple and consists of 2 phases. The first phase is called the peripheral phase and involves insertion of needles into the largest transverse diameter of the gland approximately 1 cm apart.

[a] Department of Radiation Oncology, Mount Sinai School of Medicine, Mount Sinai Hospital, 1184 5th Avenue, New York, NY 10029, USA
[b] Department of Urology, Mount Sinai School of Medicine, New York, NY, USA
* Corresponding author.
E-mail address: Richard.Stock@mountsinai.org (R.G. Stock).

Urol Clin N Am 37 (2010) 83–96
doi:10.1016/j.ucl.2009.11.013

urologic.theclinics.com

Approximately 75% of the radioactivity that is implanted is placed within the prostate via these needles. The seeds are distributed evenly throughout these needles, although needles traversing longer lengths of prostate tend to deposit 1 or 2 more seeds than shorter-length needles. The exact position of the needles and seed deposition is monitored by longitudinal live ultrasound imaging. The second phase involves the placement of interior needles (usually 5–8 needles) in such a way that the needles cover the apex and base of the gland. The remaining 25% of the activity is implanted through these needles. In the original technique, usually 3 to 4 seeds were deposited per needle. The exact placement of seeds via these needles is also monitored with longitudinal ultrasound imaging.

The final version of the Mount Sinai Hospital lookup table for activity per volume to be implanted was developed by using a quality insurance program that was based on monthly examination and review of the computed tomography (CT)-based postimplant dosimetric analyses of all implants. This quality improvement program led to an overall increase in the activity implanted per volume compared with the original MSKCC nomogram. In addition, improvements in ultrasound technology led to better visualization and more accurate placement of sources.[5] The final amount of activity implanted per volume used in the Mount Sinai lookup table was found, in a paper by Bice and colleagues,[6] to be consistent with other preplanning implant centers.

The next development in the technique of real-time ultrasound-guided seed implantation was the implementation of an intraoperative computer planning system. This system allowed for real-time capture of ultrasound prostate images. These prostate images could be captured with needles in place. This feature enabled the physician to recreate the actual implant in 3 dimensions on the computer. The program then allowed for interactive monitoring of delivered dose based on needle and seed deposition positions. In addition, it allowed for fine-tuning of needle positions and overall activity implanted. In a study by Stone and colleagues[7] intraoperative ultrasound dosimetry findings were compared with 1-month CT-based postimplant results. Although small differences existed between the intraoperative and CT dosimetry results, these data suggested that this intraoperative implant dosimetric representation system provided a close match to the actual delivered doses. It supported the concept that intraoperative dosimetry could be used to modify the implant during surgery to achieve more consistent dosimetry results.

BRACHYTHERAPY AND RADIATION DOSE

Radiation for prostate cancer is usually described by its physical prescription dose. For example, a patient receiving high-dose external beam radiotherapy (EBRT) for prostate cancer might be prescribed 81 Gy, which is typically delivered in 1.8-Gy fractions per day for 45 days. For a patient being treated with a permanent implant with ^{125}I, the typical prescription dose is 145 to 160 Gy and for those receiving palladium-103 (^{103}Pd), 125 to 130 Gy.[3,8] Patients with high-risk disease are often offered a combination of external beam irradiation and seed implantation. For these patients the dose of EBRT and the implant are reduced, usually to 45 Gy (1.8 Gy ×25) and 110 Gy for ^{125}I or 100 Gy for ^{103}Pd,[8] respectively. One of the differences between EBRT and seed implantation is the way the dose is delivered. For EBRT, frequent evaluations of treatment setup can be performed by image guidance with fiducial markers or cone beam CT to help ensure correct prostate position and treatment accuracy. On the other hand, permanent implantation is a single treatment and the delivered dose (implant quality) is determined by the posttreatment dosimetry study. This study is performed within 30 days of the implant using CT imaging and specialized software that allows calculation of the radiation dose to the prostate, rectum, urethra, and any other contiguous structures of interest. Because the modern transperineal ultrasound-guided seed implant is new, studies that report oncologic outcomes based on postimplant dose data are critically important to evaluate the efficacy and safety of the treatment.

The dose to the prostate can be described by several different parameters, for example the dose to 100%, 95%, or 90% of the prostate volume. These doses are typically termed the D100, D95, or D90. The volume of the prostate covered by the prescription dose has also been described and is designated by a "V" followed by the percentage of the dose prescribed. For example, V100 refers to the volume of the prostate covered by 100% of the prescription and V150 represents the volume covered by 150% of the prescription. The same dose parameters are also used for the critical structures. The V100 of the rectal wall represents the volume of the rectum (in cubic centimeters) covered by 100% of the prescription dose. Although not all agree, the 2 most representative descriptives of the prostate are the D90 and V150 and for the rectum the V100.[9–14] In general, a higher D90 is preferred but without increasing the V150 above 50%–75%. Because the dose deposition is highest next to the radioactive source and decreases exponentially farther away from it, the implant tends to be hotter in the middle of the gland (where the urethra is) because it is surrounded by seeds. The ideal implant technique distributes these hot nonhomogeneous regions away from the urethra and keeps the V150 below 50%–75%.

Stock was the first to describe the use of the D90 to report biochemical outcomes and dose response following ^{125}I prostate brachytherapy.[15] Patients receiving a D90 less than 140 Gy had a 4-year freedom from biochemical failure (FBF) rate of 68% compared with a rate of 92% for those receiving a D90 of 140 Gy or greater (P = .02). Several other investigators have reported similar findings.[8–11] Miles and colleagues[16] investigated 145 patients and separated them by dose. The biochemical disease-free rate for patients with a D90 greater than 140 Gy was 100% compared with 90% for those with the lower dose (P = 0.02). Recently, Kao reported on the potential for higher doses to improve results further. A total of 643 patients were treated with ^{125}I monotherapy for T1 or T2 prostate cancer with a D90 of 180 Gy or greater (median, 197 Gy; range, 180–267 Gy). Using the Phoenix definition, 5-year biochemical disease-free survival rates were 97.3% for low-risk patients and 92.8% for intermediate-/high-risk patients.[17]

Unlike the prescription dose, which represents the physical dose given to the target organ, the biologic effective dose (BED) is a measure of how the dose affects the target tissues. It also permits the calculation of a common dose (in Gy) regardless of the method or rate of the delivered radiation dose. The equation for calculating the BED for the implant is: $BED = (R_0/\lambda)\{1+[R_0/(\mu+\lambda)(\alpha/\beta)]\}$, where R_0 is the initial dose rate of implant = $(D90)(\lambda)$, λ is the radioactive decay constant = $0.693/T_{1/2}$, $T_{1/2}$ is the radioactive half-life of the isotope, μ is the repair rate constant = $0.693/t_{1/2}$, and $t_{1/2}$ is the tissue repair half-time. For EBRT the $BED = nd\,[1 + (d/\alpha/\beta)]$, where n is the number of fractions given, d is the dose per fraction, and α/β is the tissue- and effect-specific parameter associated with the linear-quadratic model. The BED for the implant is highly dependent on the D90, or the dose delivered to 90% of the gland based on the postimplant dosimetry. For patients receiving EBRT and implantation, the BED is the sum of the BED calculated for the implant and the EBRT component. When the BED is used to report dose data, the source of radiation becomes less important because all of the physical prescription doses are reduced to 1 common variable, simplifying data analysis.[18]

Stock and colleagues[18] used the BED to report the biochemical and local control rates following prostate brachytherapy. They found increasing biochemical freedom from failure (BFFF) rates as the BED increased from 100 Gy to 200 Gy. The 10-year freedom from prostate-specific antigen (PSA) failure for the BED groups (<100, >100–120, >120–140, >140–160, >160–180, >180–200, and >200) were 46%, 68%, 81%, 85.5%, 90%, 90%, and 92%, respectively (P<.0001). Recently, Taira and colleagues[19] reported similar findings, in which patients with higher BEDs had improved biochemical control. Patients with a BED more than 116 Gy had a 98.8% BFFF rate compared with 92.1% for lower doses.

The ideal treatment of prostate cancer should be the one that offers the greatest chance of local disease eradication. Historically, radiation therapy (RT) has been believed to be inferior to prostatectomy because the delivered dose was not high enough to eradicate all of the tumor. However, recent advances in prostate imaging have increased the precision of prostate brachytherapy. This development should result in a dose-response relationship for local control. Stone and colleagues[20] explored this issue by performing multicore prostate biopsies 2 years after brachytherapy in 584 men. The median PSA concentration was 7.1 ng/mL and the median follow-up was 7.1 years. There were 260 (44.5%) low-risk, 141 (24.1%) intermediate-risk, and 183 (31.4%) high-risk patients. The median BED was 186 Gy_2 (25%–75%, 158–208 Gy). Of 548 patients, 48 (8.2%) had a positive biopsy specimen at the last follow-up. The number of patients with positive biopsy results by BED group was as follows: 22 of 121 (18.2%) for patients who received less than 150 Gy_2; 15 of 244 (6.1%) for patients who received more than 150 to 200 Gy_2; and 6 of 193 (3.1%) for patients who received more than 200 Gy_2 (P<.001). These dose groups remained significant even when patients were divided into risk group. Thus, even for low-risk patients, BED around 200 Gy achieve the highest negative biopsy results. Back-converting the BED to the physical dose (using an α/β of 2) a BED of 200 Gy_2 can be achieved with postimplant D90s for ^{125}I of 188 Gy, ^{103}Pd of 167 Gy, and combination therapy with ERBT (25 fractions of 1.8 Gy) for ^{125}I of 110 Gy and for ^{103}Pd of 102 Gy.

TRIMODALITY THERAPY FOR HIGH-RISK PROSTATE CANCER

High-risk prostate cancer represents a treatment dilemma. On the one hand, patients presenting with this type of disease are at a greater risk of having microscopic systemic disease. According to the National Comprehensive Cancer Network (NCCN) risk-group stratification, patients may have Gleason scores of 8 to 10 or PSA more than 20 ng/mL. These risk features have been associated with an increased risk of microscopic system disease. On the other hand, high-risk patients also have a large local tumor burden. This finding is supported by the inclusion of T3 disease in the NCCN high-risk stratification and patients with presenting PSA of more than 20 ng/mL. These patients are also at great risk of extraprostatic disease extension.

Although radical prostatectomy has remained the gold standard for the treatment of prostate cancer, reported outcomes following this treatment of high-grade Gleason score of 8 to 10 prostate cancer have been suboptimal. Radical prostatectomy seems to have certain oncologic limitations as a surgical procedure for high-grade disease. PSA screening has decreased the incidence of locally advanced prostate cancer. Although the incidence of high-grade disease has not changed, lower PSA and lower stage have resulted in a decline in extraprostatic disease after prostatectomy. Investigators at Johns Hopkins University noted an increase in organ-confined disease in high-grade cancer from 54% in 1993 to 73% in 2007. Despite this disease-stage migration, the most recent Hopkins disease extent tables reveal rates of organ-confined disease after prostatectomy for patients with Gleason scores of 8 to 10 that range from 12% to 77% (median 39%), depending on the other prognostic variables, PSA, and clinical stage.[21] Most new patients with Gleason scores of 8 to 10 have extraprostatic disease following prostatectomy, which helps explain the high biochemical failure rates following surgery. Data from the Henri Mondor University Hospital in France on 180 patients with Gleason scores of 8 to 10, show a 7-year progression-free survival of only 37%.[22] The Mayo Clinic's experience with patients with Gleason scores of 8 to 10 reveals a 10-year progression-free survival rate of 36%.[23] Recent reports from 2 experienced and high-volume centers, MSKCC and Washington University in St Louis, Missouri, reveal biochemical control rates for patients with Gleason scores of 8 to 10 following radical prostatectomy at 10 years of 39% and 37%, respectively.[24,25] The prevailing belief that most patients with high-grade cancer primarily fail systemically has recently been challenged by the findings of SWOG 8794,[26] which tested the value of postoperative RT for poor pathologic findings. One of the conclusions of the study referring to the radical prostatectomy was "the pattern of treatment failure in high risk patients is predominantly local with a surprisingly low incidence of metastastic failure." With the increasing use of minimally invasive radical prostatectomy techniques, the risk for local recurrence seems to be greater. In 1 study, patients treated with minimally invasive versus open radical prostatectomy had greater than 3 times the odds of receiving salvage therapy within 6 months of their surgery than those treated with open prostatectomy.[27]

The treatment regimen of combined hormonal therapy, brachytherapy, and EBRT was specifically designed to enhance local control by combining the synergistic effects of hormonal therapy and radiation and dose escalation in the form of brachytherapy plus external beam irradiation. The encouraging results of the combined modality approach are derived from 2 recent advances in prostate RT: dose escalation and the use of hormonal therapy. Current regimens use neoadjuvant and concurrent hormonal therapy. The cytoreductive and synergistic qualities of hormonal therapy given with radiation have been well documented in the laboratory.[28] Numerous randomized controlled trials also document the benefit of adding hormonal therapy to RT. An update of RTOG 8610 revealed an improvement in local control (42% vs 30%), biochemical disease-free survival (24% vs 10%) and cause-specific mortality (23% vs 31%) and a reduction in distant metastases (34% vs 45%) for 4 months of hormonal therapy and 65 to 70 Gy of EBRT versus RT alone.[29] An update of RTOG 85-31 revealed a 10-year local failure rate for RT and adjuvant hormonal therapy for 23% versus 38% for the arm that received RT alone. Ten-year distant metastases rates and disease-specific mortality were 24% versus 39% and 16% versus 22% both in favor of the adjuvant hormonal arm.[30] With a median follow-up of 66 months, the European Organisation for Research and Treatment of Cancer reported an improvement in 5-year disease-specific survival (DSS) of 94% versus 79% and in overall survival of 78% versus 62%, for radiation and 3 years of adjuvant therapy versus RT alone.[31] Other prospective trials have also shown an advantage to adding hormonal therapy to radiation or to longer durations of hormonal therapy.[32,33] Although the use of hormonal therapy has not been studied in a prospective randomized fashion with brachytherapy, in a study by Merrick and colleagues[34] hormonal therapy was found to improve 10-year biochemical relapse-free survival when added to combination brachytherapy and external beam over combination therapy alone for high-risk patients with prostate cancer. In a retrospective study published by D'Amico and colleagues,[35] 1342 men treated at multiple centers received either brachytherapy alone or in combination with hormonal therapy, EBRT or both. The analysis found there was a significant reduction in the risk of prostate cancer–specific mortality (adjusted hazard ratio, 0.32; 95% confidence interval [CI], 0.14–0.73; $P = .006$) in men treated with brachytherapy and androgen-suppressive therapy and EBRT compared with neither. At Mount Sinai Hospital, the authors have used 9 months of hormonal therapy in their regimen to provide neoadjuvant therapy for 3 months before brachytherapy and concurrent hormonal therapy given during the life of the implant and during EBRT.

In addition to the effects of hormonal therapy, the current treatment benefits from dose escalation, achieved by combining low-dose-rate brachytherapy with external beam irradiation. Combination brachytherapy and external beam irradiation is a unique way of delivering extremely high doses to the prostate and lower but effective doses to the periprostatic tissues. In this way, the bulk of the disease receives the high dose from combined implant and EBRT, whereas the microscopic disease outside the gland receives a lower dose, primarily from the external beam portion of the treatment.

The importance of dose escalation, especially in high-risk disease, has been well documented. A recent report of the long-term results of the MD Anderson randomized trial of dose escalation, in which 51% of patients had Gleason scores greater than 7, documented an improvement in FBF rate of 78% for doses of 78 Gy versus 59% for the 70-Gy arm ($P = .004$).[36] In another randomized trial, reported by Zeitman and colleagues,[37] 70.2 Gy of conventional dose radiation was compared with 79.2 Gy delivered with combination photons and protons (8% of patients had Gleason scores of 8–10). FBF rate was 78.8% at 5 years for the conventional arm versus 91.3% for the high-dose arm ($P<.001$). The combination of brachytherapy and external beam irradiation results in very high BEDs. In a recent publication from Mount Sinai Hospital, combination therapy was associated with a median BED of 205 Gy_2 (range 157–266 Gy_2).[38] This dose is higher than 81 Gy (associated BED of 155 Gy_2), a common prescription dose of intensity-modulated RT.

Table 1 lists the biochemical control rates following combination therapy for high-risk patients. A recent publication from Mount Sinai Hospital reported on 181 patients with prostate cancer with Gleason scores of 8 to 10 who were treated from 1994 to 2006 with a ^{103}Pd implant (prescription dose 100 Gy), 45 Gy of EBRT, and 9 months of hormonal therapy. The median follow-up was 65 months (range 24–150 months). FBF rates were calculated using the Phoenix definition. The 8-year actuarial FBF rate, freedom from distant metastases, prostate cancer–specific survival, and overall survival were 73%, 80%, 87%, and 79%, respectively. The pretreatment PSA level significantly affected FBF rate, with 8-year rates of 72%, 82%, and 58% for patients with PSA level of 10 or less, more than 10 to 20 and more than 20 ng/mL, respectively ($P = .006$). The PSA level had no significant effect on rates of distant metastases. The Gleason score had the most significant effect on FBF rate in a multivariate analysis, and was the only factor to significantly affect rates of distant metastases; the 8-year FBF rates were 84%, 55%, and 30% for scores of 8, 9, and 10, respectively ($P = .003$). The corresponding freedom from distant metastases and prostate cancer–specific survival rates were 86%, 76%, and 30% ($P<.001$) and 92%, 80%, and 62.5% ($P = .003$), respectively.[38]

Table 1
Biochemical control rates following brachytherapy and EBRT (± hormonal therapy)

Study	Number of Patients	Biochemical Failure Definition	Rate (%)	Year
Critz & Levinson[88]	(% of 1469)	PSA > 0.2 ng/mL	61	10
Dattoli et al[44]	124	PSA > 0.2 ng/mL	72	14
Merrick et al[34]	204	PSA 0.4 ng/mL	87	10
Potters et al[42]	418	ASTRO	63	12
Stock et al[89]	360	ASTRO	83	7
Stone et al[90]	522	ASTRO	70	10
Sylvester et al[43]	114	2 increases in PSA	68	10

Abbreviation: ASTRO, American Society for Therapeutic Radiology and Oncology.

LONG-TERM OUTCOMES

It is important to track patients for many years to assess outcomes following treatment of prostate cancer, because prostate cancer is generally slow growing. Recurrences can manifest themselves years after treatment, particularly local recurrences, which tend to occur later than systemic failures.[39,40] Enthusiasm for a new prostate cancer therapy may not be warranted based on early PSA outcomes. In addition, because PSA recurrences tend to occur months to years before clinical relapse, long follow-up is needed to assess treatment end points such as distant metastases–free survival, prostate cancer-specific survival, DSS and overall survival.

In a report by Stock and colleagues,[41] 1561 patients treated at Mount Sinai Hospital were followed for 2 to 14 years. The end point examined was DSS. The DSS and overall survival rates at 10 years were 96% and 74%, respectively ($P<.0001$). A significant factor that affected DSS was Gleason score, with 10-year DSS rates of 98%, 91%, and 92% for scores of 6, 7, and 8 to 10. Multivariate analysis revealed that PSA status after treatment had the most significant effect on DSS. Ten-year rates were 100%, 52%, and 98% for patients without PSA failure, those with doubling time (DT) less than 10 months, and those with DT greater than 10 months, respectively ($P<.0001$).

Potters and colleagues[42] reported on 1449 consecutive men treated with low-dose-rate brachytherapy with a median follow-up of 82 months. The overall 12-year FBF rate (American Society for Therapeutic Radiology and Oncology definition) was 81%. DSS and overall survival rates at 12 years were 93% and 81%, respectively. Biochemical recurrence-free survival rates based on risk-group stratification were 89%, 78%, and 63% for low-, intermediate- and high-risk patients ($P = .0001$). Multivariate analysis found that D90, pretreatment PSA, and Gleason score were the only factors to significantly affect biochemical recurrence. PSA DT in patients with biochemical failure predicted for DSS with rates at 5 years of 89% and 45% for those with DTs of more than 12 months and less than 12 months, respectively ($P = .0019$).

Sylvester and colleagues[43] examined 223 patients with T1 to T3 prostate cancer treated at the Seattle Prostate Institute, Seattle, Washington, treated with brachytherapy from 1987 to 1993. Patients were treated with ^{125}I or ^{103}Pd implants following 45 Gy of external beam irradiation. The overall freedom from biochemical relapse at 15 years was 74%. Sixteen-year freedom from biochemical relapse was 88% for low-risk patients, 80% for intermediate-risk patients, and 53% for high-risk patients. Rates were 83%, 55%, and 61% for Gleason scores of 6, 7, and 8 to 10, respectively. Patients with presenting PSA levels of less than 10, more than 10 to 20, and more than 20 ng/mL had rates of 80%, 72%, and 66%, respectively. The local recurrence rate was 3.1%.

Dattoli and colleagues[44] reported on 282 patients treated with prostate brachytherapy and supplemental external beam radiation treated from 1992 to 1996 who had intermediate- or high-risk features. Patients were followed for 1 to 14 years (median 9.5 years). The overall actuarial freedom from biochemical progression at 14 years was 81%. Rates were 87% and 72% for patients with intermediate- and high-risk disease, respectively. Patients who failed biochemically were all biopsied and the local failure rate was 0%. The strongest predictor of biochemical failure was Gleason score ($P = .03$).

Taira and colleagues[19] recently reported on 463 patients treated with brachytherapy only from 1995 to 2005. The 12-year biochemical progression-free survival, DSS, and overall survival were 97%, 100%, and 75%, respectively. The 12-year biochemical progression-free survival, DSS, and overall survival for low-risk patients were 97%, 100%, and 76%, respectively, whereas the rates were 96%, 100%, and 74% for intermediate-risk patients. The biochemical progression-free survival was 98% for low-risk patients with high-quality implants versus 92% for those with less adequate implants ($P<.01$), and 98% for intermediate-risk patients with high-quality implants versus 86% for less adequate implants ($P<.01$).

BRACHYTHERAPY-ASSOCIATED MORBIDITY

Radiation-related morbidity can be acute or chronic. Urinary retention is the most common early side effect of seed implantation. Retention rates have been reported to be between 1.5% and 22% (**Table 2**).[45–57] Several investigators have identified an increased American Urological Association (AUA) symptom score as a predisposing factor to postimplant urinary retention.[49,51] Others have found that a large prostate increases the risk of retention.[50,55,56] This has led many brachytherapists to recommend neoadjuvant hormonal therapy (NHT) to shrink the enlarged gland. Stone and colleagues[58] have recently reported that men with a prostate gland larger than 50 cm^3 do not need hormonal therapy if their AUA symptom score is less than 15. A total of 395 patients with prostate cancer with glands

Table 2
Urinary retention rates following implant alone or implants with EBRT

Study	Number	Treatment	Retention Rate (%)
Blasko et al[45]	196	^{125}I	7
Vijverberg et al[46]	46	^{125}I	22
Wallner et al[47]	92	^{125}I	11
Storey et al[48]	206	^{125}I	11
Mabjeesh et al[49]	665	^{125}I	3.2
Elshaikh et al[50]	402	^{125}I	10.9
Terk et al[51]	251	^{125}I/Pd103	5
Kaye et al[52]	76	EBRT/^{125}I	5
Dattoli et al[53]	73	EBRT+PD103	7
Ragde & Korb[54]	73	EBRT/^{125}I/Pd013	10
Merrick et al[55]	170	EBRT/^{125}I/Pd013	6
Benoit et al[56]	1409	EBRT/^{125}I/Pd013	14.5
Zeitlin et al[57]	212	EBRT/^{125}I/Pd013	1.5

50 cm^3 or larger at initial evaluation were treated with either 3 months of NHT followed by implant (n = 204) or implant alone (n = 191). The mean prostate volume at baseline for the NHT patients was 72.9 cm^3 (range 50–156). After 3 months of NHT, prostate size was reduced to a mean of 54.3 cm^3 (range 21–125 cm^3, *P*<.001). The mean prostate volume for the patients without NHT was 60.6 cm^3 (range 50–120 cm^3, *P*<.001) compared with NHT patients at time of implant. Urinary retention occurred in 41 of 395 patients (10.4%). Of these 41 patients, 16 of 191 (8.4%) did not have NHT, whereas 25 of 204 (12.3%) did (*P* = .207). For patients not receiving NHT, retention occurred in 3 of 12 patients (25%) if their preimplant international prostate symptom score (IPSS) was more than 15 versus 13 of 168 (7.7%) for an IPSS less than 15 (*P* = .04, odds ratio 4.0, 95% CI 1–16). In contrast there was no difference in retention rates for NHT patients for those with an initial IPSS more than 15 versus less than 15 (2 of 25 [8%] versus 11 of 102 [10.8%], *P* = .614). This study demonstrated that hormonal therapy is not necessary in all brachytherapy patients with prostates larger than 50 cm^3 and that hormonal therapy does not increase the risk of urinary retention in patients with large prostates.

Urinary symptoms are common with permanent seed implantation, with complaints of dysuria, frequency, urgency, weak stream, and nocturia. Symptoms typically peak between 1 and 3 months after implantation, with most patients returning to baseline by 1 year (**Table 3**). Kleinberg and colleagues[59] found that nocturia was the most common acute urinary symptom following ^{125}I implantation. He noted urinary symptoms in 80% within 2 months of the implant and lasting for 1 year in 45%. Several studies have reported a doubling in symptom score in the first 1 to 3 months after implantation. Desai and colleagues[60] found that the mean total IPSS increased from 6 to 14 at 1 month post implant. It took 12 to 18 months for symptoms to return to preimplant levels. Urinary symptoms were also highly correlated to the radiation dose received by the prostate and urethra. Tanaka and colleagues[61] investigated IPSS changes and decrease in uroflow rates in 110 patients following ^{125}I brachytherapy. Mean IPSS increased from a baseline of 9 to 14.2, 17.2, 14.7, and 10.3 at 1, 3, 6, and 12 months post implantation, respectively. The corresponding changes in peak uroflow from a baseline of 13.3 cm^3/s were 11.3, 11.2, 11.7, and 12.1, respectively. The changes in IPSS and uroflow were all significant (*P*<.05) at each time frame except at 12 months. Keyes and colleagues[62] analyzed 712 ^{125}I patients for early and late urinary toxicity. The IPSS returned to baseline at a median of 12.6 months. On multivariate analysis, patients with a high baseline IPSS had a quicker resolution of their IPSS. Higher prostate D90 (dose covering 90% of the prostate), maximal postimplant IPSS, and urinary retention slowed the IPSS resolution time. Matzkin and colleagues[63] compared 2 implant techniques and assessed urinary morbidity for the 2.[63] A total of 300 men were implanted using preplanning with preloaded needles (n = 136) or intraoperative planning, using a Mick applicator (n = 164). The increased mean IPSSs were sustained for about 9 months in the preplanning group, and at about 12

Table 3
Effect of prostate brachytherapy on mean IPSS

Study	Number	Treatment	Initial IPSS	IPSS at 1 Month	IPSS at 1 Year
Lee et al[91]	31	^{125}I	8.3	18.4	10.2
Desai et al[60]	117	^{125}I	6	14	8
Merrick et al[55a]	170	EBRT/^{125}I/^{103}Pd	5.7	12	4.6
Tanaka et al[61]	110	EBRT/^{125}I	9	14.2	10.3
Matzkin et al[63bc]	300	^{125}I	8.6/7.8	17/18	8.5/11
Keyes et al[62c]	712	^{125}I	5	15	5
Niehaus et al[64c]	976	EBRT/^{125}I/^{103}Pd	5	10	4.5

[a] All patients treated with α blockers.
[b] Preplan/intraoperative planning.
[c] Data extrapolated from graph.

to 18 months they reverted to normal. The IPSSs, although similar at baseline, increased more and returned to baseline more slowly, at about 18 months, in the intraoperative planning group. Significantly better CT-based implant dosimetry parameters were noted with the intraoperative method. A positive correlation (P<.001) was found between the dosimetry parameters and symptom severity. The data from this study regarding the effects of dose on acute urinary symptoms are similar to the reports of Desai and Keyes. Higher doses result in more acute urinary symptoms; however, by 1 year to 18 months post implant most patients return to their baseline symptoms. Given that higher doses are needed to eradicate all local disease it seems a small price to pay for successful treatment.

The 2 most common isotopes used in permanent prostate brachytherapy are ^{125}I and ^{103}Pd. Brachytherapists debate the merits of one over the other, as the iodine isotope has a 60-day half-life compared with 17 days for palladium. Theoretically, iodine with a longer half-life and higher energy should cause urinary symptoms that appear more slowly and last longer than with palladium. Niehaus and colleagues[64] compared 789 palladium implants with 187 iodine implants for acute urinary morbidity. For both isotopes and all prostate size cohorts, IPSS peaked 1 month after implantation and returned to baseline at a mean of 1.9 months. Stratification of prostate size cohorts by isotope showed no significant differences in prolonged catheter dependency, IPSS resolution, or postimplant surgical intervention.

Prolonged urinary retention or severe obstructive symptoms may necessitate surgical intervention. If a transurethral resection of the prostate (TURP) needs to be performed, a safe minimum postimplant time is 6 months for ^{125}I and 2 months for ^{103}Pd. This requirement allows for enough time to pass for 90% of the radiation to be delivered. However, it is best to wait as long as possible as a postimplant TURP carries some degree of risk of incontinence. Stone and Stock[65] have shown that the prostate size continues to shrink after seed implantation, reaching 50% of its preimplant size by 5 years. It is best to manage the patient with clean intermittent catheterization and wait as long as possible for urination to return. If a TURP needs to be performed, then a minimal resection should be performed with care to preserve as much of the blood supply to the posterior urethra as possible. The bladder neck should be preserved at the 5 and 7 o'clock positions, which will maintain sufficient prostatic urethral blood supply. The apex should also be carefully resected because of the risk of damage to the external sphincter, which may have been compromised from errant distal seed deposition. Minimal cautery should be used to prevent late urethra ischemic damage. It is not unusual for a patient who has had a postimplant TURP to develop a posterior urethral stricture, which should be managed by an internal urethrotomy and self-intermittent catheterization. Eventually the scarring will resolve and the patient should be able to void without difficulty. Attempts at re-resection, with a goal of cleaning up the area, should be discouraged, as this will lead to more scarring and necrosis. Postimplant TURP rates range from 0% to 8.3% (**Table 4**).[47,48,51,53,55,56,62–68]

Several studies have demonstrated that an antecedent or postimplant TURP increases the risk of permanent urinary incontinence (**Tables 4** and **5**).[48,51,52,54,56,57,67–77] Radiation damage and

Table 4
TURP rates following prostate brachytherapy

Study	Number	Treatment	TURP Rate (%)
Wallner et al[47]	92	^{125}I	8.7
Storey et al[48]	206	^{125}I	0
Nag et al[66]	32	^{103}Pd	6.2
Terk et al[51]	251	$^{125}I/^{103}Pd$	2.4
Dattoli et al[53]	73	EBRT + ^{103}Pd	2.8
Merrik et al[55]	170	EBRT/$^{125}I/^{103}Pd$	1.2
Benoit et al[56]	1409	EBRT/$^{125}I/^{103}Pd$	8.3
Gelbum et al[67]	693	EBRT/$^{125}I/^{103}Pd$	4.0
Keyes et al[62]	712	^{125}I	1.3
Matzkin et al[63]	300	^{125}I	1.6
Niehaus et al[64]	976	EBRT/$^{125}I/^{103}Pd$	1.7
Bittner et al[68]	1014	EBRT/$^{125}I/^{103}Pd$	1.7
Stone & Stock[65]	325	^{125}I	1.8

thermal injury decreased urethral blood flow leading to superficial urethral necrosis and posterior urethral fibrosis.[54] The resulting noncompliant prostatic urethra is difficult to treat, and it is best to prevent this complication by keeping urethral doses from getting too high during the implant and by carefully performing a postimplant TURP when indicated.

For patients who do not require surgical intervention after prostate brachytherapy (1%–2%) long-term urinary morbidity has been favorable. Stone and Stock[75] analyzed 325 men implanted

Table 5
Urinary incontinence following brachytherapy

Study	Number	Procedures	Incontinence (%)
Blasko et al[69]	184	Implant	0
Talcott et al[73]	105	Implant	15
Nag et al[74]	32	Implant	19
Gelbum et al[67]	693	Implant	0.7
Wallner et al[71]	92	Implant	6
Storey et al[48]	206	Implant	10
Benoit et al[56]	2124	Implant	6.6
Zeitlin et al[57]	212	Implant	3.8
Kaye et al[52]	57	Implant	11
Stone & Stock[72]	301	Implant	0
Beyer & Priestley[70]	499	Implant	1
Anderson et al[76]	351	Implant	0.9
Talcott et al[73]	13	TURP + implant	85
Ragde & Korb[54]	48	TURP + implant	12.5
Stone & Stock[75]	43	TURP + implant	0
Kaye et al[52]	19	TURP + implant	22
Terk et al[51]	6	Implant + TURP	0
Gelbum et al[67]	28	Implant + TURP	17
Stone & Stock[75]	33	Implant + TURP	6.1
Kollmeier et al[77]	38	Implant + TURP	18

with ^{125}I and followed for a median of 7 years (range 5–15 years). All patients completed IPSS forms before and at each follow-up visit. Total IPSS and bother scores increased from a baseline of 7.1 and 1.5 to a maximum of 12.5 and 2.6, 6 months post implant. It took 3 years for symptoms to return to baseline and this situation was not changed at 7 years' follow-up. The incidence of urinary incontinence (requiring a pad) in this group was 0.7%. Other investigators have reported similar findings with long-term follow-up.[62,68] One concern is that the high interior prostate doses that are in part responsible for some of the early urinary morbidity may also result in chronic urinary complaints. Kao and colleagues[17] assessed the impact of high prostatic doses in 643 patients treated with ^{125}I monotherapy for T1 to T2 prostate cancer with a D90 of 180 Gy or greater (median 197 Gy, range 180–267 Gy). At 5 years' median follow-up the total IPSS score was no different from baseline.

Radiation injury to the rectum is uncommon following permanent seed implantation. Damage, when it occurs, is usually mild and self-limiting. Grade 1 to 2 proctitis rates range from 1% to 21.4%.[2,47,52,57,69,72,78–81] A higher incidence is expected in those patients who receive a combination of seed implant and external beam irradiation. Stone and Stock[75] followed 325 men implanted with ^{125}I (no external beam) for more than 5 years. Minor rectal bleeding was reported by 78 (24%) during the first 5 years. With longer follow-up, only 9 (2.8%) still had some minor bleeding, implying that in most bleeding resolves without interventions. Gelbum and Potters[82] reported on 825 patients treated with implant alone (^{125}I or ^{103}Pd) or an implant plus external beam irradiation. Grade 1 to 2 proctitis was noted by 16% and grade 3 by 0.5%. More severe rectal complications such as ulcer (grade 3) or fistula formation (grade 4) have been more commonly reported in patients who have had their rectal bleeding treated by biopsy or cauterization. Theodorescu and colleagues[83] reported 7 fistulas in 724 men treated with implant alone or in combination with external beam. Six of these patients had their rectal bleeding managed by biopsy and electrocautery. Gelbum and Potters[82] noted that 50% of the grade 3 rectal complications had an antecedent rectal biopsy and that the biopsied patients took twice as long to heal. Most experienced brachytherapists caution patients against biopsy and fulguration of bleeding areas in the anterior rectal wall. It is prudent to caution the patients not to have any rectal procedures performed without receiving clearance from the physicians who performed the implant.

Snyder and colleagues[10] have shown that the volume of rectum treated by the prescription dose is highly correlated to the development of grade 2 proctitis. Of 212 patients implanted with ^{125}I 22 (10.4%) developed grade 2 proctitis; 14% developed it in the first year, 72% in the second year, and 14% in the third year. No patients developed proctitis after year 3. The likelihood of developing proctitis was 5% if less than 1.3 cm^3 of anterior rectal wall received 160 Gy and no patients developed proctitis if less than 0.8 cm^3 of rectal wall received 160 Gy. Higher doses of radiation are necessary for patients with high-risk prostate cancer. These higher doses can be achieved with a combination of seed implant and external beam radiation. The anterior rectal wall invariably receives a higher dose if combination therapy is used. Sarosdy[84] noted a higher incidence of fistula formation in his patients treated with seed implant and external beam irradiation. Fecal diversion was required in 6.6% and urinary diversion in 3.2%. The median area of the anterior rectal wall covered by the prescription dose was 4.0 cm. The size of the rectal wall receiving the prescription dose in these patients was greater than described by Snyder and colleagues.[10] Recently Stone and colleagues[85] reported the long-term outcomes of rectal morbidity in 585 patients followed for a median of 5 years and treated with combination therapy. The intraoperative technique was used and the volume of the rectum receiving a prescription dose was less than 1.0 cm^3. Fecal fistulas occurred in 2 (0.34%) patients.

Brachytherapy studies demonstrate a 56% to 86% likelihood of erectile function 1 to 7 years following implantation (**Table 6**).[47,52,53,57,75,78,86,87] Stock[86] prospectively assessed erectile function in a cohort of 422 men implanted with ^{125}I or ^{103}Pd. In a multivariate analysis of pretreatment factors and treatment-related variables, the pretreatment erectile function was the most significant factor affecting postimplant potency. Men with normal erectile function before implantation had a 70% 6-year likelihood of maintaining function compared with 34% if the pretreatment function was not adequate ($P<.0001$). The only other significant variable was the radiation dose delivered. Patients receiving a dose greater than 160 Gy for ^{125}I and 120 Gy for ^{103}Pd had a poorer outcome. Age, use of NHT, and isotope selection did not influence sexual function outcomes. Taira and colleagues[87] evaluated long-term erectile function in 226 patients assessed by the International Index of Erectile Function-6 (IIEF-6). Median follow-up was 6.4 years. Pre- and postbrachytherapy potency was defined as IIEF-6 of greater than 13 without pharmacologic or

Table 6
Potency rates following prostate brachytherapy

Study	Treatment	Number	Potency Rate (%)	Years
Wallner et al[47]	^{125}I	92	86	3
Stock et al[a,86]	$^{125}I/^{103}Pd$	236	70	6
	$^{125}I/^{103}Pd$	77	34	6
Kaye et al[52]	EBRT/^{125}I	73	75	1
Dattoli et al[53]	EBRT + ^{103}Pd	73	77	3
Zeitlin et al[57]	EBRT + $^{125}I/^{103}Pd$	212	62	5
Critz et al[78]	EBRT + ^{125}I	239	76	5
Taira et al[87]	$^{125}I/^{103}Pd$	226	55.6	6.4
Stone & Stock[75]	^{125}I	236	61.5	7

[a] 236 patients had normal erectile functuon prior to implant, while 77 diminished erections.

mechanical support. The 7-year actuarial rate of potency preservation was 55.6% with median post-implant IIEF of 22 in potent patients. Potent patients were statistically younger ($P = .014$), had a higher preimplant IIEF ($P<.001$), and were less likely to be diabetic ($P = .002$). Stone and colleagues[75] analyzed 307 men with potency scores before implantation, of whom 188 (61.2%) had a score of 3 (normal erection) and 49 (16%) had a 2 (diminished, but sufficient erection). At a median 7-year follow-up, 145 (61.5%) maintained adequate erectile function (score 2–3). Preserved erectile function correlated highly with age ($P<.001$). No associations were found between potency preservation and preimplantation hormone therapy use, D90, or TURP. Potency preservation by age group 5 years after implantation was: less than 50 years, 100% (n = 8); 51 to 60 years, 81.8% (n = 48); 61 to 70 years, 60.5% (n = 124); and more than70 years, 41% (n = 56).

REFERENCES

1. Holm HH, Gammelgaard J. Ultrasonically guided precise needle placement in the prostate and seminal vesicles. J Urol 1981;18(3):385–7.
2. Torp-Pedersen S, Holm HH, Littrup PJ. Transperineal I-125 seed implantation in prostate cancer guided by transrectal ultrasound. Prog Clin Biol Res 1987; 237:143–52.
3. Stock RG, Stone NN, Wesson MF, et al. A modified technique allowing interactive ultrasound-guided three-dimensional transperineal prostate implantation. Int J Radiat Oncol Biol Phys 1995;32(1):219–25.
4. Anderson LL. Spacing nomographs for interstitial implants of I-125 seeds. Med Phys 1976;3:48.
5. Stock RG, Stone NN, Lo YC, et al. Postimplant dosimetry for (125)I prostate implants: definitions and factors affecting outcome. Int J Radiat Oncol Biol Phys 2000;48(3):899–906.
6. Bice WS Jr, Prestidge BR, Grimm PD, et al. Centralized multiinstitutional postimplant analysis for interstitial prostate brachytherapy. Int J Radiat Oncol Biol Phys 1998;41(4):921–7.
7. Stone NN, Hong S, Lo YC, et al. Comparison of intraoperative dosimetric implant representation with postimplant dosimetry in patients receiving prostate brachytherapy. Brachytherapy 2003;2: 17–25.
8. Rivardl MJ, Butler WM, Devlin PM, et al. American Brachytherapy Society recommends no change for prostate permanent implant dose prescriptions using iodine-125 or palladium-103. Brachytherapy 2007;6:34–7.
9. Stock RG, Stone NN. Importance of post implant dosimetry in permanent prostate brachytherapy. Eur Urol 2002;41:434–9.
10. Snyder KM, Stock RG, Hong SM, et al. Defining the risk of developing grade 2 proctitis following I-125 prostate brachytherapy using a rectal dose volume histogram analysis. Int J Radiat Oncol Biol Phys 2001;50:335–41.
11. Potters L, Cao Y, Calugaru E, et al. A comprehensive review of CT-based dosimetry parameters and biochemical control in patients treated with permanent prostate brachytherapy. Int J Radiat Oncol Biol Phys 2001;50:605–14.
12. Potters L, Huang D, Calugaru E, et al. Importance of implant dosimetry for patients undergoing prostate brachytherapy. Urology 2003;62:1073–7.
13. Papagikos MA, deGuzman AF, Rossi PJ, et al. Dosimetric quantifiers for low-dose-rate prostate brachytherapy: is V100 superior to D90? Brachytherapy 2005;4:252–8.
14. Morris WJ, Keyes M, Palma D, et al. Evaluation of dosimetric paramenters and disease response after

125iodine transperineal brachytherapy for low- and intermediate risk prostate cancer. Int J Radiat Oncol Biol Phys 2009;73(5):1432–8.
15. Stock RG, Stone NN, Tabert A, et al. A dose-response study for I-125 prostate implants. Int J Radiat Oncol Biol Phys 1998;41:101–8.
16. Miles EF, Nelson JW, Alkaissi AK, et al. Equivalent uniform dose, D90, and V100 correlation with biochemical control after low-dose-rate prostate brachytherapy for clinically low-risk prostate cancer. Brachytherapy 2008;7:206–11.
17. Kao J, Stone NN, Lavaf A, et al. (125)I monotherapy using D90 implant doses of 180 Gy or greater. Int J Radiat Oncol Biol Phys 2008;70:96–101.
18. Stock RG, Stone NN, Cesaretti J, et al. Biologically effective dose values for prostate brachytherapy: effects on PSA failure and post-treatment biopsies. Int J Radiat Oncol Biol Phys 2006;64:527–33.
19. Taira AV, Merrick GS, Galbreath RW, et al. Natural history of clinically staged low- and intermediate-risk prostate cancer treated with monotherapeutic permanent interstitial brachytherapy. Int J Radiat Oncol Biol Phys 2009. [Epub ahead of print].
20. Stone NN, Stock RG, Cesaretti JA, et al. Local control following permanent prostate brachytherapy: effect of high biologically effective dose on biopsy results and oncologic outcomes. Int J Radiat Oncol Biol Phys. [Epub ahead of print].
21. Makarov DV, Trock BJ, Humphreys EB, et al. Updated nomogram to predict pathologic stage of prostate cancer given prostate-specific antigen level, clinical stage, and biopsy Gleason score (Partin tables) based on cases from 2000 to 2005. Urology 2007;69:1095.
22. Rodrigues - Covarrubias F, Larre S, De La Taille A, et al. The outcome of patients with pathological Gleason score ≥ 8 prostate cancer after radical prostatectomy. BJU Int 2008;101:305.
23. Lau WK, Bergstralh EJ, Blute ML, et al. Radical prostatectomy for pathological Gleason 8 or greater prostate cancer: influence of concomitant pathological variables. J Urol 2002;167:117.
24. Donohue JF, Bianco FJ, Kuroiwa K, et al. Poorly differentiated prostate cancer treated with radical prostatectomy: long-term outcome and incidence of pathological downgrading. J Urol 2006;176:991.
25. Desireddi NV, Roehl KA, Loeb S, et al. Improved stage and grade-specific progression-free survival rates after radical prostatectomy in the PSA era. Urology 2007;70:950.
26. Swanson GP, Hussey MA, Tangen CM, et al. Predominant treatment failure in postprostatectomy patients is local: analysis of patterns of treatment failure in SWOG 8794. J Clin Oncol 2007;25:2225.
27. Hu JC, Wang Q, Pashos CL, et al. Utilization and outcomes of minimally invasive radical prostatectomy. J Clin Oncol 2008;26:2278.
28. Lee AK. Radiation therapy combined with hormone therapy for prostate cancer. Semin Radiat Oncol 2006;16:20.
29. Pilepich MV, Winter K, John M, et al. Phase III radiation therapy oncology group (RTOG) trial 86–10 of androgen deprivation adjuvant to definitive radiotherapy in locally advanced carcinoma of the prostate. Int J Radiat Oncol Biol Phys 2001;50:1243–52.
30. Pilpich MV, Winter K, Lawton CA, et al. Androgen suppression adjuvant to definitive radiotherapy in prostate carcinoma – Long term results of phase III RTOG 85–31. Int J Radiat Oncol Biol Phys 2005; 61:1285–90.
31. Bolla M, Collette L, Blank L, et al. Long-term results with immediate androgen suppression and external irradiation in patients with locally advanced prostate cancer (an EORTC study): a phase III randomized trial. Lancet 2002;360:103–8.
32. D'Amico AV, Chen MH, Renshaw AA, et al. Androgen suppression and radiation vs radiation alone for prostate cancer: a randomized trial. JAMA 2008;299:289–95.
33. Horwitz EM, Bae K, Hanks GE, et al. Ten- year follow-up of radiation therapy oncology group protocol 92–02: a phase III trial of the duration of elective androgen deprivation in locally advanced prostate cancer. J Clin Oncol 2008;26:2497–504.
34. Merrick GS, Butler WM, Wallner KE, et al. Androgen deprivation therapy does not impact cause specific survival or overall survival in high risk prostate cancer managed with brachytherapy and supplemental external beam. Int J Radiat Oncol Biol Phys 2007;68:34.
35. D'Amico AV, Moran BJ, Braccioforte MH, et al. Risk of death from prostate cancer after brachytherapy alone or with radiation, androgen suppression therapy, or both in men with high-risk disease. J Clin Oncol 2009;27(24):3923–8.
36. Kuban DA, Tucker SL, Dong L, et al. Long-term results of the M.D. Anderson randomized dose-escalation trial for prostate cancer. Int J Radiat Oncol Biol Phys 2008;70:67–74.
37. Zeitman AL, DeSilvio ML, Slater JD, et al. Comparison of conventional-dose versus high dose conformal radiation therapy in clinically localized adenocarcinoma of the prostate: a randomized controlled trial. JAMA 2005;294:1233–9.
38. Stock RG, Cesaretti JA, Hall S, et al. Outcomes for patients with high grade prostate cancer treated with a combination of brachytherapy, external beam irradiation and hormonal therapy. BJU. [Epub ahead of print].
39. Pound CR, Partin AW, Eisenberger MA, et al. Natural history of progression after PSA elevation following radical prostatectomy. JAMA 1999;281:1591–7.
40. Stock RG, Cesaretti JA, Unger P, et al. Distant and local recurrence in patients with biochemical failure

after prostate brachytherapy. Brachytherapy 2008; 7(3):217–22.
41. Stock RG, Cesaretti JA, Stone NN. Disease-specific survival following the brachytherapy management of prostate cancer. Int J Radiat Oncol Biol Phys 2006; 64(3):810–6.
42. Potters L, Morgenstern C, Calugaru E, et al. 12-year outcomes following permanent prostate brachytherapy in patients with clinically localized prostate cancer. J Urol 2008;179(Suppl 5):S20–4.
43. Sylvester JE, Grimm PD, Blasko JC, et al. 15-Year biochemical relapse free survival in clinical Stage T1-T3 prostate cancer following combined external beam radiotherapy and brachytherapy; Seattle experience. Int J Radiat Oncol Biol Phys 2007; 67(1):57–64.
44. Dattoli M, Wallner K, True L, et al. Long-term outcomes after treatment with brachytherapy and supplemental conformal radiation for prostate cancer patients having intermediate and high-risk features. Cancer 2007;110(3):551–5.
45. Blasko JC, Ragde H, Grimm PD. Transperineal ultrasound-guided implantation of the prostate: morbidity and complications. Scand J Urol Nephrol Suppl 1991;137:113–8.
46. Vijverberg PL, Blank LE, Dabhoiwala NF, et al. Analysis of biopsy findings and implant quality following ultrasonically-guided 125I implantation for localised prostatic carcinoma. Br J Urol 1993;72:470–7.
47. Wallner K, Roy J, Harrison L. Tumor control and morbidity following transperineal iodine 125 implantation for stage T1/T2 prostatic carcinoma. J Clin Oncol 1996;14:449–53.
48. Storey MR, Landgren RC, Cottone JL, et al. Transperineal 125iodine implantation for treatment of clinically localized prostate cancer: 5-year tumor control and morbidity. Int J Radiat Oncol Biol Phys 1999;43:565.
49. Mabjeesh NJ, Chen J, Stenger A, et al. Preimplant predictive factors of urinary retention after iodine 125 prostate brachytherapy. Urology 2007;70:548–53.
50. Elshaikh MA, Angermeier K, Ulchaker JC, et al. Effect of anatomic, procedural, and dosimetric variables on urinary retention after permanent iodine-125 prostate brachytherapy. Urology 2003;61:152–5.
51. Terk MD, Stock RG, Stone NN. Identification of patients at increased risk for prolonged urinary retention following radioactive seed implantation of the prostate. J Urol 1998;160:1379.
52. Kaye KW, Olson DJ, Payne JT. Detailed preliminary analysis of ^{125}Iodine implantation for localized prostate cancer using percutaneous approach. J Urol 1995;153:1020–5.
53. Dattoli M, Wallner K, Sorace R, et al. Pd-103 brachytherapy and external beam irradiation for clinically localized, high-risk prostatic carcinoma. Int J Radiat Oncol Biol Phys 1996;35:1–5.
54. Ragde H, Korb L. Brachytherapy for clinically localized prostate cancer. Semin Surg Oncol 2000;18: 45–51.
55. Merrick GS, Butler WM, Lief JH, et al. Temporal resolution of urinary morbidity following prostate brachytherapy. Int J Radiat Oncol Biol Phys 2000;47:121.
56. Benoit RM, Naslund M, Cohen JL. Complications after prostate brachytherapy in the Medicare population. Urology 2000;55:91–6.
57. Zeitlin SI, Sherman J, Raboy A, et al. High dose combination radiotherapy for the treatment of localized prostate cancer. J Urol 1998;160:91.
58. Stone NN, Marshall DT, Stone JJ, et al. Does neoadjuvant hormonal therapy improve urinary function when given to men with very large prostates undergoing prostate brachytherapy? J Urol. [Epub ahead of print].
59. Kleinberg L, Wallner K, Roy J, et al. Treatment-related symptoms during the first year following transperineal ^{125}I prostate implantation. Int J Radiat Oncol Biol Phys 1994;28:985.
60. Desai J, Stock RG, Stone NN, et al. Acute morbidity following I-125 interstitial implantation of the prostate gland. Radiat Oncol Investig 1998;6: 135–41.
61. Tanaka N, Fujimoto K, Hirao Y, et al. Variations in international prostate symptom scores, uroflowmetric parameters, and prostate volume after 125I permanent. brachytherapy for localized prostate cancer. Urology 2009;74:407–13.
62. Keyes M, Miller S, Moravan V, et al. Predictive factors for acute and late urinary toxicity after permanent prostate brachytherapy: long-term outcome in 712 consecutive patients. Int J Radiat Oncol Biol Phys 2009;73(4):1023–32.
63. Matzkin H, Kaver I, Stenger A, et al. Iodine-125 brachytherapy for localized prostate cancer and urinary morbidity: a prospective comparison of two seed implant methods—preplanning and intraoperative planning. Urology 2003;62:497–502.
64. Niehaus A, Merrick GS, Butler WM, et al. The influence of isotope and prostate volume on urinary morbidity after prostate brachytherapy. Int J Radiat Oncol Biol Phys 2006;64(1):136–43.
65. Stone NN, Stock RG. The effect of brachytherapy, external beam irradiation and hormonal therapy on prostate volume. J Urol 2007;177:925–8.
66. Nag S, Pak V, Blasko J, et al. Brachytherapy for prostate cancer. Principles and practice of brachytherapy. Armonk (NY): Futura Publ; 1997. p. 421–40.
67. Gelblum DA, Potters L, Ashley R, et al. Urinary morbidity following ultrasound-guided transperineal prostate seed implantation. Int J Radiat Oncol Biol Phys 1999;45:59.
68. Bittner N, Merrick GS, Wallner KE, et al. The impact of acute urinary morbidity on late urinary function

after permanent prostate brachytherapy. Brachytherapy 2007;6:258–66.
69. Blasko JC, Wallner K, Grimm PD, et al. PSA based disease control following ultrasound guided I-125 implantation for stage T1/T2 prostatic carcinoma. J Urol 1995;154:1096–9.
70. Beyer DC, Priestley JB. Biochemical disease-free survival following I125 prostate implantation. Int J Radiat Oncol Biol Phys 1997;37:559–63.
71. Wallner K, Lee H, Wasserman S, et al. Low risk of urinary incontinence following prostate brachytherapy in patients with prior transurethral prostate resection. Int J Radiat Oncol Biol Phys 1997;37: 565–9.
72. Stone NN, Stock RG. Prostate brachytherapy: treatment strategies. J Urol 1999;162:421.
73. Talcott JA, Clark JC, Stark P, et al. Long-term treatment-related complications of brachytherapy for early prostate cancer: a survey of treated patients. Proc Annu Meet Am Soc Clin Oncol 1999;18: 1196a.
74. Nag S, Scaperoth DD, Badalament R, et al. Transperineal palladium 103 prostate brachytherapy: analysis of morbidity and seed migration. Urology 1995;45:87–92.
75. Stone NN, Stock RG. Long-term urinary, sexual and rectal morbidity treated with I-125 prostate brachytherapy followed up for a minimum of 5 years. Urology 2007;69:339–42.
76. Anderson JF, Swanson DA, Levy LB, et al. Urinary side effects and complications after permanent prostate brachytherapy: the MD Anderson Cancer Center experience. Urology 2009;74:601–5.
77. Kollmeier MA, Stock RG, Cesaretti J, et al. Urinary morbidity and incontinence following transurethral resection of the prostate after brachytherapy. J Urol 2005;157:808–12.
78. Critz FA, Tarlton RS, Holladay DA. Prostate specific antigen-monitored combination radiotherapy for patients with prostate cancer: I-125 implant followed by external-beam radiation. Cancer 1995;75:2383.
79. Stone NN, Ratnow ER, Stock RG. Prior transurethral resection does not increase morbidity following real-time ultrasound guided prostate seed implantation. Tech Urol 2000;6:123–7.
80. Grado GL, Larson TR, Balch CS, et al. Actuarial disease-free survival after prostate cancer brachytherapy using interactive techniques with biplane ultrasound and fluoroscopic guidance. Int J Radiat Oncol Biol Phys 1998;42:289–98.
81. Hu K, Wallner K. Clinical course of rectal bleeding following I-125 prostate brachytherapy. Int J Radiat Oncol Biol Phys 1998;41:263–5.
82. Gelbum DY, Potters L. Rectal complications associated with transperineal interstitial brachytherapy for prostate cancer. Int J Radiat Oncol Biol Phys 2000; 48:119–24.
83. Theodorescu D, Gillenwater JY, Koutrouvelis PG. Prostatourethral-rectal fistula after prostate brachytherapy. Cancer 2000;89(10):2085–91.
84. Sarosdy MF. Urinary and rectal complications of contemporary permanent transperineal brachytherapy for prostate carcinoma with or without external beam radiation therapy. Cancer 2004;101:754–60.
85. Stone NN, Cesaretti JA, Rosenstein B. et al. Do high radiation doses in locally advanced prostate cancer patients treated with Pd-103 implant plus external beam irradiation cause increased urinary, rectal and sexual morbidity? Brachytherapy. [Epub ahead of print].
86. Stock RG, Kao J, Stone NN. Penile erection function after permanent radioactive seed implantation for treatment of prostate cancer. J Urol 2001;165:436–9.
87. Taira AV, Merrick GS, Galbreath RW, et al. Erectile function durability following permanent prostate brachytherapy. Int J Radiat Oncol Biol Phys 2009;75(3): 639–48.
88. Critz FA, Levinson K. 10-year disease-free survival rates after simultaneous irradiation for prostate cancer with a focus on calculation methodology. J Urol 2004;172(6 Pt 1):2232–8.
89. Stock RG, Ho A, Cesaretti JA, et al. Changing the patterns of failure for high-risk prostate cancer patients by optimizing local control. Int J Radiat Oncol Biol Phys 2006;66(2):389–94.
90. Stone NN, Potters L, Davis BJ, et al. Multicenter analysis of effect of high biologic effective dose on biochemical failure and survival outcomes in patients with Gleason score 7–10 prostate cancer treated with permanent prostate. Int J Radiat Oncol Biol Phys 2009;73(2):341–6.
91. Lee WR, McQuellon RP, Harris-Henderson K, et al. A preliminary analysis of health-related quality of life in the first year after permanent source interstitial brachytherapy for clinically localized prostate cancer. Int J Radiat Oncol Biol Phys 2000;46:27.

Neoadjuvant and Adjuvant Therapies in Prostate Cancer

Fabio A.B. Schutz, MD[a], William K. Oh, MD[b,*]

KEYWORDS

• Prostate cancer • Adjuvant therapy • Chemotherapy

Prostate cancer is the most common cancer in men in the United States and the second leading cause of cancer death, accounting for 27,360 estimated deaths in 2009.[1] The advent of prostate-specific antigen (PSA) screening has contributed to an increase in incidence since the mid-1980s.[2] It has also changed the clinical presentation from a typical patient with voiding symptoms or even low back pain caused by metastatic disease to one more commonly asymptomatic as a result of earlier diagnosis. Advances in surgical therapies, including nerve-sparing radical and robotic-assisted radical prostatectomy (RP), have paralleled advances in radiation therapy (such as intensity modulated radiation therapy [IMRT]) and chemotherapy for metastatic disease. Similarly, strategies are being developed to prevent disease recurrence and improve patient outcome after definitive local therapy. In particular, there is a great Interest in neoadjuvant and adjuvant therapies for patients at intermediate and high risk of cancer recurrence and prostate cancer–specific death.

Many studies consider biochemical recurrence as an end point to evaluate the efficacy of the neoadjuvant and adjuvant therapies, but this should be done cautiously. Prostate cancer is a disease of older men and usually has a long course. Thus a significant proportion of patients who experience biochemical recurrence may not progress or die of prostate cancer because other competing causes of death also increase with age. Therefore, careful attention to the defining characteristics of the study population and the outcomes of interest are crucial when assessing the efficacy of the adjuvant treatment options.

Risk stratification criteria in newly diagnosed prostate cancer are well established and widely used. In a large retrospective series, patients were stratified into 3 risk groups, according to pretreatment clinical staging, PSA level, and biopsy Gleason score, for patients treated with RP or radiotherapy (RT).[3] Patients presenting in the high-risk group (stage >T2b, PSA level >20 ng/dl or Gleason score 8–10) were at increased risk of developing metastatic disease and dying of prostate cancer. The relative risk of prostate cancer–specific mortality was 14.2 and 14.3 for patients submitted to RP and RT, respectively, compared with patients in the low-risk group. In the postprostatectomy setting, retrospective series have shown long-term biochemical (PSA) failure-free survival rates of 81% to 92% for organ-confined disease. However, these rates decrease significantly for patients with locally advanced disease (26% to 43% with seminal vesical involvement and 19% for lymph node positivity).[4,5]

Because high-risk patients with cancer can be readily identified by clinical criteria, many studies have attempted to use local and systemic adjuvant therapy to reduce the risk of recurrence. This review discusses neoadjuvant and adjuvant therapies in prostate cancer, including hormonal therapy (HT), chemotherapy, and postoperative radiotherapy.

[a] Lank Center for Genitourinary Oncology, Dana Farber Cancer Institute, 44 Binney Street, Boston, MA 02215, USA
[b] Division of Hematology and Medical Oncology, Tisch Cancer Institute, Mount Sinai School of Medicine, One Gustave L. Levy Place, Box 1079, New York, NY 10029, USA
* Corresponding author.
E-mail address: william.oh@mssm.edu (W.K. Oh).

Urol Clin N Am 37 (2010) 97–104
doi:10.1016/j.ucl.2009.11.012

urologic.theclinics.com

HT

Neoadjuvant HT Before RP

Since the first reports of efficacy by Huggins and colleagues[6,7] in 1941, androgen deprivation therapy (ADT) has gained widespread use in patients with metastatic prostate cancer. However, the question of which populations of patients with prostate cancer may benefit from neoadjuvant ADT continues to be poorly defined. Considering biochemical recurrence rates as a primary end point, patients with low-risk tumors (Gleason score ≤6, PSA level ≤10, stage <T2b) seem least likely to benefit from neoadjuvant ADT.

In intermediate- and high-risk patients, several randomized trials have attempted to quantify potential benefits. Most of these studies used a 3-month neoadjuvant treatment period before definitive therapy, and most of them used complete androgen blockade (CAB). A decrease in the postoperative positive surgical margins is consistently seen. However, a benefit in overall survival (OS) has not been observed in any trial.[8–10] The largest study was conducted by the European Study Group on Neoadjuvant Treatment of Prostate Cancer. A total of 402 patients were randomized between CAB for 3 months followed by RP or RP alone. A significant difference in pathologic downstaging (15% vs 7%), percentage with positive margins (27% vs 46%), and local relapse rates for cT2 patients (3% vs 11%) were observed, favoring the neoadjuvant group. However, no significant difference was observed in biochemical recurrence or OS.[9,11]

At least 2 studies have reported on the use of longer-term neoadjuvant therapy (>3 months). In the PROSIT (Protein S Italian Team) study, patients were randomized between neoadjuvant treatment with CAB for 3 or 6 months followed by RP or RP alone. The rates of positive surgical margins were significantly less in the neoadjuvant group, although not significantly different between the 2 neoadjuvant (3 and 6 months) groups (26% vs 19%, $P = .295$).[12] However, a report by the Canadian Uro-Oncology Group (CUOG) randomized 547 patients to either 3 or 8 months of neoadjuvant therapy with CAB followed by RP; a significant decrease in the positive margin rate was observed favoring those patients receiving therapy for 8 months (5% vs 17%), and the organ-confined rates (91% vs 71%) ($P<.01$). In the absence of a control group, no direct comparison could be made between neoadjuvant therapy and immediate RP.[13,14]

A meta-analysis published in 2000 analyzed the routine use of neoadjuvant HT before RP.[15] Six of the 7 studies reviewed noted a decrease in the positive surgical margin rate, but no significant improvement in survival was observed.

Although neoadjuvant ADT affects the rate of positive surgical margins, benefits in survival have not been shown. As such, the routine use of neoadjuvant HT before definitive RP is not recommended outside a clinical trial.

Adjuvant HT After RP

Several studies have attempted to address the issue of early HT in patients who have undergone definitive therapy with RP. The early use of HT in these patients was initially reported in the 1960s as having no effect on OS.[16] However, newer hormonal agents have renewed interest in hormonal manipulation in the adjuvant setting for prostate cancer, and trials addressing this issue have subsequently been undertaken.

Several trials addressing the role of adjuvant HT for patients with positive lymph nodes after RP have been reported. Myers and colleagues[17] reported the results of 62 patients with a long median follow-up (more than 10 years). The patients were divided according to DNA ploidy status and the use of adjuvant HT. Diploid (normal DNA) patients with cancer who received adjuvant HT had a statistically significant improvement in disease-free survival (DFS) and cancer-specific mortality. Although this was a small study, the benefit of early hormonal manipulation on a subset of patients was intriguing. However, further evaluation on the effect of DNA ploidy on prostate cancer has yet to be determined. A landmark study, conducted by Messing and colleagues,[18,19] randomized 98 patients with node positive disease to either androgen deprivation (ie, surgical or biochemical) or observation following RP. After a follow-up of 11.9 years a significant increase in OS (64% vs 45%) was observed in favor of the ADT group. The benefit in favor of ADT was also observed for PSA recurrence-free survival (53% vs 14%), DFS (60% vs 25%), and prostate cancer–specific survival (85% vs 51%). Some limitations of this study must be acknowledged: (1) the accrual goal of 220 patients was not attained and the few patients who were accrued took many years to enrol; (2) the pathology review was not centralized, potentially contributing to an imbalance between the 2 arms (selection bias); and (3) the control group received ADT for metastatic progression, although many patients currently receive ADT for PSA progression. However, the strength of the effect and the underlying biologic hypothesis suggest that the benefit of ADT in node positive prostate cancer is compelling.[18,19]

Regarding patients with pathologically negative lymph nodes, further investigation of the role of adjuvant ADT has been undertaken. Siddiqui and colleagues[20] reported a retrospective series from the Mayo Clinic with patients who underwent RP and had negative lymph nodes. A total of 580 patients were treated with adjuvant ADT, and 1160 were observed only. A significant benefit in 10-year biochemical systemic progression-free survival (PFS) (95% vs 90%) and cancer-specific survival (98% vs 95%) was noted, favoring ADT therapy. However, no significant difference was observed in OS (83%, for ADT and observation groups), and this was not a randomized trial.

The use of adjuvant antiandrogen therapy has also been studied. The Early Prostate Cancer (EPC) study enrolled patients with T1-4NxM0 prostate cancer in a multicenter, international, randomized clinical trial. Patients were treated with the standard of care, which was RP, radiotherapy, or watchful waiting, followed by either adjuvant high-dose bicalutamide (150 mg daily) for 2 years or placebo. There have been different reports with different populations depending on the site of the trial, but a significant improvement was noted in the PFS of patients with locally advanced prostate cancer who received bicalutamide (high risk). However, only patients treated with radiotherapy and watchful waiting had an improvement in OS.[21–23] The North American EPC trial (0023) did not enrol patients on watchful waiting, making the comparison between different sites and arms difficult. In the US trial, eligible patients (3292 patients, with ~80% post-RP and ~20% post-RT) after a median follow-up of 7.7 years showed a significant benefit in the treatment group for time to PSA progression (hazard ratio [HR] 0.80, $P<.001$), but no significant differences in mortality (12.9% vs 12.3%, respectively) or in objective progression rates (15.4% vs 15.3%, respectively) were observed.[22]

Although the treatment is still controversial, most specialists in genitourinary cancers advocate the use of adjuvant ADT in patients with lymph node positive disease who have undergone RP. The exact duration of therapy is debated although patients in Messing and colleagues' study underwent lifelong androgen deprivation. In patients without lymph node positive disease, there remains no conclusive evidence for the use of adjuvant HT after definitive therapy with RP.

Adjuvant HT After Radiation Therapy

The use of adjuvant HT for locally advanced prostate cancer or high-risk patients after RT is well established. The RTOG (Radiation Therapy Oncology Group) 85-31 trial randomized 977 patients with locally advanced prostate cancer (lymph node positive or clinical T3 disease) to receive adjuvant ADT indefinitely after definitive RT. After a follow-up of 7.6 years, a significant increase in the 10-year OS (49% vs 39%, $P = .002$), and significant decreases in local failure rate (23% vs 38%), incidence of distant metastases (24% vs 39%), and disease-specific mortality (16% vs 22%) were observed, favoring the adjuvant group.[24] This study had some limitations because 139 patients received prior RP and, in addition, the trial was conducted in the pre-PSA era, making it difficult to translate it to current practice.

A subsequent landmark trial, EORTC (European Organization for Research and Treatment of Cancer) trial 22863, reported by Bolla and colleagues,[25] enrolled 415 node negative patients with T3 or T4 tumors or high-grade (grade 3) T1 or T2 tumors, and randomized them to either adjuvant HT with goserelin for a total of 3 years or observation after definitive RT. At a median follow-up of 66 months, a significant benefit was observed for the adjuvant group in 5-year OS (78% vs 62%, $P = .0002$), cancer-specific survival (94% vs 79%), and clinical DFS (74% vs 40%).

Another trial evaluated the use of a shorter course of adjuvant HT. D'Amico and colleagues[26] randomized 206 patients with intermediate- or high-risk features (T1b–T2b tumors with PSA level 10–40 or Gleason score ≥7) to receive or not ADT (leuprolide or goserelin combined with a nonsteroidal antiandrogen flutamide) for 6 months beginning 2 months prior to definitive RT. After a median follow-up of 4.5 years, a significant advantage favoring the combination treatment group was noted in freedom from salvage ADT therapy (82 vs 57%), cancer-specific mortality (0% vs 5%), and 5-year OS (88 vs 78%, $P = .04$).

The optimal duration of the HT has been addressed specifically in 2 trials. The RTOG 92-02 trial enrolled 1554 patients with locally advanced prostate cancer (T2c–T4 with no extrapelvic lymph node involvement and PSA level ≤150). Patients were treated with 4 months of ADT (goserelin and flutamide) before and during RT, and were randomized to no further ADT or 24 months of ADT. The patients who received the long-term ADT, compared with short-term, had a significant benefit in DFS (23% vs 13%, respectively), local progression (12% vs 22%, respectively), distant metastasis (15% vs 23%, respectively), and PSA failure (52% vs 68%, respectively), but failed to show a significant increase in OS (54% vs 52%, respectively).[27] However, the EORTC trial 22961 did show a significant increase in OS for patients treated with long-term ADT. A total of 970 patients with locally advanced prostate cancer (T1c–2b pN1–2 M0 or cT2–4 cN0–2, and PSA level less than 40 times the upper limit) were randomized to short-term (6 months) or long-term (36 months) ADT. At a median follow-up of 6.4 years, the 5-year overall mortality was decreased for patients on long-term ADT compared with short-term ADT (15% vs 19%, respectively) (HR 1.42, 95.71% confidence interval [CI] 1.09–1.85).[28] Moreover, a secondary analysis from the RTOG 85-31 trial showed an association between increased survival and the length of HT. In this analysis, only 189 from 977 patients were included and they were divided into 3 groups: HT for 1 year or longer; HT for between 1 and 5 years; and HT for more than 5 years. At a median follow-up time of 9.6 years, the median duration of HT was 2.2 years, and a significant increase was observed in the 5-year (100% vs 72% and 67%) and 11-year (64% vs 42% and 33%) survivals for the group who received HT for more than 5 years, compared with those who received HT for less than 1 year, and HT for between 1 and 5 years, respectively.[29]

Adjuvant HT has become an accepted standard of care for high-risk localized prostate cancer treated with radiation therapy. In intermediate- and high-risk patients, as shown by D'Amico and colleagues, at least 6 months of total ADT before, during, and after definitive radiation therapy seems appropriate. In the high-risk patients the data regarding duration of therapy remain controversial, although it seems that a longer duration of ADT is important in improving survival.

CHEMOTHERAPY

The role of chemotherapy in advanced prostate cancer has been marked by a lack of effective drugs. Initially, a palliative benefit was shown with a combination of mitoxantrone and prednisone in patients with castration-resistant prostate cancer (CRPC), but no survival benefit was noted.[30] However, in 2004, 2 subsequent randomized phase III trials were reported (SWOG [Southwest Oncology Group] 9916 and TAX 327) comparing docetaxel to mitoxantrone in patients with CRPC. A statistically significant 2- to 2.5-month improvement in median OS in the docetaxel arm (every 3 weeks) was reported in both studies, with a reduction of 24% in the risk of death.[31,32]

The efficacy of chemotherapy in CRPC brought new options, and clinical trials have been initiated evaluating the efficacy of chemotherapeutic agents in the neoadjuvant and adjuvant setting. The ultimate goal of the (neo)adjuvant chemotherapy is to eradicate potentially micrometastatic disease, thus improving OS.

Neoadjuvant Chemotherapy

Several phase II trials proved the safety and feasibility of neoadjuvant chemotherapy with different agents and combinations, and docetaxel-based chemotherapy has been studied in this setting. Two trials in particular reported the results of single-agent use of docetaxel (without HT). Although the studies were similar in design, Dreicer and colleagues[33] studied a high-dose docetaxel for a short course (40 mg/m^2/wk, for 6 weeks), whereas Febbo and colleagues[34] studied a standard dose of docetaxel for a prolonged period (36 mg/m^2/wk, for 6 months). Both studies showed significant PSA reductions after chemotherapy of at least 50% in 24% and 58% of treated patients, respectively. No pathologic complete responses were observed. However, when neoadjuvant HT is combined with chemotherapy, some pathologic responses have been reported.[35,36]

Another area of study is the use of targeted agents. Bevacizumab is a monoclonal antibody directed against the vascular endothelial growth factor. Oh and colleagues[37] reported a phase II trial with high-risk patients with prostate cancer treated with docetaxel (70 mg/m^2), every 3 weeks for 6 cycles, and bevacizumab 15 mg/kg, every 3 weeks for 5 cycles, followed by RP. Almost all patients, except 1, presented a decline in tumor volume measured by endorectal magnetic resonance imaging, with 36% patients presenting with a decline of more than 50%.

No phase III randomized controlled trials have been completed to address outcomes when using neoadjuvant chemotherapy. Currently, the CALGB 90203 study is planning to enrol 700 high-risk patients and to compare docetaxel plus ADT followed by RP with RP alone.

Another multi-institutional phase III trial is being conducted by D'Amico and colleagues.[38] Intermediate- and high-risk patients are being treated with standard RT and concurrent ADT for 6 months, and randomized to receive docetaxel (60 mg/m^2 every 3 weeks) for 3 cycles at the start of treatment followed by weekly docetaxel (20 mg/m^2) beginning at week 1 of RT and continuing for 7 weeks.

Adjuvant Chemotherapy

Early adjuvant chemotherapy studies have reported inconclusive results. An early trial, published by the National Prostate Cancer Project (NPCP), randomized a total of 437 patients to either estramustine phosphate (600 mg/m^2 orally daily), cyclophosphamide (1 g/m^2 intravenously every 3 weeks), or observation for 2 years following definitive RT (Protocol 900) or RP (Protocol 1000). At more than 10 years' median follow-up, patients receiving estramustine had a significant improvement in PFS.[39] A second underpowered study by Wang and colleagues[40] compared HT with or without chemotherapy with mitoxantrone and prednisone in 96 patients with pT3 or T4 disease. The results significantly favored OS in the chemotherapy arm (median OS 84 months vs 41 months).

These studies led to the development of larger randomized trials. SWOG study 9921 is a phase III trial that randomized high-risk patients with prostate cancer to receive ADT for 2 years, with or without 6 cycles of mitoxantrone (12 mg/m^2 every 4 weeks) plus prednisone. A total of 983 patients were enrolled of the planned 1360, before early closure of the trial secondary to excessive numbers of acute myeloid leukemias in the mitoxantrone chemotherapy arm. Results of survival have not been reported yet, and it is unknown if there will be enough power to detect a difference in survival between the 2 arms.[41]

Another trial, TAX 3501, was designed to assess the efficacy of adjuvant docetaxel in improving survival. High-risk patients were treated with adjuvant ADT and randomized to receive immediately 6 cycles of adjuvant docetaxel (75 mg/m^2) or as a salvage treatment. However, because of poor accrual, this trial was also closed prematurely. A more recent, ongoing trial, TAX 3503, was initiated with a similar design, but is enrolling patients with increasing PSA levels (biochemical failure) after RP, and randomizing them to ADT alone followed by docetaxel when they have CRPC or ADT plus early docetaxel.

Docetaxel is also being investigated in the adjuvant setting after definitive RT. RTOG study 0521 is a phase III trial that plans to enrol 600 high-risk patients. Patients are treated with RT and ADT (LHRH agonist and oral antiandrogen) for a total of 2 years, beginning 2 months before RT, and randomized to receive adjuvant docetaxel (75 mg/m^2 every 3 weeks) for 6 cycles, beginning 1 month after the completion of RT.[38]

The use of chemotherapy, in particular docetaxel, in the neoadjuvant and adjuvant settings is promising. It is to be hoped that the current phase III trials will answer the question regarding the potential benefit of chemotherapy in improving the survival rates for high-risk patients with prostate cancer.

ADJUVANT RADIOTHERAPY

Patients with pathologic stage T3 (pT3) or positive margins are at increased risk of relapse. Recurring patients with extraprostatic extension (pT3a) are more likely to present with local relapse, particularly those with positive margins. However, those patients with seminal vesicle invasion (pT3b) tend to present with systemic relapse, irrespective of the surgical margins.[42]

Recently 2 important clinical trials have been reported that address the efficacy of adjuvant RT for patients with pT3N0 or positive margins: EORTC trial 22911 and SWOG trial 8794.

In the EORTC trial, 1005 patients with pT3 or positive margins were randomized to receive adjuvant RT (60 Gy) or observation. After a median follow-up time of 5 years, the biochemical PFS was significantly increased from 53% to 74% (*P*<.0001) in the treatment group. The clinical PFS and cumulative locoregional failure rate were also better for patients receiving adjuvant RT. However, the 5-year OS was not increased (93% vs 92%, respectively for adjuvant RT and for observation groups).[43] An update of this trial suggested that the benefit was restricted to the patients with positive margins (HR 0.38, 95% CI 0.26–0.54), compared with patients with negative margins (HR 0.88, 95% CI 0.53–1.46).[44] However, even if the adjuvant RT does not show an improvement in OS, it could delay the need for HT, thus postponing the adverse effects of ADT. On the other hand, the adverse effects of adjuvant RT may also be significant. In this trial, adjuvant RT was associated with an increase of long-term adverse effects (all grades), but the incidence of serious adverse events was rare (4.2% vs 2.6%, respectively for adjuvant RT and wait-and-see groups), and no grade 4 events were observed. Moreover, an interim analysis did not show an increase in the risk of urinary incontinence.[45]

The SWOG trial randomized 425 patients with pT3N0 prostate cancer to adjuvant RT (60–64 Gy) or usual care plus observation. After a long median follow-up, the adjuvant RT group had a significant increase in OS (15.2 vs 13.3 years; HR 0.72, 95% CI 0.55–0.96) and metastasis-free survival (14.7 vs 12.9 years; HR 0.71, 95% CI 0.54–0.94). Subset analyses have shown that this benefit was independent of the Gleason score, and included patients with or without detectable PSA post prostatectomy and those with positive margins or seminal vesicle involvement.[46] Only one-third of the observation group received salvage RT, so these results cannot be compared with the strategy of observation and salvage RT at the time of biochemical recurrence.

Regarding the strategy of salvage RT at the time of biochemical relapse, Stephenson and colleagues[47] proposed a nomogram that predicts the probability of local or distant relapse for post-prostatectomy patients with biochemical recurrence. The cutoff points in the nomogram are PSA level before salvage RT of 2 ng/mL or less, Gleason score 7 or less, presence of positive margins and a PSA doubling time (PSA-DT) greater than 10 months. The PSA level before salvage RT was a highly significant predictor of disease progression. It was observed that patients with a PSA level of less than 0.5 ng/mL at recurrence, irrespective of other factors, had a 6-year disease-free probability of 48%, compared with 26% for those treated at higher PSA levels. Even patients with other unfavorable prognostic factors, like Gleason score 8–10 and PSA-DT 10 months or less, but with a PSA level less than 0.5 ng/mL, had a 41% chance of survival after 6 years. The 41% and 48% disease control rate with early salvage RT can be compared with the relative risk reduction of biochemical recurrence observed with adjuvant RT in the previous trials.[44,46] Therefore, a direct comparison between adjuvant RT and RT at biochemical recurrence would be ideal.

SUMMARY

Adjuvant and neoadjuvant therapies in prostate cancer have been evaluated for many years and several general conclusions can be made. First, neoadjuvant and adjuvant ADT has a clear role in improving outcomes in high-risk localized prostate cancer treated with RT, but its role in intermediate-risk disease is less certain, as is the optimal duration of ADT. No definitive evidence has suggested that neoadjuvant or adjuvant ADT has a role when combined with surgery, although studies have suggested that longer durations of ADT are associated with improvements in positive margin rates. Chemotherapy is under active investigation as neoadjuvant and adjuvant therapy in high-risk prostate cancer but as yet has no proven role in decreasing risk of recurrence. Adjuvant RT after RP has been shown in recent large randomized trials to increase DFS and OS compared with no adjuvant RT. However, its benefit in all patients at risk for relapse compared with early salvage RT (eg, in the setting of an increasing PSA level) remains uncertain.

REFERENCES

1. Jemal A, Siegel R, Ward E, et al. Cancer statistics, 2009. CA Cancer J Clin 2009;59(4):225–49.
2. Vessella RL, Lange PH. Issues in the assessment of prostate-specific antigen immunoassays. An update. Urol Clin North Am 1997;24(2):261–8.
3. D'Amico AV, Moul J, Carroll PR, et al. Cancer-specific mortality after surgery or radiation for patients with clinically localized prostate cancer managed during the prostate-specific antigen era. J Clin Oncol 2003;21(11):2163–72.
4. Catalona WJ, Smith DS. Cancer recurrence and survival rates after anatomic radical retropubic prostatectomy for prostate cancer: intermediate-term results. J Urol 1998;160(6 Pt 2):2428–34.
5. Walsh PC, Partin AW, Epstein JI. Cancer control and quality of life following anatomical radical retropubic prostatectomy: results at 10 years. J Urol 1994; 152(5 Pt 2):1831–6.
6. D'Amico AV, Whittington R, Malkowicz SB, et al. Biochemical outcome after radical prostatectomy, external beam radiation therapy, or interstitial radiation therapy for clinically localized prostate cancer. JAMA 1998;280(11):969–74.
7. Kattan MW, Eastham JA, Stapleton AM, et al. A preoperative nomogram for disease recurrence following radical prostatectomy for prostate cancer. J Natl Cancer Inst 1998;90(10):766–71.
8. Labrie F, Cusan L, Gomez JL, et al. Neoadjuvant hormonal therapy: the Canadian experience. Urology 1997;49(Suppl 3A):56–64.
9. Schulman CC, Debruyne FM, Forster G, et al. 4-Year follow-up results of a European prospective randomized study on neoadjuvant hormonal therapy prior to radical prostatectomy in T2-3N0M0 prostate cancer. European Study Group on Neoadjuvant Treatment of Prostate Cancer. Eur Urol 2000;38(6):706–13.
10. Soloway MS, Pareek K, Sharifi R, et al. Neoadjuvant androgen ablation before radical prostatectomy in cT2bNxMo prostate cancer: 5-year results. J Urol 2002;167(1):112–6.
11. Witjes WP, Schulman CC, Debruyne FM. Preliminary results of a prospective randomized study comparing radical prostatectomy versus radical prostatectomy associated with neoadjuvant hormonal combination therapy in T2-3 N0 M0 prostatic carcinoma. The European Study Group on Neoadjuvant Treatment of Prostate Cancer. Urology 1997;49(Suppl 3A):65–9.
12. Selli C, Montironi R, Bono A, et al. Effects of complete androgen blockade for 12 and 24 weeks on the pathological stage and resection margin status of prostate cancer. J Clin Pathol 2002;55(7): 508–13.
13. Gleave ME, Goldenberg SL, Chin JL, et al. Randomized comparative study of 3 versus 8-month neoadjuvant hormonal therapy before radical prostatectomy: biochemical and pathological effects. J Urol 2001;166(2):500–7 [discussion: 506–7].

14. Klotz L, Gleave M, Goldenberg SL. Neoadjuvant hormone therapy: the Canadian trials. Mol Urol 2000;4(3):233–7 [discussion: 239].
15. Scolieri MJ, Altman A, Resnick MI. Neoadjuvant hormonal ablative therapy before radical prostatectomy: a review. Is it indicated? J Urol 2000;164(5):1465–72.
16. Treatment and survival of patients with cancer of the prostate. The Veterans Administration Co-operative Urological Research Group. Surg Gynecol Obstet 1967;124(5):1011–7.
17. Myers RP, Larson-Keller JJ, Bergstralh EJ, et al. Hormonal treatment at time of radical retropubic prostatectomy for stage D1 prostate cancer: results of long-term followup. J Urol 1992;147(3 Pt 2):910–5.
18. Messing EM, Manola J, Sarosdy M, et al. Immediate hormonal therapy compared with observation after radical prostatectomy and pelvic lymphadenectomy in men with node-positive prostate cancer. N Engl J Med 1999;341(24):1781–8.
19. Messing EM, Manola J, Yao J, et al. Immediate versus deferred androgen deprivation treatment in patients with node-positive prostate cancer after radical prostatectomy and pelvic lymphadenectomy. Lancet Oncol 2006;7(6):472–9.
20. Siddiqui SA, Boorjian SA, Inman B, et al. Timing of androgen deprivation therapy and its impact on survival after radical prostatectomy: a matched cohort study. J Urol 2008;179(5):1830–7 [discussion: 1837].
21. McLeod DG, Iversen P, See WA, et al. Bicalutamide 150 mg plus standard care vs standard care alone for early prostate cancer. BJU Int 2006;97(2):247–54.
22. McLeod DG, See WA, Klimberg I, et al. The bicalutamide 150 mg early prostate cancer program: findings of the North American trial at 7.7-year median followup. J Urol 2006;176(1):75–80.
23. Iversen P, Johansson JE, Lodding P, et al. Bicalutamide (150 mg) versus placebo as immediate therapy alone or as adjuvant to therapy with curative intent for early nonmetastatic prostate cancer: 5.3-year median followup from the Scandinavian Prostate Cancer Group Study Number 6. J Urol 2004;172(5 Pt 1):1871–6.
24. Pilepich MV, Winter K, Lawton CA, et al. Androgen suppression adjuvant to definitive radiotherapy in prostate carcinoma–long-term results of phase III RTOG 85-31. Int J Radiat Oncol Biol Phys 2005;61(5):1285–90.
25. Bolla M, Collette L, Blank L, et al. Long-term results with immediate androgen suppression and external irradiation in patients with locally advanced prostate cancer (an EORTC study): a phase III randomised trial. Lancet 2002;360(9327):103–6.
26. D'Amico AV, Manola J, Loffredo M, et al. 6-month androgen suppression plus radiation therapy vs radiation therapy alone for patients with clinically localized prostate cancer: a randomized controlled trial. JAMA 2004;292(7):821–7.
27. Horwitz EM, Bae K, Hanks GE, et al. Ten-year follow-up of radiation therapy oncology group protocol 92-02: a phase III trial of the duration of elective androgen deprivation in locally advanced prostate cancer. J Clin Oncol 2008;26(15):2497–504.
28. Bolla M, de Reijke TM, Van Tienhoven G, et al. Duration of androgen suppression in the treatment of prostate cancer. N Engl J Med 2009;360(24):2516–27.
29. Souhami L, Bae K, Pilepich M, et al. Impact of the duration of adjuvant hormonal therapy in patients with locally advanced prostate cancer treated with radiotherapy: a secondary analysis of RTOG 85-31. J Clin Oncol 2009;27(13):2137–43.
30. Tannock IF, Osoba D, Stockler MR, et al. Chemotherapy with mitoxantrone plus prednisone or prednisone alone for symptomatic hormone-resistant prostate cancer: a Canadian randomized trial with palliative end points. J Clin Oncol 1996;14(6):1756–64.
31. Petrylak DP, Tangen CM, Hussain MH, et al. Docetaxel and estramustine compared with mitoxantrone and prednisone for advanced refractory prostate cancer. N Engl J Med 2004;351(15):1513–20.
32. Tannock IF, de Wit R, Berry WR, et al. Docetaxel plus prednisone or mitoxantrone plus prednisone for advanced prostate cancer. N Engl J Med 2004;351(15):1502–12.
33. Dreicer R, Magi-Galluzzi C, Zhou M, et al. Phase II trial of neoadjuvant docetaxel before radical prostatectomy for locally advanced prostate cancer. Urology 2004;63(6):1138–42.
34. Febbo PG, Richie JP, George DJ, et al. Neoadjuvant docetaxel before radical prostatectomy in patients with high-risk localized prostate cancer. Clin Cancer Res 2005;11(14):5233–40.
35. Prayer-Galetti T, Sacco E, Pagano F, et al. Long-term follow-up of a neoadjuvant chemohormonal taxane-based phase II trial before radical prostatectomy in patients with non-metastatic high-risk prostate cancer. BJU Int 2007;100(2):274–80.
36. Chi KN, Chin JL, Winquist E, et al. Multicenter phase II study of combined neoadjuvant docetaxel and hormone therapy before radical prostatectomy for patients with high risk localized prostate cancer. J Urol 2008;180(2):565–70 [discussion: 570].
37. Oh WK, Febbo PG, Richie JP, et al. A phase II study of neoadjuvant chemotherapy with docetaxel and bevacizumab in patients (pts) with high-risk localized prostate cancer: a Prostate Cancer Clinical Trials Consortium trial. J Clin Oncol 2009;27:15s (Suppl; abstr 5060).
38. Available at: www.clinicaltrials.gov. Accessed September 10, 2009.

39. Schmidt JD, Gibbons RP, Murphy GP, et al. Adjuvant therapy for clinical localized prostate cancer treated with surgery or irradiation. Eur Urol 1996;29(4):425–33.
40. Wang J, Halford S, Rigg A, et al. Adjuvant mitozantrone chemotherapy in advanced prostate cancer. BJU Int 2000;86(6):675–80.
41. Flaig TW, Tangen CM, Hussain MH, et al. Randomization reveals unexpected acute leukemias in Southwest Oncology Group prostate cancer trial. J Clin Oncol 2008;26(9):1532–6.
42. Kasibhatla M, Peterson B, Anscher MS. What is the best postoperative treatment for patients with pT3bN0M0 adenocarcinoma of the prostate? Prostate Cancer Prostatic Dis 2005;8(2):167–73.
43. Bolla M, van Poppel H, Collette L, et al. Postoperative radiotherapy after radical prostatectomy: a randomised controlled trial (EORTC trial 22911). Lancet 2005;366(9485):572–8.
44. Van der Kwast TH, Bolla M, Van Poppel H, et al. Identification of patients with prostate cancer who benefit from immediate postoperative radiotherapy: EORTC 22911. J Clin Oncol 2007;25(27):4178–86.
45. Van Cangh PJ, Richard F, Lorge F, et al. Adjuvant radiation therapy does not cause urinary incontinence after radical prostatectomy: results of a prospective randomized study. J Urol 1998; 159(1):164–6.
46. Thompson IM, Tangen CM, Paradelo J, et al. Adjuvant radiotherapy for pathological T3N0M0 prostate cancer significantly reduces risk of metastases and improves survival: long-term followup of a randomized clinical trial. J Urol 2009;181(3):956–62.
47. Stephenson AJ, Scardino PT, Kattan MW, et al. Predicting the outcome of salvage radiation therapy for recurrent prostate cancer after radical prostatectomy. J Clin Oncol 2007;25(15):2035–41.

Novel Targeted Therapies for Prostate Cancer

Robyn J. Macfarlane, MD[a], Kim N. Chi, MD[a,b,c,*]

KEYWORDS

- Prostate cancer • Androgen receptor • Apoptosis
- Growth factor receptor • Chaperone proteins
- Bone targeted therapy

Prostate cancer is the most common non–skin cancer diagnosed in North America and affects 1 in 6 men. It is the second to third most common cause of cancer death in men in the Western world.[1] Patients who are diagnosed with localized prostate cancer can have an excellent long-term survival and high cure rates with standard approaches.[2] For patients with recurrent or metastatic disease, hormonal therapy in the form of medical or surgical castration can induce significant long-term remission. Despite the initial response to first-line hormonal maneuvers, development of castration-resistant disease is inevitable as shown by progressive disease in the form of increasing prostate-specific antigen (PSA) level or radiologic disease despite castrate levels of testosterone.[3,4]

Historically, the treatment arsenal for the care of patients with castration-resistant prostate cancer (CRPC) has been limited to those systemic therapies that afford some modicum of symptomatic benefit. Treatments that have been approved primarily for improved symptomatology in patients with CRPC include mitoxantrone chemotherapy,[5] radioactive isotopes,[6] and the bisphosphonate zoledronic acid.[7] Multiple trials of cytotoxic chemotherapy have been conducted in patients with metastatic CRPC, but only docetaxel has been shown to improve overall survival,[8,9] with a median improvement in overall survival of approximately 2 to 3 months compared with mitoxantrone.

Presently, there is the potential for significant change in the management of CRPC due in part to the increase in our understanding of the biologic basis for prostate cancer progression that has occurred in the last decade. The mechanisms underpinning castration resistance are varied and can be divided into those that are mediated by the androgen receptor (ie, hypersensitive, promiscuous, or amplified androgen receptor) and others that bypass it.[10,11] Further, preclinical research has elucidated mechanisms underlying malignant proliferation, angiogenesis, and metastatic potential that are implicated in prostate cancer progression. WIth the improved knowledge of prostate cancer pathogenesis comes identification of potential therapeutic targets. This article reviews the current concepts behind targeted therapy for CRPC, with a focus on novel agents that are currently in clinical trials.

ANDROGEN RECEPTOR SIGNALING

Androgens are the primary regulators of prostate cancer cell growth and proliferation, and androgen deprivation almost always results in an initial clinical response by inducing apoptosis or arrest in

[a] Division of Medical Oncology, BC Cancer Agency - Vancouver Cancer Centre, 600 West 10th Avenue, Vancouver, British Columbia, V5Z 4E6, Canada
[b] Department of Medicine, University of British Columbia, GLDHCC, Level 10, 2775 Laurel Street, Vancouver, British Columbia, V5Z 1M9, Canada
[c] Department of Urological Sciences, University of British Columbia, GLDHCC, Level 6, 2775 Laurel Street, Vancouver, British Columbia, V5Z 1M9, Canada
* Corresponding author. Division of Medical Oncology, BC Cancer Agency - Vancouver Cancer Centre, 600 West 10th Avenue, Vancouver, British Columbia, V5Z 4E6, Canada.
E-mail address: kchi@bccancer.bc.ca (K.N. Chi).

Urol Clin N Am 37 (2010) 105–119
doi:10.1016/j.ucl.2009.11.011
0094-0143/10/$ – see front matter

the G1 phase of the cell cycle. Inevitably, men will cease responding to first-line hormonal maneuvers, but it has long been recognized that second-line hormonal therapies can often be associated with a clinical response. Initially this response was presumed to be related to extragonadal production of androgens.[12] An additional factor underlying such responses may also reside within prostate cancer tissue itself. Several studies have demonstrated amplification and increased expression of androgen receptor in xenografts with hormone resistance and in prostate cancer tissues from patients with CRPC.[13–15] In vitro and in vivo, increased androgen receptor expression has been shown to be required for transformation of prostate cell lines from a hormone-sensitive to a hormone-refractory phenotype, with the effect being ligand-dependent and genotropic.[14] High androgen receptor levels were also associated with a change in the effect of bicalutamide from an androgen receptor antagonist to agonist providing a further basis for antiandrogen withdrawal affecting a positive clinical response.[14] Inhibition of the androgen receptor in hormone-refractory tumor models has also been shown to induce regression.[16] Prostate cancer cells and human tissues also possess the biochemical machinery to synthesize androgens,[17–20] invoking an autocrine/paracrine mechanism for castration-resistant progression. Ligand-independent mechanisms may occur through androgen receptor splice variants lacking the ligand binding domain that are constitutively active.[21] In light of our evolving understanding of the mechanisms of castration resistance, a strategy to develop more potent inhibitors of extragonadal androgen production and antagonists of the androgen receptor[22] has been a rational and active area for drug development. Results of clinical trials of 2 such agents targeting mechanisms of androgen receptor activation, abiraterone acetate (Couger Biotechnology Inc) and MDV3100 (Medivation Inc), have recently been reported. The early results of these clinical trials are encouraging and confirm clinically that CRPC commonly remains dependent on androgen receptor signaling.

Abiraterone acetate is an orally administered medication that inhibits the cytochrome P450 enzyme CYP17A1. This enzyme has dual function as a 17α-hydroxylase and $C_{17,20}$-lyase; both these functions are necessary to synthesize androgens from cholesterol precursors. Treatment doses at all levels studied were well tolerated in a phase I trial that enrolled patients with CRPC who were chemotherapy naive.[23] Reported toxicities were largely anticipated in light of the mechanism of action of abiraterone with mineralcorticoid excess (hypertension, hypokalemia, edema). In most cases these were easily controlled by administration of an aldosterone antagonist (eplerenone) or corticosteroids. PSA decreases of 30% or more and 50% or more were observed in 66% and 57% of patients, respectively. High rates of response have been observed in several phase II trials of abiraterone in patients with CRPC who were chemotherapy naive and who had progressed after docetaxel therapy. A phase II trial recently reported data from 27 chemotherapy-naive patients with CRPC, and PSA decreases of more than 50% from baseline were observed in 85% of patients.[24] In another early report of a phase II trial of 47 patients who had previously received docetaxel, 51% of patients were noted to have a PSA decrease of 50% or more.[25] Of 35 patients with measurable disease, 6 (17%) had a partial response. Seventeen patients remained on therapy for more than 6 months and the median duration of treatment was an impressive 167 days. An improvement in performance status was seen in 23% of patients compared with baseline. Treatment was well tolerated with only grade 1 to 2 adverse events reported. Data from another phase II trial suggest that patients who have previously received cytotoxic chemotherapy, but who have not received prior high dose ketoconazole (which also suppresses steroidogenesis through P450-dependent enzymes), may have increased rates of response and time to PSA progression compared with those who have been exposed to ketoconazole.[26]

A randomized, double-blind, placebo-controlled trial of abiraterone and prednisone has completed accrual of a planned enrolment of 1158 patients with CRPC who are progressing after docetaxel (http://clinicaltrials.gov identifier: NCT00638690). Patients were randomized 2:1 in favor of abiraterone, and the trial is powered to detect a difference in median overall survival of 15 months in the abiraterone-prednisone group versus 13 months in the placebo-prednisone group (hazard ratio [HR] = 0.80). A second phase III trial with abiraterone has been initiated in patients with CRPC who are chemotherapy naive and asymptomatic or minimally symptomatic (not requiring opiate analgesics). The primary end points for this study are overall survival and progression-free survival with an estimated enrolment of 1000 patients (NCT00887198).

MDV3100 is a potent novel small androgen receptor antagonist that prevents nuclear translocation and DNA binding of androgen receptor, and, unlike bicalutamide, possesses no agonistic activity. A first-in-man, multicenter phase I/II dose escalation study has been reported and shows encouraging clinical results. Treatment has been well tolerated and early results indicate that at 12 weeks, 57% of chemotherapy-naive patients and 45% of chemotherapy-pretreated patients had a 50% or greater decrease in PSA compared with baseline. Data to date suggest a dose response, especially in patients previously treated with chemotherapy.[27] Given this, 160 mg/d has been selected as the dosage for a phase III trial in which approximately 1200 patients with CRPC who have progressed after docetaxel will be randomized 2:1 in favor of MDV3100 versus placebo (NCT00974311). The primary end point of the trial is overall survival.

VASCULAR ENDOTHELIAL GROWTH FACTOR AND RECEPTOR

Growth beyond a few millimeters and the ability to metastasize are dependent on a malignant tumor's ability to recruit new vasculature in a process known as angiogenesis. Several mediators of angiogenesis have been identified, including vascular endothelial growth factor (VEGF) which signals through VEGF receptors (VEGFR) 1 and 2 to promote angiogenesis. Elevated VEGFR, notably VEGFR-2, has been associated with progression of prostate cancer in the TRAMP model and is also over expressed in human prostate cancers.[28] In patients with metastatic CRPC, increased plasma VEGF as a continuous or dichotomous variable has been correlated with poor prognosis and disease progression.[29] Antitumor effects have been observed with inhibition of the VEGF/VEGFR pathways in experimental models of prostate cancer.[30] The combination of VEGF inhibition with chemotherapy may result in an indirect antitumor effect by enhancing permeability via vascular normalization.[31] Given this sound preclinical rationale, targeting of the VEGF pathway is a reasonable therapeutic approach for patients with prostate cancer and 3 such agents are currently in phase III trials: bevacizumab (Genentech), aflibercept (Sanofi-Aventis) and sunitinib (Pfizer Inc).

Bevacizumab is a monoclonal antibody directed against VEGF-A and causes potent inhibition of VEGFR signaling and angiogenesis. Bevacizumab has reported single agent activity in renal cell cancer,[32] and is approved for use in combination with chemotherapy for patients with metastatic colorectal, breast, and lung cancers. Bevacizumab-associated toxicities include hypertension, thromboembolism, hemorrhage, gastrointestinal perforation, and proteinuria. The *Cancer and Leukemia Group B* (CALGB) has conducted a phase II trial of bevacizumab in combination with docetaxel-estramustine chemotherapy in patients with metastatic CRPC.[33] A PSA decrease of more than 50% from baseline occurred in 81% of patients, and the median time to progression (for objective disease or PSA) was in the 9 months range. Overall survival for the group was 21 months. A phase III randomized placebo-controlled trial evaluating the effects on overall survival from docetaxel, prednisone, and bevacizumab versus docetaxel and prednisone has fully accrued the planned 1020 subjects and results are awaited (NCT00110214). Bevacizumab has also been tested in combination with docetaxel and RAD001 (an inhibitor of mTOR) in chemotherapy-naive patients,[34] and in combination with satraplatin (an oral chemotherapy) in patients previously treated with docetaxel.[35] Both combinations were reasonably well tolerated, but more later-phase data will be required to establish efficacy and to determine whether either of these combinations will find a role in the standard treatment of CRPC.

Aflibercept (VEGF Trap) is a recombinantly produced fusion protein consisting of human VEGF receptor extracellular domains fused to the Fc portion of human immunoglobulin (Ig) G1. Aflibercept is a potent inhibitor of VEGF-A, VEGF-B, and other VEGF family members like placental growth factor that bind to VEGFR-1 and VEGFR-2, by binding and inactivating these circulating factors.[36] Given the similar mechanism of action, the adverse events are comparable with those seen with bevacizumab. Phase I trials have demonstrated the safety of aflibercept in combination with docetaxel.[37] A phase III, randomized, double-blind, placebo-controlled trial is underway for patients with metastatic CRPC (NCT00519285).

Sunitinib is an orally administered multitargeted tyrosine kinase inhibitor including the receptor kinase activity of VEGFR, platelet-derived growth factor receptor, and KIT. Sunitinib has been shown to significantly improve progression-free survival in metastatic renal cell cancer and is therefore approved for use.[38] A phase II study investigating sunitinib in patients with metastatic CRPC has been presented.[39] This trial determined progression based on clinical and radiological (ie, non-PSA based) parameters, with the primary objective being to determine whether sunitinib therapy was associated with a clinical progression-free survival of 12 weeks in more than 30% of patients. All patients had received 1 or 2 prior chemotherapies including docetaxel. A 12-week progression-free survival was attained in 78.9% of patients. Forty-seven percent of patients discontinued therapy because of toxicity and there were 2 early deaths. A phase III study has been initiated that will randomize patients with CRPC progressing after docetaxel to receive sunitinib or placebo in a 2:1

fashion (in favor of sunitinib). The primary end point is overall survival, and a planned 819 patients will be enrolled (NCT00676650). More recently, a phase II study was presented looking at sunitinib in combination with docetaxel as a first-line treatment in 55 patients with metastatic CRPC.[40] Although the PSA response rate was encouraging with 31 (56%) patients showing a PSA response, the combination resulted in an increase in adverse events with a rate of febrile neutropenia of 15% and dose reductions were required for sunitinib (26% of patients) and docetaxel (33% of patients).

Other VEGFR targeted agents have also been studied in prostate cancer. Sorafenib is an orally administered multitargeted kinase inhibitor and has inhibitory action against Raf kinase, PDGFR, VEGFR-2 and -3, and c-kit pathways. Sorafenib has proven efficacy for treatment of advanced renal cell carcinoma[41] and hepatocellular carcinoma.[42] In prostate cancer, phase II trials of single agent sorafenib used in the pre- or post-docetaxel setting have reported modest activity with a low rate of PSA responses and a median progression-free survival of 2 to 4 months.[43,44] However, discordant responses in these trials were seen with increasing PSA levels but improved scans or symptoms, suggesting that PSA may not be reliable as a marker of an antitumor effect with sorafenib. Interest has also been garnered surrounding the hypothesis that sorafenib may potentiate the effects of docetaxel. A phase I dose-escalation study recently reported that the combination of docetaxel and sorafenib was well tolerated with no dose-limiting toxicity observed at the doses tested; the recommended dose of sorafenib was 400 mg twice daily given continuously with standard dose docetaxel 75 mg/m^2 every 3 weeks. There was, however, a high rate of febrile neutropenia (8 of 24 patients) and uncomplicated neutropenia (5 of 24 patients).[45] Preliminary results of a phase II study using docetaxel and sorafenib as first-line treatment in men with CRPC also showed discordant PSA/clinical response.[46] A similar finding was reported recently in a phase II study in which patients who had progressed on docetaxel or mitoxantrone were rechallenged with the same chemotherapy on which they had progressed in addition to sorafenib.[47] Fourteen patients were evaluable at the time of reporting. Of these, 11 (73%) had stable disease radiographically for a median time of 6.7 months. Six of 14 (42%) patients had a decrease in PSA level after adding sorafenib. PSA responses did not correlate with radiographic changes or clinical benefit.

Cediranib is an orally administered small molecule that potently inhibits VEGFR tyrosine kinase. A phase II study using cediranib after progression on docetaxel has recently been reported. The primary end point was progression-free survival as determined by clinical and radiographic criteria (ie, not PSA level). Twenty-three of 34 enrolled patients were evaluable; of those, 13 showed tumor shrinkage and 4 met the criteria for partial response. As with the previous studies, PSA levels did not correlate well with imaging responses.[48]

APOPTOSIS

Resistance to apoptosis or programmed cell death is another mechanism attributed to prostate cancer progression and treatment resistance. The *bcl-2* gene (B-cell leukemia-lymphoma gene 2) is the prototype of a class of oncogenes that contributes to neoplastic progression by enhancing tumor cell survival through inhibition of apoptosis. Bcl-2 is a mitochondrial membrane protein that was initially identified in follicular lymphoma. By heterodimerizing with Bax and other proapoptotic regulators it prevents release of cytochrome *c* and subsequent activation of the apoptotic cascade. The selective and competitive dimerization between pairs of these antagonists and agonists of the Bcl-2 family of proteins determines how a cell responds to an apoptotic signal. Over-expression of *bcl-2* has been shown to be associated with treatment resistance. In prostate cancer, *bcl-2* has been found to be expressed in clinical samples of androgen-dependent and -independent disease,[49] and experimental and clinical studies report that increased expression of *bcl-2* confers, or is associated with, the development of androgen independence and treatment resistance.[50,51] G3139 (Genta, Inc) is an 18-mer phosphorothioate antisense oligonucleotide complimentary to the first 6 codons of the initiating sequence of the human *bcl-2* mRNA. In preclinical prostate cancer models, G3139 and other *bcl-2* antisense oligonucleotides have shown significant activity in inhibiting expression of *bcl-2*, delaying time to the development of androgen independence, and enhancing the effects of chemotherapy by increased apoptosis.[51] Phase I trials with prolonged infusions of G3139 as a single agent or in combination with chemotherapy have shown good tolerability.[52,53] Initial results have been reported from a randomized phase II trial in 115 patients with CRPC, which was conducted by the European Organisation for Research and Treatment of Cancer (EORTC).[54] Patients randomized to receive combination therapy received a median of 2 fewer cycle of treatment (6 vs 8 cycles), and the PSA response rate was numerically lower in the combination therapy arm (37% vs 46%). Further trials for this agent in CRPC are not known to be planned.

One possible explanation for a lack of clinical benefit being observed with G3139 is that there are several prosurvival bcl-2 family members. The specific targeting of only 1 member may simply be insufficient to overcome apoptotic resistance exerted by the other bcl-2 family members. This hypothesis is supported by preclinical testing in which enhanced regressions in cancer models treated with combined targeting of antiapoptotic bcl-2 family members was observed.[55] AT101 (Ascenta Therapeutics, Inc) is a small molecule inhibitor of multiple antiapoptotic Bcl-2 family members (Bcl-2, Bcl-X_L, Bcl-W, Mcl-1) derived from gossypol, which is a natural compound from cotton seeds. AT101 has single agent and combination activity in vitro and in vivo. In a single agent phase II trial with 23 chemotherapy-naive patients with CRPC, 2 (9%) had decreases in PSA level of 50% or more that were confirmed and 5 (22%) additional patients had decreases in PSA level ranging from 3% to 54%.[56] Adverse events included diarrhea, fatigue, nausea, anorexia, and small bowel obstruction necessitating dose reduction. A phase I/II trial of AT101 in combination with standard docetaxel and prednisone with escalating doses of AT101 has been completed and a recommended phase II dose was identified with several PSA responses observed.[57] Based on the promising early clinical data, a randomized phase II trial is currently ongoing. The accrual goal is 220 patients with chemotherapy-naive metastatic CRPC, and the trial is designed to evaluate docetaxel with or without AT101 with a primary end point of overall survival (NCT00571675).

CHAPERONE PROTEINS

The heat shock protein-90 (Hsp90) molecular chaperone complex is essential for androgen receptor stability and maturation, and has been identified as a potential therapeutic target for CRPC. Hsp90 also acts as a chaperone to several other client proteins associated with malignant progression (Akt, Raf-1, HER-2, and hypoxia-inducible factor-1α).[58] Hsp90 is an ATP-dependent chaperone, and several specific inhibitors have been developed against its ATPase activity. Small molecule inhibitors of histone deacetylase (HDAC) can also result in the loss of Hsp90 ATP binding activity through acetylation and subsequent degradation of androgen receptor.[59–62] HDAC inhibitors are also of interest as the frequently occurring TMPRSS2:ETS gene fusions in prostate cancer[63] may result in epigenetic reprogramming including upregulation of HDAC-1 and downregulation of its targets[64] with resultant susceptibility to HDAC inhibition.[65]

17-Allylamino-17-demethoxygeldanamycin (17-AAG) is a benzoquinone ansamycin antibiotic. In preclinical models it has exhibited antitumor activity and is presumed to act by binding to the Hsp90 ATP binding site. Phase I trials have demonstrated the safety of the agent in humans, however a recent phase II trial in patients with CRPC reported only minimal clinical activity.[66] Similarly, HDAC inhibitors in phase II trials involving patients with CRPC have yet to demonstrate any clinically significant activity.[67] Despite these early failures, other Hsp90 and HDAC inhibitors continue to be evaluated.

Clusterin is another chaperone protein of interest. Clusterin exists as an intracellular truncated 55-kDa nuclear form (nCLU) which is proapoptotic[68] and a 75- to 80-kDa secreted heterodimer disulfide-linked glycoprotein (sCLU), which has been shown to be antiapoptotic.[69] Clusterin has been defined mostly in its role of inhibiting apoptosis. Clusterin expression is induced after therapeutic stress and functions as a cytoprotective chaperone similar to an ATP-independent small heat shock protein, and is transcriptionally activated by heat shock factor-1.[70] Clusterin's ability to inhibit apoptosis has also been shown to act through inhibition of activated Bax, a critical proapoptotic Bcl-2 family member.[69] Furthermore, over-expression of clusterin leads to activation of the PI-3Kinase/Akt pathway through the megalin cell surface receptor.[71] Clusterin expression increases in response to cell stress induced by a variety of factors in xenograft models and forced over-expression of clusterin confers resistance to radiation, hormone treatment, and chemotherapy, whereas inhibition of clusterin expression enhances apoptotic death from these treatment modalities.[72] Clusterin has been associated with androgen-independent progression in preclinical models of prostate cancer.[51] Clusterin is over-expressed in a variety of human cancers including prostate, in which its expression increases after castration and with castration-resistant disease.[73]

OGX-011 (OncoGenex Pharmaceuticals Inc) is a second-generation phosphorothioate antisense molecule with a prolonged tissue half-life. OGX-011 has been shown to significantly decrease sCLU expression through inhibition of clusterin mRNA translation in vitro and in vivo. Phase I trials have established that OGX-011 can inhibit clusterin expression in prostate cancer tissues in humans and that standard doses of chemotherapy can be delivered with OGX-011 at biologically active doses.[74,75] A randomized phase

II trial of OGX-011 with mitoxantrone or docetaxel in patients with CRPC that had previously progressed on or within 3 months of completing docetaxel reported tolerability but also interesting antitumor activity.[76] In patients treated with the combination of mitoxantrone and OGX-011, 27% had a decrease in PSA level of more than 50% from baseline, and median overall survival was 11.4 months. In those subjects who received OGX-011 with docetaxel, 40% had a 50% decrease in PSA level from baseline and a median overall survival of 14.7 months. Another phase II study with OGX-011 randomized 82 patients with chemotherapy-naive metastatic CRPC to receive first-line docetaxel with or without OGX-011.[77] Decreases in PSA level were similar between groups, although there appeared to be fewer patients with progression as best response and a longer time to progression in the doceaxtel/OGX-011 combination therapy group. Mature results from this study reported a median overall survival of 16.9 months for the docetaxel group and 23.8 months for those subjects treated with docetaxel/OGX-011 combination.[78] In a multivariate analysis factors significantly associated with an improved overall survival were an Eastern Collaborative Oncology Group (ECOG) performance status of 0 versus 1, presence of bone or lymph node metastases only versus other metastases, and treatment arm assignment to OGX-011 plus docetaxel versus docetaxel alone (HR = 0.49, 95% CI 0.28–0.85). A phase III trial is being planned to compare docetaxel/OGX-011 versus docetaxel in patients with metastatic CRPC with a primary end point of overall survival.

INSULINLIKE GROWTH FACTOR-1 RECEPTOR

The insulinlike growth factor (IGF) axis is composed of 2 peptide growth factors (IGF-I and -II), 2 transmembrane receptors (IGF-IR and -IIR), 6 IGF binding proteins (IGFBP-1 to -6), and IGFBP proteases. Among their many actions, IGFs regulate cellular processes of proliferation, differentiation, and apoptosis, and as a result have been implicated as having a critical role in the development of several malignancies. In a metaregression analysis, elevated concentrations of IGF-I and risk of prostate cancer have been correlated, and high plasma IGF-I and low IGFBP-3 have been associated with more advanced stage prostate cancer.[79,80] IGF-IR, IGF-I and -II, and IGFBP-2 have all been reported to be over expressed in human primary prostate cancer compared with normal prostate tissue. Levels are also increased in advanced and metastatic disease.[81] An increasing body of evidence has linked activation of the IGF axis with androgen-independent progression of prostate cancer.[82] These findings have made targeting the IGF axis an attractive concept for prostate cancer. Using a variety of methods to block IGF signaling, preclinical studies have supported this theory.[83]

Humanized monoclonal antibodies specific to IGF-IR, selected to have limited agonistic effect or affinity to the homologous insulin receptor, have entered clinical testing. Testing in prostate cancer has been initiated with 2 humanized monoclonal therapeutic antibodies against IGF-IR: CP-751,871 (Pfizer Inc) and IMC-A12 (ImClone Systems Inc). Both agents have been well tolerated in early clinical studies. The tolerability of the regimen was demonstrated in a phase I trial of the combination of CP-751,871 and docetaxel. A randomized phase II of docetaxel with or without CP-751,871 has been conducted and results are pending (NCT00313781). A single agent phase II study with IMC-A12 in asymptomatic, chemotherapy-naive patients with CRPC was reported recently. Thirty-one patients were enrolled, and the trial was designed to assess safety and antitumor activity. The most common adverse events related to IMC-A12 were fatigue and hyperglycemia; the hyperglycemia was asymptomatic and easily managed in most cases. Other related events included thrombocytopenia, hyperkalemia, and pneumonia. Nineteen of the 31 patients had disease stability for 6 months or more, and 5 patients continue on IMC-A12.[84] Further studies are planned.

PHOSPHATIDYLINOSITOL-3-KINASE (PI3K)-AKT SIGNALING PATHWAY

An important signal transduction pathway downstream of growth factor receptors like IGF-1R is the PI3K-Akt (also known as protein kinase B) pathway. After activation by receptor tyrosine kinases, PI3Ks catalyze the transfer of a phosphate group to generate phosphatidylinositol-3,4,5 trisphosphate (PIP3) from phosphatidylinositol-4,5 bisphosphate (PIP2). PIP3 serves to recruit Akt to the inner cell membrane where it is activated. Activation of Akt leads to phosphorylation of several downstream targets such as mTOR (mammalian target of rapamycin) and others that have an effect on critical cellular functions including proliferation, growth, apoptosis, glucose homeostasis, nutrient response, and DNA damage. PTEN is a tumor suppressor gene whose product is a lipid phosphatase that negatively regulates the PI3K-Akt pathway by regenerating PIP2 from PIP3.[85,86] The rationale in prostate cancer for targeting the PI3K-Akt pathway is based on evidence that it contributes to castration-resistant progression through mechanisms including activation of the androgen receptor and androgen responsive genes.[87,88] PTEN is also frequently deleted in prostate cancer and has been identified as a negative prognostic factor.[89]

Targeting mTOR as an important downstream effector of the PI3K/Akt pathway is a rational approach. The mTOR inhibitor sirolimus, also known as rapamycin, is an immunosuppressive agent used after solid organ transplant and as an antiproliferative agent in patients with coronary artery stents. A small phase I study using rapamycin in 13 patients with CRPC showed some low level of activity,[90] and additional trials using other mTOR inhibitors as single agents or in combination in patients with prostate cancer are ongoing (eg, deforolimus [NCT00110188], temsirolimus [NCT00919035], everolimus [NCT00629525]). One concern is that mTOR inhibition may induce feedback activation of Akt signaling through IGF-1R.[91] Thus, combined blockade of IGF-1R signaling and mTOR inhibition is a rational approach and is being tested in the phase I setting (eg, NCT00730379). Alternatively, upstream targeting of PI3K and Akt directly is an attractive prospect and several inhibitors are in early phase clinical development.

BONE TARGETING

Therapies directed toward the biologic underpinnings of bone progression are a rational treatment direction given the propensity for prostate cancer to metastasize to bone. Bisphosphonates are an established treatment for patients with metastatic CRPC and studies continue to define their use for earlier disease. Additional agents targeting bone metastases–related biologic targets are also under clinical development.

RANK Ligand

Receptor activator of nuclear factor kappa B (RANK) and its ligand (RANK-L) have been identified as mediators that increase osteoclastogenesis. RANK-L is a member of the tumor necrosis factor (TNF) superfamily and is expressed by osteoblasts. RANK-L binding to RANK is necessary and sufficient to stimulate osteoclast cell differentiation, proliferation, and to inhibit osteoclast apoptosis. The effects of RANK are blocked by the secretory glycoprotein osteoprotegerin (OPG), which is a decoy receptor for RANK-L and thus functions to hinder the ability of RANK-L to stimulate bone resorption. The interplay between OPG, RANK-L, and RANK is critical in the pathogenesis of bone metastases[92] and implicated in advanced prostate cancer.[93,94]

Denosumab (Amgen Inc) is a fully humanized monoclonal antibody specifically directed against RANK-L that can be administered via subcutaneous injection. Denosumab has proven activity in reducing bone resorption and increasing bone density compared with placebo or bisphosphonates in patients with physiologic and treatment-related bone loss.[95,96] Treatment with denosumab is well tolerated, with little difference in related adverse event rates between denosumab treated patients and those treated with placebo. Osteonecrosis of the jaw is an infrequent but significant toxicity associated with bisphosphonate usage that can occur in up to 5% to 10% of patients, but seems dependent on the length of exposure.[97] A randomized, double-blind, placebo-controlled trial of denosumab versus zoledronic acid in patients with bone metastatic CRPC has completed accrual. The primary end point of the trial is incidence of skeletal-related events and final results are expected to be reported after 2010 (NCT00321620).

Endothelin-1

Endothelins (ET) are peptides containing 21 amino acids that were first described as potent vasoconstrictors but were later identified as being elevated in men with metastatic prostate cancer and as mediators of the osteoblastic response of bone to metastatic disease.[98] Three forms of ET have been described (ET-1, -2, -3) which bind to 2 receptors, ET receptor A and B (ET-A, ET-B). ET-1 preferentially binds to ET-A where, in addition to mediating a vasoconstriction response, ET-A signaling has been associated with proliferation, antiapoptotic effects, and pain. ET-B functions as a decoy receptor and clearance mechanism for ET-1, thus mitigating its effects. ET-1 production by metastatic prostate cells in bone has been shown to be stimulated by osteoblasts, which are in turn stimulated by ET-1 to proliferate, thereby stimulating new bone formation and osteoblastic metastases, contributing to a vicious cycle of progression.[99]

Atrasentan (Abbott Laboratories) is an orally bioavailable competitive inhibitor of ET-1 binding with 1800-fold selectivity to the ET-A receptor compared with ET-B. Treatment with atrasentan is well tolerated and side effects are related to vasodilation and include peripheral edema, rhinitis, and headache. There have been rare incidences of heart failure, and hypotension and hyponatremia were dose limiting in phase I trials. In a randomized, double-blind, phase II study,

288 patients with metastatic CRPC received atrasentan at a lower dose (2.5 mg), higher dose (10 mg), or placebo.[87] A nonsignificant increase in time to progression was observed in the intention to treat population for the group on the 10-mg dose (183 vs 137 days). This result achieved statistical significance when only per protocol evaluable patients were considered (196 vs 129 days, $P = .021$, n = 244). Changes in bone deposition and turnover markers were lower in the patients treated with atrasentan. A multinational, double-blind, placebo-controlled trial was subsequently undertaken.[100] Eight-hundred and nine patients were randomized to placebo or atrasentan 10 mg/d. There was evidence of biologic effect with atrasentan, with a delay in the increase in bone alkaline phosphates as a marker of bone deposition, however the primary end point of time to progression was not significantly different, with most patients progressing at the first disease assessment at 12 weeks into the study. As progression was overwhelmingly defined on radiographic changes, as opposed to clinical/symptomatic progression, it is unclear whether the study design allowed for a true assessment of the clinical effects of atrasentan, as the changes in imaging may have reflected progression that had occurred between baseline scanning and start of study drug or just after start of study drug. A second phase III trial in patients with nonmetastatic CRPC with progression as the primary end point was also performed. Similarly, biologic effects were observed with a decrease in bone alkaline phosphatase, however time to progression was not different statistically.[101] Development of atrasentan continues in combination with docetaxel. A phase I/II trial has been performed in patients with CRPC with a maximum tolerated dose of docetaxel identified as being 70 to 75 mg/m^2 with atrasentan given at 10 mg/d.[102] Drug-related grade 3 to 4 toxicities included a fairly high febrile neutropenia rate of 16% to 25%. Confirmed PSA responses were 23% and median overall survival was 17.6 months, both of which are lower than expected from prior studies with docetaxel. A phase III trial involving 930 patients with metastatic CRPC and a primary end point of overall survival is being conducted by the Southwest Oncology Group, comparing docetaxel and prednisone versus docetaxel, prednisone, and atrasentan (NCT00134056).

ZD4054 (AstraZeneca) is a more specific inhibitor of ET-A with no reported binding to ET-B, and thus a potentially more active agent as the mitigating effects of ET-B on ET-1/ET-A signaling remain unhampered. A randomized phase II trial was performed comparing patients who had received ZD4054 at a 10 mg/d, 15 mg/d, or placebo.[103] No difference was observed in the primary end point of progression, however an overall survival difference emerged in favor of the ZD4054 10 mg and 15 mg treatment groups (24.5 and 23.5 months respectively, vs 17.3 months for placebo). Three phase III trials are now enrolling comparing ZD4054 to placebo in patients with CRPC and no clinical metastases (NCT00626548), with bone metastases but with minimal or no symptoms (NCT00554229), and in patients receiving docetaxel chemotherapy (NCT00617669).

Src Family Kinases

Src is the prototypical member of the Src family of nonreceptor tyrosine kinases. Src is involved in signal transduction downstream of multiple cell surface receptors including EGFR, PDGFR, VEGFR, and integrins, and thus is implicated in multiple cellular processes including differentiation, proliferation, adhesion, and migration. Src, related kinases, and their upstream cell surface receptors have been implicated in prostate cancer progression and are frequently over expressed in CRPC. Increases in the activity of Src family kinases have been correlated with the presence of distant metastases and poor outcomes.[104] Src signaling is important for normal functioning of osteoclasts, bone resorption, and osteoblast proliferation and bone deposition, and implicated in bone metastases progression.[105]

Dasatinib (Bristol-Myers-Squibb Co) was clinically developed for its activity against the Bcr-Abl tyrosine kinase associated with chronic myelogenous leukemia. Dasatinib was subsequently shown to have activity against Src family kinases resulting in direct antitumor effects in preclinical models of prostate cancer suppressing cell adhesion, migration, and invasion.[106] Phase II trials using dasatinib in a twice daily[107] and once daily[108] dosing regimen have been performed in patients with prostate cancer. Only 1 patient in each of the trials had a PSA response of more than 50% decrease, however lesser decreases were noted and decreases in bone turnover markers (serum bone alkaline phosphatase and urinary *N*-telopepetide) were also observed, providing proof of principal biologic activity data. A phase I/II study of docetaxel and dasatinib revealed the combination to be safe and tolerable. PSA responses were observed in 13 of 32 patients (41%), and of 31 patients with bone scans 30 had best response of improved (32%) or stable (65%) disease at 6 weeks or more.[109] A randomized phase III study of docetaxel with or without dasatinib is now being conducted with a primary end point of overall survival and planned accrual of more than 1300 patients (NCT00744497). AZD-0530 (AstraZeneca) is another orally administered Src-kinase inhibitor in clinical trials. A phase II study is being conducted randomizing patients with bone metastases from breast or prostate cancer to receive AZD-0530 or zoledronic acid (NCT00558272). The primary objective of this study is to compare changes in markers of bone turnover.

Radiopharmaceuticals

Radiopharmaceuticals are indicated for patients with multifocal painful bone metastases, or for those patients who have persistent pain despite adequate attempts at palliation with external-beam radiation. Samarium-153-ethylene diamine tetramethylene phosphonic acid ([^{153}Sm]EDTMP) is a bone targeted radiopharmaceutical that has previously been assessed for its palliative properties as a single agent. In 2 randomized, placebo-controlled trials [^{153}Sm]EDTMP was found to result in improved pain control that was durable compared with placebo.[110,111] Transient myelosuppression was the most common toxicity associated with treatment. Preclinical data support the synergism of docetaxel and [^{153}Sm]EDTMP, and early phase studies have recently been reported evaluating the safety and efficacy of this combination.[112–114] Therapy with docetaxel and [^{153}Sm]EDTMP was tolerable with reversible marrow toxicity as the most common adverse event. In a phase II study, 43 patients with CRPC who had achieved a response or stabilization after 4 cycles of docetaxel/estramustine were given consolidation docetaxel (20 mg/m^2) for 6 weeks and [^{153}Sm]EDTMP during week 1. PSA response rate was 77%, and the pain response rate was 69%. The 1- and 2-year survival rates were 77% and 56%, respectively. Pain, as assessed by visual analog scale, was affected favorably in the long-term.[114] These data suggest that the combination of docetaxel and [^{153}Sm]EDTMP is safe and may have more activity than either agent alone.[115]

The α-emitter radium-223 (^{223}Ra) is a new bone-seeking radionuclide studied as a single-agent therapy in a randomized, multicentre, phase II study. Patients with CRPC and bone pain needing external-beam radiotherapy were assigned to 4 intravenous (IV) injections of ^{223}Ra (33 patients) or placebo (31 patients), given every 4 weeks. The primary end points were change in bone alkaline phosphatase concentration and time to skeletal-related events. There was an improvement in the median bone alkaline phosphatase during treatment (−65.6% [95% CI −69.5 to −57.7]) versus 9.3% (3.8–60.9) in the ^{223}Ra group and placebo groups, respectively (P<.0001) but no statistical difference in the time to first skeletal-related event. The HR for overall survival, adjusted for baseline covariates, was 2.12 (1.13–3.98, P = .020) in favor of ^{223}Ra.[116] Based on these results, a phase III study is underway in patients with CRPC with a primary end point of overall survival and a planned enrolment of 750 patients. Patients are required to be symptomatic with no chemotherapy planned for 6 months and not eligible for docetaxel (NCT00699751).

CYTOTOXIC AGENTS

The epothilones are a newer class of cytotoxic agents produced from the myxobacterium *Sorangium cellulosum*, which, like taxanes, inhibit the function of microtubules as their primary mechanism of action; this results in arrest of mitotic activity at the G2/M phase of the cell cycle. To date, epothilones A to F have been identified and characterized. In preclinical cell lines, it has been established that the epothilones are more potent in their anticancer effects than the taxanes.[117] Given their increased water solubility, epothilones do not require preparation in cremaphore, the causative agent in most hypersensitivity reactions in patients being treated with paclitaxel.[118] Several epothilones have been clinically tested in the chemotherapy-naive and post docetaxel setting of CRPC.

Ixabepilone (BMS-247,550, Bristol-Myers-Squibb) is a semisynthetic derivative of epothilone B. One randomized phase II study comparing ixabepilone (given every 3 weeks) to mitoxantrone and prednisone in the postdocetaxel population found no significant difference in PSA response rate or in median survival between the 2 arms.[119] A second phase II study evaluated weekly ixabepilone in 69 patients, 37 of whom had had previous exposure to taxanes. The rate of neutropenia was lower than that reported in the every 3 weeks regimen (14% vs 54%), but there was a 13% rate of grade 3/4 neuropathy or fatigue reported among patients who had previously been treated with docetaxel. PSA response was observed in 22% of patients and objective response was seen in 27%.[120] More recently, ixabepilone has been tested in combination with mitoxantrone and prednisone in patients progressing after docetaxel. A phase II multicentre study has been presented in abstract form. Patients received ixabepilone (35 mg/m^2) and mitoxantrone (12 mg/m^2) IV every 2 weeks and prednisone 5 mg orally twice daily. Support with G-CSF was given prophylactically. Of the 37 patients evaluable for response, 14 (38%) have had a decrease in PSA level of more than 50%, and 19 (51%) have had a decrease in PSA level of more than 30%. Fifteen patients had measurable disease, and, of those, 2 (13%) have had an objective response as defined by RECIST (*Response Evaluation Criteria in Solid Tumors*). The most common grade 3/4 toxicities included neutropenia (17%), thrombocytopenia (8%), fatigue, and pneumonia.[121]

Epothilone B (patupilone, EPO906, Novartis) has also been studied in phase II trials. One such trial looked at once weekly administration of patupilone in 37 patients, 29 of whom had had treatment with 1 prior chemotherapy regimen. PSA responses were observed in 22% of evaluable patients. Grade 3/4 diarrhea was seen in 19% of patients.[122] Based on preclinical data that dosing every 3 weeks was more efficacious and less toxic, a phase II study was conducted using that schedule in patients having progressed after docetaxel. Eighty-three patients were enrolled and there was minimal hematologic toxicity with no hematologic grade 3/4 adverse events observed. Grade 3/4 fatigue was seen in 16%, diarrhea in 13%, and anorexia in 5%. PSA response (defined as a confirmed >50% decrease from baseline) was seen in 45% of evaluable patients; decrease in PSA level of more than 30% was seen in 56%. Median progression-free survival for PSA and non-PSA outcomes (measurable disease, symptomatic progression, or death) was 7.6 months and 5.6 months, respectively.[123] Based on the encouraging tolerability and the promising data on progression-free survival, the investigators of this study encouraged further study of patupilone in this population.

Sagopilone (ZK-EPO, Bayer) is the first fully synthetic epothilone that has been produced and tested in a phase II study enrolling chemotherapy-naive patients with CRPC. Fifty-three patients were enrolled of whom 42% had a decrease in PSA level of more than 50%. Of those patients who had measurable disease (N = 39), 1 had a complete response, and 9 (26%) had partial response. Median progression-free survival was 6.4 months. Grade 3 neuropathy occurred in 19% of patients, and fatigue was the other most commonly reported grade 3 adverse event.[124] Based on the tolerability of sagopilone and the observation that the decrease in PSA level and progression-free survival approximated that of the current standard of care (docetaxel and prednisone), the investigators concluded that further study of this agent is warranted.

SUMMARY

In the last 2 decades, there has been an increasing understanding of the biologic underpinnings of cancer in general, and prostate cancer specifically, relating to androgen-independent progression, factors affecting cell proliferation and survival, and mediators of metastases. Coupled with rational drug design and more sophisticated trial end points, a large number of therapeutic agents have entered clinical trials in the last decade, which promises to significantly change our management of patients with CRPC in the near future. Any benefits that emerge in the late stage castration-resistant state with these agents would provide a strong rationale to bring them forward as combination strategies and to earlier disease settings.

REFERENCES

1. Jemal A, Siegel R, Ward E, et al. Cancer statistics. CA Cancer J Clin 2008;58:71–96.
2. D'Amico AV, Whittington R, Malkowicz SB, et al. Biochemical outcome after radical prostatectomy, external beam radiation therapy, or interstitial radiation therapy for clinically localized prostate cancer. JAMA 1998;280:969–74.
3. Scher HI, Halabi S, Tannock I, et al. Design and end points of clinical trials for patients with progressive prostate cancer and castrate levels of testosterone: recommendations of the prostate cancer clinical trials working group. J Clin Oncol 2008;26:1148–59.
4. Heidenreich A, Aus G, Bolla M, et al. EAU guidelines on prostate cancer. Eur Urol 2008;53:68–80.
5. Tannock IF, Osoba D, Stockler MR, et al. Chemotherapy with mitoxantrone plus prednisone or prednisone alone for symptomatic hormone-resistant prostate cancer: a Canadian randomized trial with palliative end points. J Clin Oncol 1996;14:1756–64.
6. Oosterhof GO, Roberts JT, de Reijke TM, et al. Strontium(89) chloride versus palliative local field radiotherapy in patients with hormonal escaped prostate cancer: a phase III study of the European Organisation for Research and Treatment of Cancer, Genitourinary Group. Eur Urol 2003;44:519–26.
7. Saad F, Gleason DM, Murray R, et al. A randomized, placebo-controlled trial of zoledronic acid in patients with hormone-refractory metastatic prostate carcinoma. J Natl Cancer Inst 2002;94:1458–68.
8. Petrylak DP, Tangen CM, Hussain MH, et al. Docetaxel and estramustine compared with mitoxantrone and prednisone for advanced refractory prostate cancer. N Engl J Med 2004;351:1513–20.
9. Tannock IF, de Wit R, Berry WR, et al. Docetaxel plus prednisone or mitoxantrone plus prednisone for advanced prostate cancer. N Engl J Med 2004;351:1502–12.

10. Debes JD, Tindall DJ. Mechanisms of androgen-refractory prostate cancer. N Engl J Med 2004; 351:1488–90.
11. Feldman BJ. The development of androgen-independent prostate cancer. Nat Rev Cancer 2001;1: 34–5.
12. Fossa SD, Slee PH, Brausi M, et al. Flutamide versus prednisone in patients with prostate cancer symptomatically progressing after androgen-ablative therapy: a phase III study of the european organization for research and treatment of cancer genitourinary group. J Clin Oncol 2001;19:62–71.
13. Linja MJ, Savinainen KJ, Saramaki OR, et al. Amplification and overexpression of androgen receptor gene in hormone-refractory prostate cancer. Cancer Res 2001;61:3550–5.
14. Chen CD, Welsbie DS, Tran C, et al. Molecular determinants of resistance to antiandrogen therapy. Nat Med 2004;10:33–9.
15. Mohler JL, Gregory CW, Ford OH 3rd, et al. The androgen axis in recurrent prostate cancer. Clin Cancer Res 2004;10:440–8.
16. Snoek R, Cheng H, Margiotti K, et al. In vivo knockdown of the androgen receptor results in growth inhibition and regression of well-established, castration-resistant prostate tumors. Clin Cancer Res 2009;15:39–47.
17. Titus MA, Schell MJ, Lih FB, et al. Testosterone and dihydrotestosterone tissue levels in recurrent prostate cancer. Clin Cancer Res 2005;11:4653–7.
18. Stanbrough M, Bubley GJ, Ross K, et al. Increased expression of genes converting adrenal androgens to testosterone in androgen-independent prostate cancer. Cancer Res 2006;66:2815–25.
19. Holzbeierlein J, Lal P, LaTulippe E, et al. Gene expression analysis of human prostate carcinoma during hormonal therapy identifies androgen-responsive genes and mechanisms of therapy resistance. Am J Pathol 2004;164:217–27.
20. Locke JA, Guns ES, Lubik AA, et al. Androgen levels increase by intratumoral de novo steroidogenesis during progression of castration-resistant prostate cancer. Cancer Res 2008;68:6407–15.
21. Hu R, Dunn TA, Wei S, et al. Ligand-independent androgen receptor variants derived from splicing of cryptic exons signify hormone-refractory prostate cancer. Cancer Res 2009;69:16–22.
22. Attar RM, Jeur-Kunkel M, Balog A, et al. Discovery of BMS-641988, a novel and potent inhibitor of androgen receptor signaling for the treatment of prostate cancer. Cancer Res 2009; 69(16):6522–30.
23. Attard G, Reid AH, Yap TA, et al. Phase I clinical trial of a selective inhibitor of CYP17, abiraterone acetate, confirms that castration-resistant prostate cancer commonly remains hormone driven. J Clin Oncol 2008;26:4563–71.
24. Ryan C, Efstathios E, Smith M, et al. Phase II multicenter study of chemotherapy (chemo)-naive castration-resistant prostate cancer (CRPC) not exposed to ketoconazole (keto), treated with abiraterone acetate (AA) plus prednisone [abstract]. J Clin Oncol 2009;27:5046.
25. Reid AH, Attard G, Danila D, et al. A multicenter phase II study of abiraterone acetate (AA) in docetacel pretreated castration-resistant prostate cancer (CRPC) patients (pts) [abstract]. J Clin Oncol 2009;27:5047.
26. Danila DC, de Bono J, Ryan CJ, et al. Phase II multicenter study of abiraterone acetate (AA) plus prednisone therapy in docetaxel-treated castration-resistant prostate cancer (CRPC) patients (pts): impact of prior ketoconazole (keto) [abstract]. J Clin Oncol 2009;27:5048.
27. Scher HI, Beer TM, Higano CS, et al. Antitumor activity of MDV3100 in a phase I/II study of castration-resistant prostate cancer (CRPC) [abstract]. J Clin Oncol 2009;27:5011.
28. Huss WJ, Hanrahan CF, Barrios RJ, et al. Angiogenesis and prostate cancer: identification of a molecular progression switch. Cancer Res 2001;61:2736–43.
29. George DJ, Halabi S, Shepard TF, et al. Prognostic significance of plasma vascular endothelial growth factor levels in patients with hormone-refractory prostate cancer treated on cancer and leukemia group B 9480. Clin Cancer Res 2001;7: 1932–6.
30. Melnyk O, Zimmerman M, Kim KJ, et al. Neutralizing anti-vascular endothelial growth factor antibody inhibits further growth of established prostate cancer and metastases in a pre-clinical model. J Urol 1999;161:960–3.
31. Jain RK, Tong RT, Munn LL. Effect of vascular normalization by antiangiogenic therapy on interstitial hypertension, peritumor edema, and lymphatic metastasis: insights from a mathematical model. Cancer Res 2007;67:2729–35.
32. Yang JC, Haworth L, Sherry RM, et al. A randomized trial of bevacizumab, an anti-vascular endothelial growth factor antibody, for metastatic renal cancer. N Engl J Med 2003;349(5):427–34.
33. Picus J, Halabi S, Rini B, et al. The use of bevacizumab (B) with docetaxel (D) and estramustine (E) in hormone refractory prostate cancer (HRPC): Initial results of CALGB 90006 [abstract]. Proc Am Soc Clin Oncol 2003;22:1578.
34. Gross ME, Soscia J, Sakowsky S, et al. Phase I trial of RAD001, bevacizumab, and docetaxel for castration-resistant prostate cancer (CRPC) [abstract]. J Clin Oncol 2009;27:5154.
35. Vaishampayan UN, Heilbrun LK, Heath EI, et al. Phase II trial of bevacizumab and oral satraplatin and prednisone in docetaxel pretreated metastatic

castrate resistant prostate cancer [abstract]. J Clin Oncol 2009;27:e16028.
36. Verheul HM, Hammers H, van Erp K, et al. Vascular endothelial growth factor trap blocks tumor growth, metastasis formation, and vascular leakage in an orthotopic murine renal cell cancer model. Clin Cancer Res 2007;13:4201–8.
37. Isambert N, Freyer G, Zanetta S, et al. A phase I dose escalation and pharmacokinetic (PK) study of intravenous aflibercept (VEGF trap) plus docetaxel (D) in patients (pts) with advanced solid tumors: preliminary results [abstract]. J Clin Oncol 2008;26:3599.
38. Motzer RJ, Hutson TE, Tomczak P, et al. Sunitinib versus interferon alfa in metastatic renal-cell carcinoma. N Engl J Med 2007;356:115–24.
39. Periman PO, Sonpavde G, Bernold DM, et al. Sunitinib malate for metastatic castration resistant prostate cancer following docetaxel-based chemotherapy [abstract]. J Clin Oncol 2008;26:5157.
40. Zurita AJ, Liu G, Hutson T, et al. Sunitinib in combination with docetaxel and prednisone in patients with metastatic hormone-refractory prostate cancer [abstract]. J Clin Oncol 2009;27:5166.
41. Escudier B, Eisen T, Stadler WM, et al. TARGET Study Group Sorafenib in advanced clear-cell renal-cell carcinoma. N Engl J Med 2007;356(2):125–34.
42. Llovet JM, Ricci S, Mazzaferro V, et al. SHARP Investigators Study Group Sorafenib in advanced hepatocellular carcinoma. N Engl J Med 2008;359(4):378–90.
43. Chi KN, Ellard SL, Hotte SJ, et al. A phase II study of sorafenib in patients with chemo-naive castration-resistant prostate cancer. Ann Oncol 2008;19(4):746–51.
44. Aragon-Ching JB, Jain L, Gulley JL, et al. Final analysis of a phase II trial using sorafenib for metastatic castration-resistant prostate cancer. BJU Int 2009;103(12):1636–40.
45. Mardjuadi F, Medioni J, Kerger J, et al. A phase I study of sorafenib in association with docetaxel-prednisone in chemonaive metastatic castration-resistant prostate cancer [abstract]. J Clin Oncol 2009;27:5153.
46. Cetnar JP, Rosen MA, Vaughn DJ, et al. Phase II study of sorafenib and docetaxel in men with metastatic castration resistant prostate cancer [abstract]. J Clin Oncol 2009;27:e16055.
47. Nabhan C, Tolzein K, Lestingi TM, et al. Effect of sorafenib on chemotherapy resistance and refractoriness in castration-resistant prostate cancer [abstract]. J Clin Oncol 2009;27:e16105.
48. Karakunnel JJ, Gulley JL, Arlen P, et al. Cediranib (AZD2171) in docetaxel-resistant, castration-resistant prostate cancer [abstract]. J Clin Oncol 2009;27:5141.
49. Krajewska M, Krajewski S, Epstein JI, et al. Immunohistochemical analysis of bcl-2, bax, bcl-X, and mcl-1 expression in prostate cancers. Am J Pathol 1996;148:1567–76.
50. Raffo AJ, Perlman H, Chen MW, et al. Overexpression of bcl-2 protects prostate cancer cells from apoptosis in vitro and confers resistance to androgen depletion in vivo. Cancer Res 1995;55:4438–45.
51. Miyake H, Nelson C, Rennie PS, et al. Testosterone-repressed prostate message-2 is an antiapoptotic gene involved in progression to androgen independence in prostate cancer. Cancer Res 2006;60:170–6.
52. Chi KN, Gleave ME, Klasa R, et al. A phase I dose-finding study of combined treatment with an antisense bcl-2 oligonucleotide (genasense) and mitoxantrone in patients with metastatic hormone-refractory prostate cancer. Clin Cancer Res 2001;7:3920–7.
53. Tolcher AW, Chi K, Kuhn J, et al. A phase II, pharmacokinetic, and biological correlative study of oblimersen sodium and docetaxel in patients with hormone-refractory prostate cancer. Clin Cancer Res 2005;11:3854–61.
54. Sternberg CN, Dumez H, Van Poppel H, et al. Multicenter randomized EORTC trial 30021 of docetaxel + oblimersen and docetaxel in patients (pts) with hormone refractory prostate cancer (HRPC) [abstract]. The Prostate Cancer Symposium (ASCO, ASTRO, SUO); 2007:144.
55. Yamanaka K, Rocchi P, Miyake H, et al. A novel antisense oligonucleotide inhibiting several antiapoptotic bcl-2 family members induces apoptosis and enhances chemosensitivity in androgen-independent human prostate cancer PC3 cells. Mol Cancer Ther 2005;4:1689–98.
56. Liu G, Wilding G, Somer B, et al. An open-label, multicenter, phase II study of single-agent AT-101 in men with hormone refractory prostate cancer (HRPC) and rising prostate-specific antigen (PSA) levels who have not received prior chemotherapy [abstract]. Prostate Cancer Symposium (ASCO, ASTRO, SUO); 2007:258.
57. MacVicar GR, Greco A, Reeves J, et al. An open-label, multicenter, phase I/II study of AT-101 in combination with docetaxel and prednisone in men with castrate-resistant prostate caner [abstract]. J Clin Oncol 2009;27:5062.
58. Banerji U. Heat shock protein 90 as a drug target: some like it hot. Clin Cancer Res 2009;15:9–14.
59. Edwards A, Li J, Atadja P, et al. Effect of the histone deacetylase inhibitor LBH589 against epidermal growth factor receptor-dependent human lung cancer cells. Mol Cancer Ther 2007;6:2515–24.
60. Pratt WB, Galigniana MD, Morishima Y, et al. Role of molecular chaperones in steroid receptor action. Essays Biochem 2004;40:41–58.

61. Marrocco DL, Tilley WD, Bianco-Miotto T, et al. Suberoylanilide hydroxamic acid (vorinostat) represses androgen receptor expression and acts synergistically with an androgen receptor antagonist to inhibit prostate cancer cell proliferation. Mol Cancer Ther 2007;6:51–60.
62. Welsbie DS, Xu J, Chen Y, et al. Histone deacetylases are required for androgen receptor function in hormone-sensitive and castrate-resistant prostate cancer. Cancer Res 2009;69:958–66.
63. Tomlins SA, Rhodes DR, Perner S, et al. Recurrent fusion of TMPRSS2 and ETS transcription factor genes in prostate cancer. Science 2005;310:644–8.
64. Iljin K, Wolf M, Edgren H, et al. TMPRSS2 fusions with oncogenic ETS factors in prostate cancer involve unbalanced genomic rearrangements and are associated with HDAC1 and epigenetic reprogramming. Cancer Res 2006;66:10242–6.
65. Bjorkman M, Iljin K, Halonen P, et al. Defining the molecular action of HDAC inhibitors and synergism with androgen deprivation in ERG-positive prostate cancer. Int J Cancer 2008;123:2774–81.
66. Heath EI, Hillman DW, Vaishampayan U, et al. A phase II trial of 17-allylamino-17-demethoxygeldanamycin in patients with hormone-refractory metastatic prostate cancer. Clin Cancer Res 2008;14:7940–6.
67. Hussain M, Dunn R, Rathkopf D, et al. Suberoylanilide hydroxamic acid (vorinostat) post chemotherapy in hormone refractory prostate cancer (HRPC) patients (pts): a phase II trial by the prostate cancer clinical trials consortium (NCI 6862). J Clin Oncol 2007;25:5132.
68. Leskov KS, Klokov DY, Li J, et al. Synthesis and functional analyses of nuclear clusterin, a cell death protein. J Biol Chem 2003;278:11590–600.
69. Zhang H, Kim JK, Edwards CA, et al. Clusterin inhibits apoptosis by interacting with activated bax. Nat Cell Biol 2005;7:909–15.
70. Humphreys DT, Carver JA, Easterbrook-Smith SB, et al. Clusterin has chaperone-like activity similar to that of small heat shock proteins. J Biol Chem 1999;274:6875–81.
71. Ammar H, Closset JL. Clusterin activates survival through the phosphatidylinositol 3-kinase/Akt pathway. J Biol Chem 2008;283:12851–61.
72. Gleave M, Chi KN. Knock-down of the cytoprotective gene, clusterin, to enhance hormone and chemosensitivity in prostate and other cancers. Ann N Y Acad Sci 2005;1058:1–15.
73. July LV, Akbari M, Zellweger T, et al. Clusterin expression is significantly enhanced in prostate cancer cells following androgen withdrawal therapy. Prostate 2002;50:179–88.
74. Chi KN, Eisenhauer E, Fazli L, et al. A phase I pharmacokinetic and pharmacodynamic study of OGX-011, a 2′-methoxyethyl antisense oligonucleotide to clusterin, in patients with localized prostate cancer. J Natl Cancer Inst 2005;97:1287–96.
75. Chi KN, Siu LL, Hirte H, et al. A phase I study of OGX-011, a 2′-methoxyethyl phosphorothioate antisense to clusterin, in combination with docetaxel in patients with advanced cancer. Clin Cancer Res 2008;14:833–9.
76. Saad F, Hotte SJ, North SA, et al. A phase II randomized study of custirsen (OGX-011) combination therapy in patients with poor-risk hormone refractory prostate cancer (HRPC) who relapsed on or within six months of 1st-line docetaxel therapy [abstract]. J Clin Oncol 2008;26:5002.
77. Chi KN, Hotte SJ, Yu E, et al. A randomized phase II study of OGX-011 in combination with docetaxel and prednisone or docetaxel and prednisone alone in patients with metastatic hormone refractory prostate cancer (HRPC) [abstract]. J Clin Oncol 2007;25:5069.
78. Chi KN, Hotte SJ, Yu E, et al. Mature results of a randomized phase II study of OGX-011 in combination with docetaxel/prednisone versus docetaxel/prednisone in patients with metastatic castration-resistant prostate cancer [abstract]. J Clin Oncol 2009;27:5012.
79. Renehan AG, Zwahlen M, Minder C, et al. Insulin-like growth factor (IGF)-I, IGF binding protein-3, and cancer risk: systematic review and meta-regression analysis. Lancet 2004;363:1346–53.
80. Chan JM, Stampfer MJ, Ma J, et al. Insulin-like growth factor-I (IGF-I) and IGF binding protein-3 as predictors of advanced-stage prostate cancer. J Natl Cancer Inst 2008;94:1099–106.
81. Hellawell GO, Turner GD, Davies DR, et al. Expression of the type 1 insulin-like growth factor receptor is up-regulated in primary prostate cancer and commonly persists in metastatic disease. Cancer Res 2002;62:2942–50.
82. Krueckl SL, Sikes RA, Edlund NM, et al. Increased insulin-like growth factor I receptor expression and signaling are components of androgen-independent progression in a lineage-derived prostate cancer progression model. Cancer Res 2004;64:8620–9.
83. Wu JD, Odman A, Higgins LM, et al. In vivo effects of the human type I insulin-like growth factor receptor antibody A12 on androgen-dependent and androgen-independent xenograft human prostate tumors. Clin Cancer Res 2005;11:3065–74.
84. Higano C, Alumkal J, Ryan CJ, et al. A phase II study evaluating the efficacy and safety of single agent IMC A12, a monoclonal antibody, against the insulin-like growth factor-1 receptor, as monotherapy in patients with metastatic, asymptomatic castration-resistant prostate cancer [abstract]. J Clin Oncol 2009;27:5142.

85. Vivanco I, Sawyers CL. The phosphatidylinositol 3-kinase AKT pathway in human cancer. Nat Rev Cancer 2002;2:489–501.
86. Gera JF, Mellinghoff IK, Shi Y, et al. AKT activity determines sensitivity to mammalian target of rapamycin (mTOR) inhibitors by regulating cyclin D1 and c-myc expression. J Biol 2004;279:2737–46.
87. Mousses S, Wagner U, Chen Y, et al. Failure of hormone therapy in prostate cancer involves systematic restoration of androgen responsive genes and activation of rapamycin sensitive signaling. Oncogene 2007;20(41):6718–23.
88. Wang Y, Mikhailova M, Bose S, et al. Regulation of androgen receptor transcriptional activity by rapamycin in prostate cancer cell proliferation and survival. Oncogene 2008;27(56):7106–17.
89. Yoshimoto M, Joshua AM, Cunha IW, et al. Absence of TMPRSS2:ERG fusions and PTEN losses in prostate cancer is associated with a favorable outcome. Mod Pathol 2008;21(12):1451–60.
90. Amato RJ, Jac J, Mohammad T, et al. Pilot study of rapamycin in patients with hormone-refractory prostate cancer. Clin Genitourin Cancer 2008; 6(2):97–102.
91. Wan X, Harkavy B, Shen N, et al. Rapamycin induces feedback activation of akt signaling through an IGF-1R-dependent mechanism. Oncogene 2007;26:1932–40.
92. Hofbauer LC, Schoppet M. Clinical implications of the osteoprotegerin/RANKL/RANK system for bone and vascular diseases. JAMA 2004;292: 490–5.
93. Chen G, Sircar K, Aprikian A, et al. Expression of RANKL/RANK/OPG in primary and metastatic human prostate cancer as markers of disease stage and functional regulation. Cancer 2006;107: 289–98.
94. Brown JM, Vessella RL, Kostenuik PJ, et al. Serum osteoprotegerin levels are increased in patients with advanced prostate cancer. Clin Cancer Res 2001;7:2977–83.
95. Ellis GK, Bone HG, Chlebowski R, et al. Randomized trial of denosumab in patients receiving adjuvant aromatase inhibitors for nonmetastatic breast cancer. J Clin Oncol 2008;26:4875–82.
96. Bone HG, Bolognese MA, Yuen CK, et al. Effects of denosumab on bone mineral density and bone turnover in postmenopausal women. J Clin Endocrinol Metab 2008;93:2149–57.
97. Bamias A, Kastritis E, Bamia C, et al. Osteonecrosis of the jaw in cancer after treatment with bisphosphonates: incidence and risk factors. J Clin Oncol 2005;23:8580–7.
98. Nelson JB, Hedican SP, George DJ, et al. Identification of endothelin-1 in the pathophysiology of metastatic adenocarcinoma of the prostate. Nat Med 1995;1:944–9.
99. Carducci MA, Jimeno A. Targeting bone metastasis in prostate cancer with endothelin receptor antagonists. Clin Cancer Res 2006;12:6296–300.
100. Carducci MA, Saad F, Abrahamsson PA, et al. A phase 3 randomized controlled trial of the efficacy and safety of atrasentan in men with metastatic hormone-refractory prostate cancer. Cancer 2007;110:1959–66.
101. Nelson JB, Love W, Chin JL, et al. Phase 3, randomized, controlled trial of atrasentan in patients with nonmetastatic, hormone-refractory prostate cancer. Cancer 2008;113:2478–87.
102. Armstrong AJ, Creel P, Turnbull J, et al. A phase I-II study of docetaxel and atrasentan in men with castration-resistant metastatic prostate cancer. Clin Cancer Res 2008;14:6270–6.
103. James ND, Caty A, Borre M, et al. Safety and efficacy of the specific endothelin-A receptor antagonist ZD4054 in patients with hormone-resistant prostate cancer and bone metastases who were pain free or mildly symptomatic: a double-blind, placebo-controlled, randomised, phase 2 trial. Eur Urol 2008;55(5):1112–23.
104. Tatarov O, Mitchell TJ, Seywright M, et al. Src family kinase activity is up-regulated in hormone-refractory prostate cancer. Clin Cancer Res 2009; 15(10):3540–9.
105. Fizazi K. The role of src in prostate cancer. Ann Oncol 2007;18:1765–73.
106. Nam S, Kim D, Cheng JQ, et al. Action of the src family kinase inhibitor, dasatinib (BMS-354825), on human prostate cancer cells. Cancer Res 2005;65:9185–9.
107. Yu EY, Wilding G, Posadas E, et al. Dasatinib in patients with hormone-refractory progressive prostate cancer: a phase II study [abstract]. J Clin Oncol 2008;26:5156.
108. Yu E, Massard C, Gross M, et al. A phase II study of once-daily dasatinib for patients with castration-resistant prostate cancer [abstract]. J Clin Oncol 2009;27:5147.
109. Araujo J, Armstrong AJ, Braud EL, et al. Dasatinib and docetaxel combination treatment for patients with castration-resistant progressive prostate cancer: a phase I/II study [abstract]. J Clin Oncol 2009;27:5061.
110. Serafini AN, Houston SJ, Resche I, et al. Palliation of pain associated with metastatic bone cancer using samarium-153 lexidronam: a double-blind placebo-controlled clinical trial. J Clin Oncol 1998;16(4):1574–81.
111. Sartor O, Reid RH, Hoskin PJ, et al. Samarium-153-lexidronam complex for treatment of painful bone metastases in hormone-refractory prostate cancer. Urology 2004;63(5):940–5.
112. Eisenberger MA, Lin J, Sinibaldi J, et al. Phase I trial with a combination of docetaxel and

^{153}Sm-EDTMP in patients with castration-resistant prostate cancer [abstract]. J Clin Oncol 2009;27: 5155.
113. Morris MJ, Pandit-Taskar N, Stephenson RD, et al. Phase I/II study of docetaxel and 153-sm for castrate metastatic prostate cancer: summary of dose-escalation cohorts and first report of the expansion cohort [abstract]. J Clin Oncol 2009;27:5057.
114. Fizazi K, Beuzeboc P, Lumbroso J, et al. Phase II trial of consolidation docetaxel and samarium-153 in patients with bone metastases from castration-resistant prostate cancer. J Clin Oncol 2009;27:2429–35.
115. Bellmunt J, Rosenberg JE, Choueiri TK. Recent progress and pitfalls in testing novel agents in castration-resistant prostate cancer. Eur Urol 2009;56(4):606–8.
116. Nilsson S, Franz L, Parker C, et al. Bone-targeted radium-223 in symptomatic, hormone-refractory prostate cancer: a randomised, multicentre placebo-controlled phase II study. Lancet Oncol 2007;8(7):587–94.
117. Altmann KH. Recent developments in the chemical biology of epothilones. Curr Pharm Des 2005; 11(13):1595–613.
118. Julien B, Shah S. Heterologous expression of epothilone biosynthetic genes in *Myxococcus xanthus*. Antimicrobial Agents Chemother 2002;46(9):2772–8.
119. Rosenberg JE, Weinberg VK, Kelly WK, et al. Activity of second-line chemotherapy in docetaxel-refractory hormone-refractory prostate cancer patients: randomized phase 2 study of ixabepilone or mitoxantrone and prednisone. Cancer 2007;110(3): 556–63.
120. Wilding G, Chen Y, DiPaola RP, et al. Updated results on phase II study of a weekly schedule of BMS-247550 for patients with castrate refractory prostate cancer [abstract]. J Clin Oncol 2008;26: 5070.
121. Small E, Harzstark A, Weinberg VK, et al. Ixabepilone, mitoxantrone, and prednisone in patients with metastatic castration-resistant prostate cancer refractory to docetaxel-based therapy: a phase II study of the DOD prostate cancer clinical trials consortium [abstract]. J Clin Oncol 2009;27:5058.
122. Hussain A, Dipaola RS, Baron AD, et al. A phase IIa trial of weekly EPO906 in patients with hormone-refractory prostate cancer [abstract]. J Clin Oncol 2004;22:4563.
123. Beardsley EK, Saad F, Eigl B, et al. A phase II study of patupilone in patients with metastatic castration-resistant prostate cancer who have progressed after docetaxel [abstract]. J Clin Oncol 2009;27: 5139.
124. Beer TM, Smith DC, Hussain A, et al. Phase II study of first-line sagopilone combined with prednisone in patients with metastatic castration-resistant prostate cancer [abstract]. J Clin Oncol 2009;27: 5059.

Immunotherapy for Prostate Cancer: An Emerging Treatment Modality

Charles G. Drake, MD, PhD[a,b,*]

KEYWORDS

- Prostate cancer • Vaccine
- T cell • Lymphocyte • CTLA4 • PD-1

Renal cell carcinoma and melanoma have traditionally been thought of as immune-responsive tumors, because rare spontaneous remissions of both tumor types are occasionally observed, and because both tumor types show some degree of responsiveness to nonspecific immunologic stimulation in the form of intravenous interleukin 2 (IL-2).[1,2] Indeed, the prostate gland was originally believed to be immunologically privileged based on a paucity of lymphatic drainage,[3] and animal studies suggest that in the absence of tumorigenesis, the prostate gland is ignored by the immune system.[4] Prostate cancer, however, represents a different immunologic milieu, and several groups showed that prostate tumors contain infiltrating lymphocytes. In some, but not all of these studies, the presence of prostate-infiltrating lymphocytes seems to correlate with improved prognosis.[5,6] In addition, the CD4 and CD8 T cells that infiltrate the prostate gland are oligoclonal in their T-cell receptor sequences,[7,8] suggesting that these cells are responding in a specific manner to their cognate antigen. CD8 T-cell infiltration seems to be more prevalent in prostate cancer than in prostatic intraepithelial neoplasia, again suggesting the likelihood of an ongoing antitumor T-cell response (Gurel and colleagues, unpublished data, 2009).

In light of these observations, it seems possible that prostate cancer might represent a better target for immunologic intervention than previously believed. Other characteristics of the disease contribute to its attractiveness as an immunotherapy target. Perhaps foremost among these is that prostate cancer is initially responsive to hormonal manipulation, and that androgen ablation results in a clear increase in the inflammatory infiltrate in the gland.[7,9] The apoptotic response of prostate cancer to androgen ablation also results in a profound reduction of tumor burden, and a decrease in levels of the immunosuppressive factors associated with bulky disease. Secondarily, although not a perfect tumor maker, circulating levels of prostate-specific antigen (PSA) can be used to guide treatment decisions. In addition, the prostate gland is unique among secretory organs, providing various antigens that could be potentially targeted immunologically. Prostate cancer tends to be a slow-growing disease,[10] and the time from initial biochemical relapse to metastatic disease is typically in the range of 7 to 8 years.[11] This extended disease course allows more time for clinical intervention than is available for other tumor types, and also may allow adequate time for a patient's immune system to be sufficiently activated and mediate an antitumor response.

Consulting: Amplimmune Inc, BMS Inc, Dendreon Inc, IRX, Medarex Inc, Sanofi Aventis.
Stock ownership: Amplimmune Inc.
[a] Departments of Oncology, Immunology, and Urology, Johns Hopkins Sidney Kimmel Comprehensive Cancer Center, 1650 Orleans Street CRB I #410, Baltimore, MD 21231, USA
[b] The Brady Urological Institute, Johns Hopkins University, Baltimore, MD, USA
* Departments of Oncology, Immunology, and Urology, Johns Hopkins Sidney Kimmel Comprehensive Cancer Center, 1650 Orleans Street CRB I #410, Baltimore, MD 21231.
E-mail address: cdrake@jhmi.edu

Urol Clin N Am 37 (2010) 121–129
doi:10.1016/j.ucl.2009.11.001

If prostate tumors are infiltrated with CD8 T cells, why then does the immune system not attack and eliminate evolving prostate tumors more frequently? Numerous mechanisms are involved,[12] but one major concern is that the lymphocytes that infiltrate prostate cancer display an exhausted or nonfunctional phenotype. In this respect, the majority (approximately 80%) of the CD8 T cells in the prostate gland express the cell-surface molecule programmed-death 1 (PD-1), which has been associated with a lack of lytic function in several chronic infectious diseases and tumor types,[13] and with poor outcome in renal cell cancer and bladder cancer.[14,15] Antibody-mediated blockade of the PD-1/B7-1 interaction has been shown to restore CD8 T-cell function in human immunodeficiency virus,[16] hepatitis C virus,[17] and in a murine model of chronic infection.[18] Similar results have been observed in animal models of cancer[19] and in cancer-specific human CD8 T cells.[20] So, blocking the interaction of PD-1 and its ligand using a monoclonal antibody restores CD8 T-cell lytic function in several infectious disease and tumor models, and might represent 1 technique by which to augment an antitumor immune response. But many other immunosuppressive characteristics are associated with prostate cancer, including increased circulating levels of transforming growth factor β (TGF-β), which directly suppresses CD8 T-cell activation and function.[21] Other cells in the prostate that potentially downregulate CD8 lytic function include CD4 regulatory T cells (Treg), and immunosuppressive macrophages and myeloid suppressor cells.[22–25]

ACTIVE IMMUNOTHERAPY FOR PROSTATE CANCER

In the past, tumor immunology has generally focused on the concept of activating or educating antitumor lymphocytes, in a manner similar to that used to initiate an immune response against an infectious agent (ie, a vaccine), but this terminology, and the term "vaccine", are probably inappropriate in this context. First, nearly all vaccines for infectious diseases are administered in a preventative setting (ie, in a milieu in which the target antigens [or pathogens] are completely absent). In this context, the immune system has not been previously exposed to the antigens involved, and it is facile to generate a potent, antigen-directed immune response that leads to immunologic memory. In contrast, cancer vaccines are nearly always administered in the context of an evolving or progressive tumor; in this case the immune system has generally been exposed to the target antigen for a considerable time, but has failed to mount an effective response. Thus, cancer vaccines are administered in the setting of ongoing tolerance, a situation in which it is more challenging to generate any response at all, much less a productive immune response leading to long-lasting immunologic memory. For this reason, it is probably more appropriate to refer to approaches designed to activate an immune response against cancer as "immunotherapy," because, like chemotherapy, these approaches are intended to provide therapy for existing tumors. These stimulatory approaches are generally active in nature, in contrast with the passive administration of antitumor antibodies, which also falls under the broader rubric of tumor immunotherapy. Many immunotherapy approaches have been tested in prostate cancer; these approaches all share the common goal of inducing a specific T-cell response directed against the tumor.[26–29] In the case of the prostate-infiltrating lymphocytes described earlier, the goal of active immunotherapy for prostate cancer is to activate the specific cells preexisting in the gland and to recruit and expand additional pools of tumor-specific lymphocytes that can then traffic to prostate tumors and lyse their targets.

DNA Vaccines

One approach with considerable promise for immunotherapy of prostate tumors involves using DNA-based constructs to activate a specific antitumor immune response. This approach was highlighted in a recent study by McNeel and colleagues.[30] These investigators used a DNA vaccine directed against prostatic acid phosphatase (PAP) to treat 22 men with biochemically recurrent prostate cancer (so-called D0 disease). As is nearly always the case for immunotherapy, the treatment was well tolerated, and appeared to result in a T-cell and antibody response to the target antigen. Decreases in the rate of increase of PSA were noted, although the overall clinical significance of such changes is not without controversy. DNA-based immunotherapy vectors are straightforward to synthesize, and this trial therefore provides a foundation on which future trials evaluating additional target antigens may be based.

Viral Vectors: ProstVac VF

Another approach to immunotherapy that has been applied to prostate cancer and other tumor types involves viral vectors, in particular attenuated vaccinia strains. These vectors have the advantage of being capable of incorporating a large target payload, and straightforward synthesis and production.[31] In the context of prostate cancer, a strategy targeting PSA has been systematically developed over the past decade. Because this platform has been extensively reviewed elsewhere,[32] only a few points regarding this agent are discussed in this article. Early in the development of vaccinia-based vectors, it was noted that additional immunization did not seem to result in additional immunity directed against the targeted antigen, but rather at the viral components of the vector itself. Thus, a heterologous prime-boost strategy was designed, in which vaccinia and fowlpox vectors incorporating PSA were synthesized. In a randomized phase II trial, it was shown that vaccinia priming, followed by a series of fowlpox booster treatments, resulted in an optimal immune response as revealed by correlative laboratory studies.[33] Long-term follow-up of that trial has suggested a trend toward increased progression-free survival in men treated with the optimal immunotherapy sequence.[34] An additional refinement to the vaccinia-PSA approach was based on laboratory studies showing that the addition of a triad of costimulatory molecules (B7-1, LFA3, ICAM-1) to the immunizing agent resulted in a significant augmentation of immune responses.[35] The resulting product, ProstVac VF, was partially developed by the Therion Corporation, which launched a 2:1 randomized trial comparing ProstVac VF with placebo in approximately 120 men with asymptomatic, metastatic, castrate-resistant prostate cancer (CRPC) (TBC-PRO-002). Data from this trial were originally presented in 2006, but at that time there was no statistical difference between the treatment groups in the primary end point (time to progression), or a secondary survival end point.[36] However, long-term follow-up data from these patients were recently presented, and a statistically significant survival advantage was evident, with a median overall survival of 24.5 months in the immunotherapy group versus 16 months in the control group. Because overall survival was a secondary end point in this trial, those data should be considered hypothesis generating. Nevertheless, a phase III trial of this agent is in the planning stages for 2010 initiation (http://www.bavarian-nordic.com/prostvac). In addition to these trials, ProstVac VF has been combined with an impressive number of conventional therapies for prostate cancer, as discussed later. This developmental pathway illustrates several general principles surrounding immunotherapy for prostate cancer. First and perhaps foremost is the slow pace of disease; in the absence of reliable surrogate clinical end point trials take significant time to mature. Secondly, the vaccinia prime, fowlpox boost strategy exemplifies the notion of a heterologous prime-boost immunization scheme (heterologous strategies are rarely used in cancer immunotherapy).

Cell-Based Immunotherapy (GVAX Prostate and Onyvax-P)

A third approach to active immunotherapy for prostate cancer that has proceeded to phase III and phase II randomized clinical trials involves the use of allogeneic prostate cancer cells as immunotherapy vectors. Because cancer cells themselves are generally not sufficiently immunogeneic to mediate protection in murine models, for optimal immunity cancer cells must be either engineered to express a proinflammatory cytokine or administered along with a potent immune stimulator (ie, an adjuvant).[37] The first approach is exemplified by GVAX prostate, which used the cell lines PC3 and LnCaP transfected to secrete GM-CSF.[38] In clinical studies, these cells are irradiated to prevent ongoing division, then injected intradermally. Phase II studies of GVAX prostate were promising,[39,40] and in 2004 a large, randomized phase III trial comparing GVAX prostate with standard docetaxel chemotherapy every 3 weeks in men with minimally symptomatic, metastatic CRPC was launched. This trial, VITAL-1, completed accrual in July, 2007; an interim safety analysis performed in January, 2008 supported trial continuation. A second randomized phase III trial of GVAX prostate was launched in July, 2005; in this trial GVAX prostate was combined with docetaxel to treat men with more advanced disease (ie, patients with symptomatic metastatic CRPC). Although docetaxel chemotherapy is generally administered along with prednisone at a daily dose of 10 mg, prednisone was omitted from the GVAX plus docetaxel treatment arm because of its immunosuppressive properties. The control arm was standard docetaxel combined with prednisone every 3 weeks. This trial (VITAL-2) was halted early because an interim analysis showed an imbalance of deaths in the immunotherapy arm (67 vs 47). The mechanism for this imbalance has yet to be explained, but it did not seem to result from a failure of randomization. Based on these data, an unplanned early futility analysis was designed and completed for the fully accrued VITAL-1 trial.[41] At the time the analysis was conducted, only 371 deaths had occurred, fewer than the prespecified 400 required for 80% power, but the analysis suggested that VITAL-1 had less than a 30% chance of reaching its primary end point of a 20% improvement in survival, and further patient follow-up was halted. The Kaplan-Meier survival curves for VITAL-1 show a clear crossover at 21 months; after this time point patients on the immunotherapy arm show a superior survival. Thus, it remains theoretically possible that further follow-up of these study patients could reveal a late treatment effect, similar to that seen with ProstVac VF in the TBC-PRO-002 trial. Further clinical development of the GVAX prostate platform has been discontinued by the manufacturer (Cell Genesys Inc). Comparison of the GVAX prostate clinical experience with that of ProstVac VF (TBC-PRO-002) and with Sipuleucel-T (see later discussion) suggests that, in asymptomatic metastatic prostate cancer, a positive result in a randomized clinical trial is more likely when the trial design compares immunotherapy with placebo, rather than with docetaxel chemotherapy. In addition, the unexpected imbalance in deaths in VITAL-2 suggests that combining immunotherapy with other treatment modalities may prove complex, and that randomized phase II trials should be considered before initiating phase III studies.

Another cell-based immunotherapy approach for prostate cancer involves 3 allogeneic prostate cancer cell lines chosen to represent different disease states (Onyvax-P, Onyvax Inc). Specifically, the product includes an immortalized normal human prostate epithelial cell line (ONYCAP23), a transformed cell line from a well-differentiated prostate cancer (P4E6), and the androgen-dependent cell line LnCaP, which was derived from a lymph node metastasis.[42] In clinical trials, the cell lines are first administered as 2 doses of irradiated cells at 2-week intervals along with bacillus Calmette-Guérin as an adjuvant, followed by monthly boosts of the cell lines alone. A phase II trial of Onyvax-P in men with CRPC showed the treatment to be well tolerated and showed a decrease in the PSA velocity in 11 of the 26 patients treated.[43] The current status of Onyvax-P is uncertain, as previously ongoing phase II trials are now closed to accrual (http://www.clincaltrials.gov).

Active Cellular Immunotherapy (Sipuleucel-T)

The active immunotherapy that is most likely closest to approval by the US Food and Drug Administration (FDA) for prostate cancer involves an approach that is different from those described earlier. To manufacture Sipuleucel-T (Dendreon Inc, Seattle, WA, USA), patients undergo plasmapheresis, and a personalized immunotherapy product is produced by culturing a patient's peripheral blood monocytes with a proprietary protein that couples GM-CSF with a target antigen (PAP). This approach has the theoretic advantage of removing antigen-presenting cells (and lymphocytes) from an immunosuppressive patient environment as the cells are activated. In addition, the discrete target antigen facilitates immune monitoring. Phase I and phase III trials of Sipuleucel-T have been reported, with encouraging results.[44–46] FDA approval of this agent is pivotal on a large (>500 patients) randomized placebo-controlled phase III trial (IMPACT), which completed accrual in October, 2007, and which was reported to meet its primary (survival) end point in April, 2009 (http://www.dendreon.com). Thus, when considered along with the TBC-PRO-002 trial of ProstVac VF already described and an earlier phase III trial of Sipuleucel-T (D9901[46]), 3 randomized trials of immunotherapy for metastatic prostate cancer have reported a survival benefit. In all 3 cases the comparator arm was a placebo treatment. Although a placebo comparator might seem unwarranted given that docetaxel chemotherapy every 3 weeks is approved by the FDA for metastatic CRPC in symptomatic and asymptomatic patients, both of these trials enrolled only asymptomatic men, and controversy exists regarding the optimal timing of chemotherapeutic intervention in metastatic prostate cancer.[47]

COMBINING CONVENTIONAL THERAPY WITH ACTIVE IMMUNOTHERAPY

Androgen Ablation

One of the more interesting combination regimens for prostate cancer involves the administration of immunotherapy along with androgen ablation. The clinical rationale for this hypothesis stems from a demonstration of an increased T-cell infiltrate in the prostate glands of men who had undergone androgen ablation before radical prostatectomy.[7] The infiltrating CD4 T cells showed evidence of oligoclonality, suggestive of an antigen-driven immune response. The author obtained similar results in an animal model of prostate cancer, and showed that androgen ablation appeared to mitigate systemic CD4 T-cell tolerance significantly.[4] Further animal studies explored the relative timing of immunotherapy and androgen ablation, and showed that an optimal combinatorial effect is obtained when immunotherapy is administered before androgen ablation.[48] In addition to mitigating T-cell tolerance and promoting T-cell infiltration into the prostate gland, androgen ablation also mediates regrowth of the thymus, the organ in which T cells are produced, and thymic regrowth is accompanied by an increase in T-cell production.[49] Given these considerable data, it is perhaps surprising that more clinical trials have not been performed with this combination.[50] An initial trial was performed by Sanda and colleagues[51] several years ago; ProstVac (without TRICOM or the heterologous prime-boost developed later), was administered to a small number of patients with biochemically relapsed disease. Using a more developed version of ProstVac VF, Madan and colleagues[52] studied sequencing the androgen-receptor antagonist nilutamide in a phase II trial. These results (although derived from only a few patients) mirrored the results obtained by Kast and colleagues in animal studies; patients who received the ProstVac VF vector before secondary androgen manipulation with nilutamide appeared to have an increased survival compared with those who were treated with immunotherapy after androgen manipulation. In the Dendreon P-11 study, men with biochemically relapsed prostate cancer received Sipuleucel-T after androgen ablation. Although final study results have yet to be reported, an initial presentation of these data suggested that this particular combination did not seem to affect the time to PSA recurrence, which was the primary trial end point. Additional clinical trials are warranted, but the results obtained thus far strongly suggest that the precise sequence of the 2 modalities may be of critical importance.

Chemotherapy

Two large phase III randomized controlled trials demonstrated that docetaxel chemotherapy significantly prolongs survival in men with metastatic CRPC,[53,54] and several trials have combined docetaxel chemotherapy with an additional agent in an effort to improve on this documented survival benefit. Agents tested in this manner include antiangiogenesis agents, mTOR inhibitors, endothelin inhibitors, and others[55]; it followed that immunotherapy might be tested in a similar manner. As discussed earlier, the Cell Genesys VITAL-2 trial compared the combination of GVAX prostate plus docetaxel (without prednisone) with docetaxel plus prednisone in men with symptomatic CRPC, and interim analysis suggested a potential adverse outcome in the men treated with combination therapy. In contrast, a phase II trial comparing docetaxel plus ProstVac VF with ProstVac VF alone showed a prolongation of progression-free survival in the group who received combination treatment, and found that docetaxel did not seem to impair an immunotherapy-mediated immune response.[56] In addition to combination with standard docetaxel, preclinical and clinical data suggest that low-dose cyclophosphamide may enhance an immunotherapy-induced antitumor immune response, most likely through transient depletion of Treg.[57,58] Recent studies by the author's group in an autochronous murine model of prostate cancer confirm these results and reinforce the notion that chemotherapy and immunotherapy must be delivered in a precise sequence for optimal efficacy.[59]

Radiotherapy

Radiotherapy is a conventional methodology for treating localized and recurrent prostate cancer, and several studies showed that radiotherapy has significant proinflammatory effects: upregulation of the proapoptotic molecules Fas and FasL on tumor cells and increasing levels of class I MHC (important for T-cell-mediated tumor lysis).[60] Several preclinical studies directly support the notion of combining radiotherapy for prostate cancer with immunotherapy.[61,62] The combination of active immunotherapy and radiotherapy has been evaluated clinically, once again using the ProstVac VF platform.[63] Thirteen of the 17 patients randomized to the combination radiotherapy/immunotherapy arm in this trial showed an increased T-cell response to the target antigen (PSA), supporting the notion of combining radiotherapy with immunotherapy for prostate cancer. In addition, an ongoing phase III trial of the immune modulator ipilimumab (see later discussion) in patients who have failed docetaxel chemotherapy includes a low dose of radiotherapy in an effort to enhance tumor antigen presentation.

IMMUNE MODULATORS (BRAKES AND ACCELERATORS)

Anti-CTLA4 (Ipilimumab, Tremilimumab)

Although the prostate glands of patients with cancer contain a CD4 and CD8 T-cell infiltrate, phenotypic analyses of these cells[8,64,65] and numerous murine studies[66–70] are consistent with the notion that these infiltrating cells are nonfunctional in lytic function. Several T-cell molecules seem to contribute to this lack of function, most notably CTLA4, which interacts with B7 family molecules on antigen-presenting cells to downregulate T-cell function. In animal studies, CTLA4 blockade was shown to augment an antitumor response initiated by cell-based immunotherapy,[71] and the CTLA4 blocking monoclonal antibody ipilimumab (Medarex Inc, Princeton, NJ, USA) has been evaluated clinically in prostate cancer in several phase I and phase II studies.[72,73] Notably, PSA and radiological responses have been observed following treatment with single-agent ipilimumab, prompting initiation of the multi-institution, randomized phase III trial of this agent described earlier. A study combining anti-CTLA4 with GVAX prostate has also been conducted; initial results were encouraging, suggesting PSA responses in 4 of the first 6 patients treated, with further follow-up accruing.

Additional Brakes and Accelerators (PD-1, OX40)

PD-1 is a cell-surface molecule expressed on activated and exhausted CD8 T cells; expression of B7-H1 (the major PD-1 ligand) in various tumor types is associated with a poor outcome.[13,74] Blockade of PD-1 with a monoclonal antibody augments antitumor immunity in several murine studies and a phase I trial of a novel, fully human monoclonal antibody specific for PD-1 has completed accrual. This agent was shown to be well tolerated, and clinical responses were observed in several tumor types. The author and others found that most prostate-infiltrating CD8 T cells seem to express PD-1, suggesting that PD-1 blockade might have efficacy in prostate cancer.[8,75] Although limited space does not permit a full discussion in this article, several other cell-surface markers on CD8 T cells are important in activation and initiation of CD8 lytic function, most notably OX40,[76] and several preclinical studies show synergy between OX40 engagement and other antitumor treatment modalities.[70]

MONOCLONAL ANTIBODIES

Anti-PSMA

In several tumor types, monoclonal antibodies directed against cell-surface proteins expressed on cancer cells have had a major effect on morbidity and mortality. Thus, trastuzumab and rituximab (Rituxan) are now standard therapies for patients with Her-2 expressing breast cancer and CD20 expressing lymphoma. Efforts to target prostate cancer cells directly using monoclonal antibody therapy have focused on the cell-surface molecule known as prostate-specific membrane antigen (PSMA),[77] and a modified (human IgG1) monoclonal antibody designated J591.[78] To deliver a cytotoxic payload to prostate tumor cells, this antibody has been conjugated to lutetium-177 (^{177}Lu) or yttrium-90 (^{90}Y), two β-emitting radionuclides with distinct properties. ^{177}Lu is a mixed β and γ emitter; the fraction of total energy released as γ irradiation (15%) can be used for imaging with a standard γ camera. In contrast, ^{90}Y is a pure β emitter, and a separate radiolabeled antibody must be used for imaging and dosimetry purposes. ^{177}Lu is a lower-energy β emitter, with an optimal tumor treatment size of 1.2 to 3.0 mm, whereas modeling of the higher energy ^{90}Y shows an optimal tumor treatment size in the 28- to 42-mm range. Because both agents have theoretic advantages and disadvantages, phase I trials in prostate cancer were performed with each. In the ^{90}Y trial, 29 patients with CRPC were treated, and a recommended dose determined.[79] Consistent with the documented specificity of PSMA, metastatic sites were well targeted, and several PSA responses were observed, providing evidence of clinical activity. The ^{177}Lu trial showed similar targeting, and 21 of 35 treated patients had evidence of biologic activity.[80] A randomized phase II trial of ^{177}Lu anti-PSMA in men with non-metastatic prostate cancer has been designed in concordance with the hypothesis that immunotherapy for prostate cancer will prove most successful in patients with a minimal disease burden; this trial is now accruing.

SUMMARY

If Sipuleucel-T is approved for the treatment of metastatic CRPC in 2010, it will be the first antigen-specific immunotherapy to be approved by the FDA for the treatment of solid tumors. This might be viewed as a watershed moment for immunotherapy, and a vindication of prostate cancer as an immune target. From a therapeutic standpoint it is relevant that only a small handful of agents have been approved by the FDA for the treatment of metastatic CRPC, highlighting the significance of the pivotal trial results. In other ways, data from the potentially pivotal D9902B (IMPACT) trial illustrate some of the hurdles facing the development of immunotherapy. This trial was, of necessity, conducted in the metastatic castrate-resistant setting, a paradox in light of copious experimental data suggesting that immunotherapy is most likely to be efficacious in a setting of minimal residual disease. Moving agents like Sipuleucel-T, ProstVac VF, and others earlier in the disease process is attractive, but hampered by a lack of surrogate end points in prostate cancer that reliably predict survival (or other clinical benefits). In addition, the IMPACT trial used Sipuleucel-T as a single agent, again out of an understandable regulatory necessity. Yet, it is also clear that from significant experimental data that single-agent immunotherapy (much like single-agent chemotherapy) is of incremental benefit in patients with advanced disease. Thus, an obvious future development path for this agent (and others) involves combinatorial approaches administered earlier in the course of disease. The ongoing development of immune checkpoint blocking agents like anti-CTLA4 (ipilimumab, tremilimumab) and anti-PD-1 (Medarex Inc, Princeton, NJ, USA) suggests one route toward combination therapy. Conventional treatments for prostate cancer, especially androgen ablation with its multiple stimulatory immunologic mechanisms, are natural partners for combination with immunotherapy, and several trials combining androgen ablation with active immunotherapy for prostate cancer have been undertaken. Combinations involving radiotherapy and chemotherapy are also supported by preclinical data, but the recent clinical trial experience combining GVAX prostate with docetaxel chemotherapy highlights the importance of completing careful (and perhaps randomized) phase II trials before initiation of larger phase III studies. Despite the inherent complexity involved, the field must move forward with data-driven combination approaches to achieve the ultimate goal of inducing long-term remission in most patients with prostate cancer.

REFERENCES

1. Fyfe G, Fisher RI, Rosenberg SA, et al. Results of treatment of 255 patients with metastatic renal cell carcinoma who received high-dose recombinant interleukin-2 therapy. J Clin Oncol 1995;13:688–96.
2. Atkins MB, Lotze MT, Dutcher JP, et al. High-dose recombinant interleukin 2 therapy for patients with metastatic melanoma: analysis of 270 patients treated between 1985 and 1993. J Clin Oncol 1999;17:2105–16.
3. Whitmore WF, Gittes RF. Studies on the prostate and testis as immunologically privileged sites. Cancer Treat Rep 1977;61:217–22.
4. Drake CG, Doody AD, Mihalyo MA, et al. Androgen ablation mitigates tolerance to a prostate/prostate cancer-restricted antigen. Cancer Cell 2005;7:239–49.
5. Vesalainen S, Lipponen P, Talja M, et al. Histological grade, perineural infiltration, tumour-infiltrating lymphocytes and apoptosis as determinants of long-term prognosis in prostatic adenocarcinoma. Eur J Cancer 1994;30A:1797–803.
6. McArdle PA, Canna K, McMillan DC, et al. The relationship between T-lymphocyte subset infiltration and survival in patients with prostate cancer. Br J Cancer 2004;91:541–3.
7. Mercader M, Bodner BK, Moser MT, et al. T cell infiltration of the prostate induced by androgen withdrawal in patients with prostate cancer. Proc Natl Acad Sci U S A 2001;98:14565–70.
8. Sfanos KS, Bruno TC, Meeker AK, et al. Human prostate-infiltrating CD8+ T lymphocytes are oligoclonal and PD-1+. Prostate 2009;69:1694–703.
9. Gannon PO, Poisson AO, Delvoye N, et al. Characterization of the intra-prostatic immune cell infiltration in androgen-deprived prostate cancer patients. J Immunol Methods 2009;348:9–17.
10. Coffey DS, Isaacs JT. Prostate tumor biology and cell kinetics–theory. Urology 1981;17:40–53.
11. Pound CR, Partin AW, Eisenberger MA, et al. Natural history of progression after PSA elevation following radical prostatectomy. JAMA 1999;281:1591–7.
12. Drake CG, Jaffee E, Pardoll DM. Mechanisms of immune evasion by tumors. Adv Immunol 2006;90:51–81.
13. Chen L. Co-inhibitory molecules of the B7-CD28 family in the control of T-cell immunity. Nat Rev Immunol 2004;4:336–47.
14. Thompson RH, Gillett MD, Cheville JC, et al. Costimulatory B7-H1 in renal cell carcinoma patients: indicator of tumor aggressiveness and potential therapeutic target. Proc Natl Acad Sci U S A 2004; 101:17174–9.
15. Inman BA, Sebo TJ, Frigola X, et al. PD-L1 (B7-H1) expression by urothelial carcinoma of the bladder and BCG-induced granulomata: associations with localized stage progression. Cancer 2007;109: 1499–505.
16. Freeman GJ, Wherry EJ, Ahmed R, et al. Reinvigorating exhausted HIV-specific T cells via PD-1-PD-1 ligand blockade. J Exp Med 2006;203:2223–7.
17. Penna A, Pilli M, Zerbini A, et al. Dysfunction and functional restoration of HCV-specific CD8 responses in chronic hepatitis C virus infection. Hepatology 2007;45:588–601.
18. Barber DL, Wherry EJ, Masopust D, et al. Restoring function in exhausted CD8 T cells during chronic viral infection. Nature 2006;439:682–7.
19. Curiel TJ, Wei S, Dong H, et al. Blockade of B7-H1 improves myeloid dendritic cell-mediated antitumor immunity. Nat Med 2003;9:562–7.
20. Blank C, Kuball J, Voelkl S, et al. Blockade of PD-L1 (B7-H1) augments human tumor-specific T cell responses in vitro. Int J Cancer 2006;119:317–27.
21. Shariat SF, Kim JH, Andrews B, et al. Preoperative plasma levels of transforming growth factor beta(1) strongly predict clinical outcome in patients with bladder carcinoma. Cancer 2001;92:2985–92.
22. Miller AM, Lundberg K, Ozenci V, et al. CD4+ CD25high T cells are enriched in the tumor and peripheral blood of prostate cancer patients. J Immunol 2006;177:7398–405.
23. Yokokawa J, Cereda V, Remondo C, et al. Enhanced functionality of CD4+CD25(high)FoxP3+ regulatory T cells in the peripheral blood of patients with prostate cancer. Clin Cancer Res 2008;14:1032–40.
24. Getnet D, Maris CH, Hipkiss EL, et al. Tumor recognition and self-recognition induce distinct transcriptional profiles in antigen-specific CD4 T cells. J Immunol 2009;182:4675–85.
25. Ostrand-Rosenberg S, Sinha P. Myeloid-derived suppressor cells: linking inflammation and cancer. J Immunol 2009;182:4499–506.

26. McNeel DG, Malkovsky M. Immune-based therapies for prostate cancer. Immunol Lett 2005;96:3–9.
27. Gulley JL, Madan RA, Arlen PM. Enhancing efficacy of therapeutic vaccinations by combination with other modalities. Vaccine 2007;(25 Suppl 2):B89–96.
28. Fong L, Small EJ. Immunotherapy for prostate cancer. Curr Oncol Rep 2007;9:226–33.
29. Slovin SF. Pitfalls or promise in prostate cancer immunotherapy–which is winning? Cancer J 2008; 14:26–34.
30. McNeel DG, Dunphy EJ, Davies JG, et al. Safety and immunological efficacy of a DNA vaccine encoding prostatic acid phosphatase (PAP) in patients with stage D0 prostate cancer. J Clin Oncol 2009;27: 425–30.
31. Acres B, Bonnefoy JY. Clinical development of MVA-based therapeutic cancer vaccines. Expert Rev Vaccines 2008;7:889–93.
32. Madan RA, Arlen PM, Mohebtash M, et al. Prostvac-VF: a vector-based vaccine targeting PSA in prostate cancer. Expert Opin Investig Drugs 2009;18: 1001–11.
33. Kaufman HL, Wang W, Manola J, et al. Phase II randomized study of vaccine treatment of advanced prostate cancer (E7897): a trial of the Eastern Cooperative Oncology Group. J Clin Oncol 2004;22: 2122–32.
34. Kaufman HL, Wang W, Manola J, et al. Phase II prime/boost vaccination using poxviruses expressing PSA in hormone dependent prostate cancer: follow-up clinical results from ECOG 7897 [abstract]. Proc Am Soc Clin Oncol 2005;24:4501a.
35. Hodge JW, Sabzevari H, Yafal AG, et al. A triad of costimulatory molecules synergize to amplify T-cell activation. Cancer Res 1999;59:5800–7.
36. Kantoff PW, Glode LM, Tannenbaum SI, et al. Randomized, double-blind, vector-controlled study of targeted immunotherapy in patients (pts) with hormone-refractory prostate cancer (HRPC) [abstract]. J Clin Oncol 2006;24:100S.
37. Dranoff G, Jaffee E, Lazenby A, et al. Vaccination with irradiated tumor cells engineered to secrete murine granulocyte-macrophage colony-stimulating factor stimulates potent, specific, and long-lasting anti-tumor immunity. Proc Natl Acad Sci U S A 1993;90:3539–43.
38. Simons JW, Sacks N. Granulocyte-macrophage colony-stimulating factor-transduced allogeneic cancer cellular immunotherapy: the GVAX vaccine for prostate cancer. Urol Oncol 2006;24:419–24.
39. Higano CS, Corman JM, Smith DC, et al. Phase 1/2 dose-escalation study of a GM-CSF-secreting, allogeneic, cellular immunotherapy for metastatic hormone refractory prostate cancer. Cancer 2008; 113:975–84.
40. Small EJ, Sacks N, Nemunaitis J, et al. Granulocyte macrophage colony-stimulating factor–secreting allogeneic cellular immunotherapy for hormone-refractory prostate cancer. Clin Cancer Res 2007; 13:3883–91.
41. Higano C, Saad F, Somer B, et-al. A phase III trial of GVAX immunotherapy for prostate cancer versus docetaxel plus prednisone in asymptomatic, castration-resistant prostate cancer (CRPC). In: Genitourinary Cancer Symposium 2009, Abstract 150, 2009.
42. Doehn C, Bohmer T, Jocham D. Technology evaluation: Onyvax-P, Onyvax. Curr Opin Mol Ther 2005;7: 511–9.
43. Michael A, Ball G, Quatan N, et al. Delayed disease progression after allogeneic cell vaccination in hormone-resistant prostate cancer and correlation with immunologic variables. Clin Cancer Res 2005; 11:4469–78.
44. Burch PA, Breen JK, Buckner JC, et al. Priming tissue-specific cellular immunity in a phase I trial of autologous dendritic cells for prostate cancer. Clin Cancer Res 2000;6:2175–82.
45. Small EJ, Fratesi P, Reese DM, et al. Immunotherapy of hormone-refractory prostate cancer with antigen-loaded dendritic cells. J Clin Oncol 2000; 18:3894–903.
46. Small EJ, Schellhammer PF, Higano CS, et al. Placebo-controlled phase III trial of immunologic therapy with sipuleucel-T (APC8015) in patients with metastatic, asymptomatic hormone refractory prostate cancer. J Clin Oncol 2006;24:3089–94.
47. Schurko B, Oh WK. Docetaxel chemotherapy remains the standard of care in castration-resistant prostate cancer. Nat Clin Pract Oncol 2008;5:506–7.
48. Koh YT, Gray A, Higgins SA, et al. Androgen ablation augments prostate cancer vaccine immunogenicity only when applied after immunization. Prostate 2009;69:571–84.
49. Roden AC, Moser MT, Tri SD, et al. Augmentation of T cell levels and responses induced by androgen deprivation. J Immunol 2004;173:6098–108.
50. Aragon-Ching JB, Williams KM, Gulley JL. Impact of androgen-deprivation therapy on the immune system: implications for combination therapy of prostate cancer. Front Biosci 2007;12:4957–71.
51. Sanda MG, Smith DC, Charles LG, et al. Recombinant vaccinia-PSA (PROSTVAC) can induce a prostate-specific immune response in androgen-modulated human prostate cancer. Urology 1999; 53:260–6.
52. Madan RA, Gulley JL, Schlom J, et al. Analysis of overall survival in patients with nonmetastatic castration-resistant prostate cancer treated with vaccine, nilutamide, and combination therapy. Clin Cancer Res 2008;14:4526–31.
53. Tannock IF, de Wit R, Berry WR, et al. Docetaxel plus prednisone or mitoxantrone plus prednisone for advanced prostate cancer 1. N Engl J Med 2004; 351:1502–12.

54. Petrylak DP, Tangen CM, Hussain MH, et al. Docetaxel and estramustine compared with mitoxantrone and prednisone for advanced refractory prostate cancer 2. N Engl J Med 2004;351:1513–20.
55. Bradley DA, Hussain M. Promising novel cytotoxic agents and combinations in metastatic prostate cancer. Cancer J 2008;14:15–9.
56. Arlen PM, Gulley JL, Parker C, et al. A randomized phase II study of concurrent docetaxel plus vaccine versus vaccine alone in metastatic androgen-independent prostate cancer. Clin Cancer Res 2006; 12:1260–9.
57. Machiels JP, Reilly RT, Emens LA, et al. Cyclophosphamide, doxorubicin, and paclitaxel enhance the antitumor immune response of granulocyte/macrophage-colony stimulating factor-secreting whole-cell vaccines in HER-2/neu tolerized mice. Cancer Res 2001;61:3689–97.
58. Laheru D, Lutz E, Burke J, et al. Allogeneic granulocyte macrophage colony-stimulating factor-secreting tumor immunotherapy alone or in sequence with cyclophosphamide for metastatic pancreatic cancer: a pilot study of safety, feasibility, and immune activation. Clin Cancer Res 2008;14: 1455–63.
59. Wada S, Yoshimura K, Hipkiss EL, et al. Cyclophosphamide augments antitumor immunity: studies in an autochthonous prostate cancer model. Cancer Res 2009;69:4309–18.
60. Chakraborty M, Abrams SI, Coleman CN, et al. External beam radiation of tumors alters phenotype of tumor cells to render them susceptible to vaccine-mediated T-cell killing. Cancer Res 2004;64:4328–37.
61. Demaria S, Kawashima N, Yang AM, et al. Immune-mediated inhibition of metastases after treatment with local radiation and CTLA-4 blockade in a mouse model of breast cancer. Clin Cancer Res 2005;11: 728–34.
62. Harris TJ, Hipkiss EL, Borzillary S, et al. Radiotherapy augments the immune response to prostate cancer in a time-dependent manner. Prostate 2008; 68:1319–29.
63. Gulley JL, Arlen PM, Bastian A, et al. Combining a recombinant cancer vaccine with standard definitive radiotherapy in patients with localized prostate cancer. Clin Cancer Res 2005;11:3353–62.
64. Bronte V, Kasic T, Gri G, et al. Boosting antitumor responses of T lymphocytes infiltrating human prostate cancers. J Exp Med 2005;201:1257–68.
65. Sfanos KS, Bruno TC, Maris CH, et al. Phenotypic analysis of prostate-infiltrating lymphocytes reveals TH17 and Treg skewing. Clin Cancer Res 2008;14: 3254–61.
66. Anderson MJ, Shafer-Weaver K, Greenberg NM, et al. Tolerization of tumor-specific T cells despite efficient initial priming in a primary murine model of prostate cancer. J Immunol 2007;178:1268–76.
67. Bai A, Higham E, Eisen HN, et al. Rapid tolerization of virus-activated tumor-specific CD8+ T cells in prostate tumors of TRAMP mice. Proc Natl Acad Sci U S A 2008;105:13003–8.
68. Lees JR, Charbonneau B, Hayball JD, et al. T-cell recognition of a prostate specific antigen is not sufficient to induce prostate tissue destruction. Prostate 2006;66:578–90.
69. Degl'Innocenti E, Grioni M, Boni A, et al. Peripheral T cell tolerance occurs early during spontaneous prostate cancer development and can be rescued by dendritic cell immunization. Eur J Immunol 2005;35:66–75.
70. Redmond WL, Gough MJ, Weinberg AD. Ligation of the OX40 co-stimulatory receptor reverses self-Ag and tumor-induced CD8 T-cell anergy in vivo. Eur J Immunol 2009;39:2184–94.
71. Hurwitz AA, Foster BA, Kwon ED, et al. Combination immunotherapy of primary prostate cancer in a transgenic mouse model using CTLA-4 blockade. Cancer Res 2000;60:2444–8.
72. Small EJ, Tchekmedyian NS, Rini BI, et al. A pilot trial of CTLA-4 blockade with human anti-CTLA-4 in patients with hormone-refractory prostate cancer. Clin Cancer Res 2007;13:1810–5.
73. Fong L, Kwek SS, O'Brien S, et al. Potentiating endogenous antitumor immunity to prostate cancer through combination immunotherapy with CTLA4 blockade and GM-CSF. Cancer Res 2009;69:609–15.
74. Keir ME, Butte MJ, Freeman GJ, et al. PD-1 and its ligands in tolerance and immunity. Annu Rev Immunol 2008;26:677–704.
75. Ebelt K, Babaryka G, Frankenberger B, et al. Prostate cancer lesions are surrounded by FOXP3+, PD-1+ and B7-H1+ lymphocyte clusters. Eur J Cancer 2009;45:1664–72.
76. Weinberg AD, Vella AT, Croft M. OX-40: life beyond the effector T cell stage. Semin Immunol 1998;10: 471–80.
77. Silver DA, Pellicer I, Fair WR, et al. Prostate-specific membrane antigen expression in normal and malignant human tissues. Clin Cancer Res 1997;3:81–5.
78. Ross JS, Gray KE, Webb IJ, et al. Antibody-based therapeutics: focus on prostate cancer. Cancer Metastasis Rev 2005;24:521–37.
79. Milowsky MI, Nanus DM, Kostakoglu L, et al. Phase I trial of yttrium-90-labeled anti-prostate-specific membrane antigen monoclonal antibody J591 for androgen-independent prostate cancer. J Clin Oncol 2004;22:2522–31.
80. Bander NH, Milowsky MI, Nanus DM, et al. Phase I trial of 177lutetium-labeled J591, a monoclonal antibody to prostate-specific membrane antigen, in patients with androgen-independent prostate cancer. J Clin Oncol 2005;23:4591–601.

Blood and Tissue Biomarkers in Prostate Cancer: State of the Art

Michelangelo Fiorentino, MD, PhD[a,b], Elisa Capizzi, MSc[b], Massimo Loda, MD[a,b,*]

KEYWORDS

- Prostate cancer • Tissue biomarkers
- Blood biomarkers • Molecular pathology

The prevalence of prostate cancer (PCa) is high and increases with age. PCa is the most common noncutaneous cancer in American men, with an estimate of 192,280 new cases diagnosed in 2009 but with only 27,360 deaths, and a leading cause of male cancer-related death, second only to lung cancer, representing 10% of all cancer deaths in men in the United States (http://www.cancer.org/docroot/STT/STT_0.asp).

Multiple factors contribute to the high incidence and prevalence of PCa. Risk factors include age, family history, environmental exposures, and race. Prostate-specific antigen (PSA) screening has impacted the detection of PCa and is directly responsible for a dramatic decrease in stage at diagnosis, with over 80% of PCa being localized to the prostate. Gleason score and stage at the time of diagnosis remain the mainstays to predict prognosis, in the absence of more accurate and reliable tissue or blood biomarkers.[1] Because of PSA screening, however, these parameters are beginning to lose discriminatory power for patients with organ-confined disease and intermediate tumor differentiation. As a result, most men diagnosed today in this post-PSA screening era are being overtreated, and those men with the most aggressive form of the disease-metastatic PCa are inadequately treated.

Despite extensive research efforts, very few biomarkers of PCa have been introduced to date in clinical practice. Even screening with PSA has recently been questioned.[2,3]

In the 1980s and 1990s the search for diagnostic or prognostic markers in human solid tumors focused predominantly on immunohistochemical markers. The vast majority of these, however, never found a clinical application probably as a result of underpowered databases, lack of validation sets, and inappropriate end points (eg, PSA failure instead of death), or the introduction confounders in statistical analyses such as inappropriate case selection or too many biomarkers analyzed at once. The application from 2005 by the major biomedical journals of the REMARK recommendations for reporting tumor marker studies has radically changed this approach, leading to a general reduction in the number of studies describing immunohistochemical markers.[4] At the same time, a steady increase in the number of studies dealing with prognostic or diagnostic circulating blood/serum tumor biomarkers has been observed, reflecting the need for new and

This work was supported by the National Cancer Institute [RO1CA131945, PO1CA89021, P50 CA90381, PO1 CA55075, R01 CA136578], and the Prostate Cancer Foundation.

[a] Center for Molecular Oncologic Pathology, Departments of Pathology and Medical Oncology, Dana-Farber Cancer Institute, Brigham and Women's Hospital, Harvard Medical School, D1536, 44 Binney Street, Boston, MA 02115, USA

[b] Laboratory of Molecular Oncologic Pathology, Addarii Institute of Oncology, S.Orsola-Malpighi Hospital, Bologna, Italy

* Corresponding author. Dana-Farber Cancer Institute, D1536, 44 Binney Street, Boston, MA 02115.

E-mail address: massimo_loda@dfci.harvard.edu (M. Loda).

Urol Clin N Am 37 (2010) 131–141
doi:10.1016/j.ucl.2009.11.006

urologic.theclinics.com

noninvasive tests to predict the behavior of PCa. A thorough analysis of all tissue and serum biomarkers in prostate cancer cannot be easily synthesized and goes beyond the scope of this article. Therefore, the authors focus here on the most recently reported tissue and circulating biomarkers for PCa whose application in clinical practice is either current or expected in the near future.

TISSUE BIOMARKERS

Investigation of immunohistochemical biomarkers in solid tumors has rapidly progressed alongside the development of tissue microarray (TMA) and imaging technologies. The use of TMA allows the simultaneous analysis of hundreds of cases, resulting in a more uniform staining procedure while reducing costs.[5] The development of automated image analysis systems with high throughput and more precise quantitation is now progressively replacing the subjective, semiquantitative manual scoring previously performed by pathologists. Computerized image analysis allows the translation of the number of tumor cells expressing the biomarker and its intensity of immunostaining into numerical data, more amenable to large-scale bioinformatic analyses.[6] Furthermore, the application to in situ histologic techniques of antibody or probes conjugated with nanoparticles (quantum dots) permits the simultaneous use of multiple biomarkers in tissue or TMA sections.[7] These important technical advances have recently made immunohistochemical biomarkers more reliable and quantifiable in most solid tumors, including PCa. The TMA technology also allows one to ascertain the power of single biomarkers in much larger series of formalin-fixed, paraffin-embedded (FFPE) archival tumor samples. The application of tissue biomarkers to the largest cohorts of PCa patients traditionally studied by epidemiologists has led to the establishment of the new discipline of pathoepidemiology. Pathoepidemiology combines the information from tumor registries and cancer statistics with the knowledge of morphology, biomarker expression, and molecular genetics. The access to these well-annotated cohorts of patients is particularly valuable in the field of PCa, where patients must be followed for decades rather than years to obtain meaningful prognostic information.

Technologies of genome-wide scanning such as gene expression profiling, comparative genomic hybridization (CGH), and single nucleotide polymorphism (SNP) arrays are now also applicable to nucleic acids extracted from archival tissues.[8] Genome-wide analyses are now able to quickly unravel expression signatures, specific genomic losses or gains, and the activation or silencing of entire cell pathways on large series of PCa patients.

To provide a panoramic view of the most promising tissue biomarkers, this article describes the immunohistochemical prognostic markers and targets of therapy belonging to the following broad categories: biomarkers of pathway activation, chromosome 8 aberrations, TMPRSS2-ERG fusion, tumor metabolism, stem cell markers, and SNP analysis/gene expression profiling/genomic comparative hybridization.

Pathway Activation Markers

Signal trafficking regulation through major cell hubs is central in the processes of tumor initiation and progression, and represents a major target for tumor-specific therapies. In prostate adenocarcinoma, the phosphatidylinositol 3-kinase (PI3K) is the most frequently activated signal transduction pathway.[9] In contrast, aberrant activation of the MAPK pathway seems less frequently involved, possibly due to absence of Ras and Raf mutations.[10] In PCa the most common mechanism of PI3K pathway activation is the deletion of the gene encoding the phosphatase and tensin homologue (PTEN) protein, whose inactivation in turns leads to phosphorylations of AKT and of the S6 ribosomal subunit, which are therefore powerful biomarkers of PI3K activation.[11] Upregulation of the PI3K/AKT/mTOR pathway is estimated to occur in about 50% of PCa, but not only through loss of PTEN. In addition, PTEN deletions seem to be more frequent in metastatic than in organ-confined disease.[12,13] Immunohistochemistry can easily detect the activation of the major components of the PI3K pathway using antibodies against specific phosphorylation sites of the AKT, mTOR, and S6 proteins. Decreased expression of PTEN can be identified by immunohistochemistry as well, while its genetic inactivation may be determined by fluorescence in situ hybridization (FISH) or by genome-wide analyses such as array CGH (aCGH). In humans, down-regulation of PTEN and consequent activation of the PI3K pathway members in PCa tissue samples has been correlated to higher Gleason grade, advanced stage, and development of androgen resistance.[11,14,15] Immunohistochemical detection of phospho-AKT in PCa tissue also predicts early biochemical recurrence and poor outcome.[16,17] Of note, in mice inhibition of mTOR with rapamycin analogues results in complete reversal of the neoplastic prostate phenotype driven by activated AKT1.[18] Several phase 1 and 2 clinical trials with specific agents targeting key activated proteins in the PI3K pathway are ongoing in PCa patients, including selective inhibitors of p110, AKT1, and mTOR.[19] The TMPRSS2-ERG translocation (see later discussion) is found in upwards of 60% of prostate cancers and is androgen driven.[20] Because this translocation results in similar downstream effects to MAPK activation, PCa displaying the fusion may be considered MAPK active. The combination of androgen blockade with tyrosine kinase inhibitors targeting the PI3K or the MAPK pathway may represent alternative therapeutic choices in PCa. Selection of patients for these therapeutic regimens therefore becomes very important. Such selection can only occur through the use of selective biomarkers.

Chromosome 8 Aberrations and MYC

Losses of 8p and gains of 8q represent 2 of the most common chromosome aberrations in PCa.[21] In particular, the 8p locus seems to be the most commonly deleted region in PCa, occurring in 30% of organ-confined tumors and in about half of advanced cases. Single genomic losses at 8p represent early events in prostate carcinogenesis, as demonstrated by the occurrence of frequent 8p deletions in experimental prostate intraepithelial neoplasia (PIN).[22] In humans, most PIN lesions are also associated with loss of heterozygosity at chromosome 8p21, where the *NKX3.1* gene, encoding a validated tumor suppressor gene, resides. *NKX3.1* is an androgen-regulated homeodomain transcription factor that regulates the proliferation rate of prostate luminal epithelial cells.[23,24] The development of PIN lesions in NKX3.1-deficient mice has been recently associated with alterations of the PTEN/AKT axis.[25] Haploinsufficiency of NKX3.1 might extend the proliferative stage of regenerating luminal cells, leading to epithelial hyperplasia and dysplasia. NKX3.1 has been used as a biomarker, with conflicting results to date.[26]

On the other hand, 8q is the most commonly gained region in advanced PCa.[27] Genetic polymorphisms at 8q are consistently associated with prostate cancer risk across multiple ethnic groups, with the highest susceptibility at the 8q24 region.[28] Specific genetic variants at 8q24 have also been correlated with higher Gleason grade and more aggressive prostate cancer behavior.[29] The coding region closest to 8q24 is the well-known oncogene MYC. Although many attempts have been made to correlate polymorphism at 8q24 with MYC upregulation, none to date has clearly demonstrated a relationship with MYC increased transcription.[30] MYC is a well-known regulator of proliferation and biologic activity in prostate cancer cells, and its amplification is associated with the presence of PIN and poor clinical outcome of PCa.[31] In addition, transgenic expression of MYC results in PIN as well as invasive cancers in the prostate.[32] Nuclear overexpression of the MYC protein has been shown in PIN, suggesting a role for MYC in early prostate carcinogenesis.[33]

TMPRSS2-ERG Fusion

One of the most important recent findings in PCa is the discovery of the TMPRSS2-ERG fusion. The fusion of the 5′ untranslated region of the androgen-regulated TMPRSS2 gene with the transcription factor ERG leads to the aberrant expression of ERG in an androgen-dependent manner.[34] TMPRSS2-ERG gene fusion is rare in normal prostate tissue whereas it is consistently detectable in PIN, in organ-confined as well as in metastatic hormone refractory PCa.[35] The presence of the TMPRSS2-ERG fusion has been associated, in some studies, with high tumor stage, presence of lymph node metastases, and poor outcome.[36,37] These reports, together with the finding that the fusion occurs in both PIN and adjacent invasive cancer cells apparently as an "all or none" phenomenon in individual invasive clones within the same prostate, led to the hypothesis that the TMPRSS2-ERG rearrangement might define, from the early steps of carcinogenesis, a subset of more aggressive PCa. Unfortunately, attempts to correlate the fusion status with high Gleason score or with outcome have given conflicting results in subsequent studies.[38–40] This issue is further complicated by the presence of a growing number of different translocations involving the ETS transcription factor family.[41] Further work is required to understand the role that this prevalent translocation plays in prostatic carcinogenesis and its relationship to the biologic behavior of prostate adenocarcinoma.

Biomarkers of Altered Lipid Metabolism in Prostate Cancer

More than 80 years ago the Nobel prize winner Otto Warburg proposed that tumorigenicity of cancer cells derived from their ability to switch from oxidative phosphorylation to glycolysis to satisfy their high energetic needs.[42] The products of the glycolytic pathway and of the subverted metabolic pathways may provide the substrate for the structural need in the tumor cell enhanced proliferative state. Lipogenesis is therefore a distinctive feature of tumor cells.[43–45] Cancer cells synthesize de novo large amounts of fatty acids and cholesterol irrespective of the circulating lipid levels, and benefit from this increased lipid synthesis in terms of growth advantage, self survival, and drug resistance. Numerous studies have shown that inactivation of most lipogenic enzymes, such as ATP citrate lyase (ACL), fatty acid synthase (FASN), and acetyl-CoA carboxylase, results in either cytostatic or cytotoxic effects in tumor cells.[46–48] Cholesterol is critical for the composition and stabilization of cell membranes while fatty acids may also be required for post-transcriptional regulation of key signal transduction proteins through posttranslational modifications such as palmitoylation and myristoylation. Fatty acid synthase (FASN) is the only enzyme that is able to synthesize fatty acids de novo in normal and cancer cells, and its main enzymatic product palmitic acid is responsible for the acylation (palmitoylation) of key regulatory switches in most signal transduction pathways. FASN was proposed as the first bona fide candidate metabolic oncogene in the prostate.[49] The mere forced expression of FASN is able to transform immortalized prostate epithelial cells, to form invasive tumors in immunodeficient mice while transgenic mice expressing FASN in the prostate develop PIN.[50] The proposed mechanisms of FASN oncogenicity include structural needs of synthesized lipids, protection from endoplasmic reticulum stress, inhibition of the intrinsic (mitochondrial) pathway of apoptosis, and palmitoylation of Wnt-1 with subsequent stabilization of β-catenin and activation of the pathway.[50–52] Natural and irreversible inhibitors of FASN are able to reduce cell proliferation and induce cell death in PCa cell lines, and to reduce the volume of PCa xenograft tumors in mice.[53,54] FASN can be therefore considered an excellent and promising biomarker and therapeutic target in prostate cancer.

Caveolae are plasma membrane microdomains rich in cholesterol, similar to lipid rafts but characterized by the presence of a protein family named caveolins. Both lipid rafts and caveolae are cholesterol- and sphingolipid-enriched microdomains in cell membranes that regulate phosphorylation cascades originating from membrane-bound proteins. Altered cholesterol synthesis results in changes in membrane cholesterol and, in turn, in Akt signaling in both normal and malignant cells.[55] Caveolins possess a key regulatory activity in cell molecular transport and cell trafficking. The most studied member of this family, Caveolin-1, has been involved in prostate cancer initiation and progression and identified as a marker of aggressive PCa. Caveolin-1 knockout in the PCa TRAMP mouse model significantly reduces prostate tumor size and the development of metastases.[56] This effect might be at least in part mediated by FASN, which is downstream of Caveolin-1.[57] Caveolin 1 may therefore be an important biomarker of aggressive behavior in prostate cancer.

Stem Cell Markers

Identification and isolation of cancer stem cells (CSCs) in solid tumors, including PCa, has been an area of intense research effort in the last 10 years. A growing body of literature supports the CSCs hypothesis as a model to explain intratumoral heterogeneity and the development of resistance to therapy.[58]

CSCs (also known as tumor-initiating cells, TICs) are characterized by unlimited renewal potential when injected into immunodeficient mice in which neoplasms recapitulating the heterogeneity of the original tumor form at high efficiency.[59,60] CSC phenotype is usually defined by a panel of multiple rather than single surface markers. In PCa these cells have been identified as $CD44^{+}/\alpha2\beta1^{high}/CD133^{+}$ and androgen receptor negative.[61] This phenotype was widely employed to select and isolate putative CSCs from prostate cell lines, xenografts, and biopsies of human tumors to test their invasive property and to identify a specific CSC genetic signature.[62]

$CD44^{+}/CD24^{-}$ cells isolated from LNCaP cells possess increased clonogenic properties, form tumors in NOD/SCID mice, and show a gene signature of invasiveness originally identified in breast tumors.[63,64] There is also experimental evidence that a subpopulation of $CD44^{+}$ CSC-like cells is able to invade Matrigel, suggesting that basement membrane invasion is a characteristic trait of these putative prostate CSCs.[65] It is intriguing that in human PCa tissues all the cells with neuroendocrine differentiation are $CD44^{+}$, suggesting a role for such cells in the resistance to androgen therapy and tumor recurrence.[66] Additional studies are required to better identify putative prostate CSCs in PCa tissue samples. To the authors' knowledge there are no conclusive studies that have characterized the molecular phenotype and the clinical significance of CSCs in PCa patients. Based on current knowledge, it seems most plausible that prostate CSCs originate from cells in different stages of prostate epithelial cell differentiation, providing an alternative explanation for the well-known morphologic and biologic heterogeneity of human PCa.[67]

Reliable recognition of prostate CSCs and development of novel markers for their identification might help the development of therapies specifically targeted at the CSCs compartment.

Single Nucleotide Polymorphism Analysis, Gene Expression Profiling, and Comparative Genomic Hybridization

SNP array technology allows genome-wide and high-throughput analysis of DNA polymorphisms with the intent of comparing different cancers, exploring tumor-normal differences, and assessing polymorphic alleles with predictive behavior. SNP is therefore the method of choice to assess genetic variants and allelic imbalances. Although in the prostate no susceptibility genes comparable to BRCA1 in breast or APC in colon have been discovered so far, multiple germ-line polymorphisms have been correlated to increased individual risk of developing PCa.[68] In addition to susceptibility studies, SNP arrays have been used to distinguish genetic subsets of PCa with different clinical behavior.[69] Progression of PCa toward metastasis and high Gleason grade in the primary tumor were recently correlated to gains of 8q, 1q, 3q, and 7q, whereas androgen ablation therapy was characterized by gains at 2p and 10q using SNP array analysis.[70] In another large control study based on SNP arrays, germ-line deletion at 2p24.3 was strongly associated with aggressive PCa.[71] Germline polymorphisms within genes encoding for androgen-metabolizing proteins have been also correlated to response rate in PCa patients treated with hormone therapy.[72]

aCGH is the best technology to detect DNA copy number alterations in cancer compared with normal tissues.[73] Deletions in 8p, 13q, 6q and gains in 8q and 7q, and specific losses at 10q24 (PTEN) and gains at Xq12 (AR) are the most common copy number alterations in PCa. Loss of 8p and gain of 11q13 have been associated with advanced stage and biochemical recurrence, respectively.[74] Of note, intermediate risk PCa was characterized by copy number alterations previously associated with high-risk disease.[75] The progressive optimization of the aCGH on DNA extracted from FFPE tissues will extend the applications of this technique with further expansion into clinical practice.[76]

Gene expression profiling of up to 26K genes is now available also for RNA extracted from FFPE tissues.[77,78] Expression-based models have been correlated to patient outcome and to biochemical recurrence in PCa.[79,80] A case-control study comparing men who had just PSA failure with those who developed metastatic PCa after radical prostatectomy showed that the 2 groups could be separated by an expression model containing 17 genes with a specific enrichment in the 8q24 locus.[81] Unfortunately, the high number of genes used in constructing these predictive models and the variable cutoffs employed to estimate the signal to noise ratio in each model, together with the complex bioinformatic algorithms required to deconvolute and interpret the data, have prevented the routine use of gene expression analyses in clinical practice, although these may become useful adjuncts to the commonly used Partin tables or Kattan nomograms.[8] Once the RNA extraction techniques from FFPE tissues are optimized and the relevant gene signatures applied, this technology will likely become necessary for stratification, prognostication, and assessment of predictive behavior in PCa patients.

BLOOD BIOMARKERS

The focus of molecular diagnostics is rapidly moving from tissues to bodily fluids, and particularly to blood. Detection of biomarkers with diagnostic and prognostic significance in bodily fluids may in the near future provide valuable clinical information while avoiding unnecessary invasive procedures. The current technological advances allow reliable extraction and separation of circulating tumor cells (CTCs) in the blood and of tumor-derived nucleic acids and proteins in plasma, urine, sputum, and stools. Enhanced tumor invasion during the metastatic process, active secretion of proteins by highly vascularized tumors, or passive release of cellular breakdown materials in areas of necrosis could all result in tumor-specific nucleic acid or protein material in the bloodstream or in other fluids. PCa is relatively poorly vascularized, with little or no necrotic areas. Therefore, the presence of tumor cells or tumor-derived material in the blood of PCa patients probably reflects increased tumor invasiveness. Tumor-specific DNA mutations, genomic instability and epigenetic changes, detection of aberrant proteins, exploration of tumor-specific transcriptome signatures, and microRNA expression profiles may all represent valuable biomarkers that can be found in bodily fluids in cancer patients.

While not addressing the paramount role that PSA plays as a serum biomarker, the authors now focus on 2 intriguing and novel blood biomarkers in PCa: the detection and characterization of the free tumor plasma DNA (FPDNA) and the isolation of CTCs.

Free Plasma DNA

It has been known since the 1950s that free plasma DNA (FPDNA) circulates in the blood of normal individuals while increases in FPDNA may occur in pathologic conditions including autoimmune diseases, liver cirrhosis, major traumas, and malignant tumors.[82,83] The detection of circulating free plasma DNA seems to be a promising and noninvasive test for early tumor detection, assessment of disease recurrence, and monitoring of therapy.[84–86] Increased FPDNA levels have been observed in patients with several epithelial malignancies, including PCa, when compared with healthy subjects.[87,88] In addition, FPDNA has been recently correlated with both tumor stage and the presence of CTCs, suggesting a role of FPDNA as candidate biomarker for the monitoring of PCa patients.[89–91]

An important concern for the application of FPDNA tests are false positives, particularly in patients with autoimmune or inflammatory diseases and a recent history of trauma or surgical procedures.[83] To hone in on the tumor origin of circulating DNA, specific genetic aberrations (eg, loss of heterozygosity and microsatellite analysis) or epigenetic alterations (eg, gene promoter hypermethylation) should be identified in FPDNA. Such alterations have been successfully reported in blood and bone marrow samples.[92,93] However, discrepancies between genetic aberrations in the primary tumor DNA and in FPDNA have been reported, and might be ascribed to tumor heterogeneity with various populations of cells with diverse genetic alterations undergoing lysis.[92,94] Further clinical validation of these findings may unravel a role for FPDNA as a valuable new biomarker for monitoring the metastatic progression in PCa patients.

Circulating Tumor Cells and Disseminating Tumor Cells

The occurrence of a metastatic, castration-resistant tumor represents the major cause of PCa-related mortality. Metastatic spread has been typically considered a late process in malignant progression, but several studies have recently suggested that dissemination of primary cancer cells to distant sites might be an early event in tumorigenesis. In addition, tumor cells can bypass the lymph node filter and disseminate directly through the bloodstream to distant organs.[95] These findings led to the development of different assays for the detection of disseminated tumor cells (DTCs) in bone marrow (BM) and CTCs in the peripheral blood. The 2 main techniques employed are the immunologic and the polymerase chain reaction (PCR)-based molecular approach.[96] In the immunologic approach, immunochemistry using monoclonal antibodies against surface epithelial antigen is the most widely applied technique. This method is easy to perform and enables the evaluation of cell size and morphology, but sensitivity and specificity are antibody dependent. Real-time reverse transcription (RT)-PCR–based assays are extremely sensitive and able to detect aberrations at a single cell level. Prostate-specific transcripts such as PSA, prostate-specific membrane antigen, and prostate stem cell antigen are usually used as single or multiplexed surrogate markers in blood CTCs using RT-PCR or quantitative real-time PCR (qPCR). The major problem of the molecular approach is the false positive rate due to illegitimate transcripts and heterogeneous expression of target markers. The introduction of a cancer cell-enrichment step during the CTC isolation process and the establishment of a reliable cutoff value for analysis may overcome these problems.[97] Most clinical reports on DTC focused on BM, the most common metastatic site in PCa. Some investigators reported significant correlations between the presence of DTCs and clinical-pathologic parameters such as high Gleason grade or metastatic disease.[98,99] In addition, the presence of DTC in the BM at the time of diagnosis represents an independent negative prognostic parameter in patients with localized PCa.[100] Because BM aspiration is invasive, uncomfortable for the patients, and not suitable for repeated analysis, recent efforts have focused on the detection of CTCs in the peripheral blood. CTCs can now be easily detected by PCR in the blood at the time of diagnosis before, during, and after therapy, and their increased number has been positively associated with high Gleason score and stage.[101] In addition, the detection of PSA mRNA by qPCR has been significantly correlated to time to progression and overall survival.[102] Technical limitations of the PCR technique and the need for a more standardized method for the detection of CTCs in the peripheral blood led to the development of new technologies. The CellSearch (Veridex) is a device recently approved by the Food and Drug Administration for the monitoring of metastatic breast, colon, and prostate cancer able to isolate single CTCs by immunomagnetic enrichment followed by fluorimetric count (http://www.accessdata.fda.gov/cdrh_docs/reviews/K073338.pdf). Data generated using this automated system showed that CTCs could be detected in 55% to 62% of patients with castration-resistant prostate cancer (CRCP).[103,104] A baseline CTC count of 5 cells/7.5 mL or more of blood before therapy represents a powerful predictor of poor overall survival (OS).[105] In addition, the study of CTC dynamics following therapy showed that the CTC count predicts clinical outcome better than the algorithms based on PSA.[102] Patients whose CTC counts decreased from 5 cells or more at baseline to less than 5 cells after treatment had a better OS compared with those showing an increase during therapy.[106] By contrast, in patients with organ-confined PCa the number of detectable CTCs appears low and does not correlate with known prognostic factors.[107] Further molecular characterization of CTCs or DTCs in cancer patients could provide additional information on cancer biology and could improve the management of the disease by selecting effective targeted therapy in the individual patient context. Recent studies show that both high- and low-resolution techniques such as FISH or CGH could be performed on isolated cancer cells to obtain a genomic profile of CTCs/DTCs that could be related to prognosis and response to therapy.[108–110] The ultimate goal of the research on DTC/CTC is their propagation in vitro after isolation from cancer patients. Such an approach could provide a tool to test personalized oncologic treatments directly on the cells responsible for tumor progression of each specific patient.

SUMMARY

The clinical nomograms based on Gleason grade, tumor stage, and serum PSA are still the best predictors of PCa outcome. The biotechnological advancements achieved in the last decade represent a remarkable source for new prognostic and predictive tissue and serum molecular biomarkers. To introduce new biomarkers in the clinical practice of PCa the 3 following requirements must be necessarily satisfied: (1) the value of each biomarker must be tested in large annotated series of patients with reliable validation sets; (2) the statistical analyses must be robust, taking into account all the possible confounders and the patient selection; (3) the tissues utilized for biomarker validation and for the extraction of protein or nucleic acids must be reviewed by pathologists for the precise assessment of tumor areas, pathologic parameters, and tissue preservation. Pathoepidemiology is the first example of the useful interconnection of 2 apparently distant branches of medicine, with preventive, diagnostic, and clinical overlap that will ultimately benefit prostate cancer patients.

REFERENCES

1. Stark JR, Perner S, Stampfer MJ, et al. Gleason score and lethal prostate cancer: does 3 + 4 = 4 + 3? J Clin Oncol 2009;27(21):3459–64.
2. Schröder FH, Hugosson J, Roobol MJ, et al. Screening and prostate-cancer mortality in a randomized European study. N Engl J Med 2009;360(13):1320–8.
3. Andriole GL, Crawford ED, Grubb RL 3rd, et al. Mortality results from a randomized prostate-cancer screening trial. N Engl J Med 2009;360(13):1310–9.
4. McShane LM, Altman DG, Sauerbrei W, et al. Reporting recommendations for tumor marker prognostic studies. J Clin Oncol 2005;23(36):9067–72.
5. Camp RL, Neumeister V, Rimm DL. A decade of tissue microarrays: progress in the discovery and validation of cancer biomarkers. J Clin Oncol 2008;26(34):5630–7.
6. Wells WA, Barker PE, MacAulay C, et al. Validation of novel optical imaging technologies: the pathologists' view. J Biomed Opt 2007;12(5):051801.
7. Byers RJ, Di Vizio D, O'connell F, et al. Semiautomated multiplexed quantum dot-based in situ hybridization and spectral deconvolution. J Mol Diagn 2007;9(1):20–9.
8. Febbo PG. Genomic approaches to outcome prediction in prostate cancer. Cancer 2009; 115(Suppl 13):3046–57.
9. Lee JT Jr, Steelman LS, McCubrey JA. Phosphatidylinositol 3′-kinase activation leads to multidrug resistance protein-1 expression and subsequent chemoresistance in advanced prostate cancer cells. Cancer Res 2004;64(22):8397–404.
10. Lee JT, Lehmann BD, Terrian DM, et al. Targeting prostate cancer based on signal transduction and cell cycle pathways. Cell Cycle 2008;7(12):1745–62.
11. Sarker D, Reid AH, Yap TA, et al. Targeting the PI3K/AKT pathway for the treatment of prostate cancer. Clin Cancer Res 2009;15(15):4799–805.
12. Yoshimoto M, Cunha IW, Coudry RA, et al. FISH analysis of 107 prostate cancers shows that PTEN genomic deletion is associated with poor clinical outcome. Br J Cancer 2007;97(5):678–85.
13. Sircar K, Yoshimoto M, Monzon FA, et al. PTEN genomic deletion is associated with p-Akt and AR signalling in poorer outcome, hormone refractory prostate cancer. J Pathol 2009;218(4):505–13.
14. McMenamin ME, Soung P, Perera S, et al. Loss of PTEN expression in paraffin-embedded primary prostate cancer correlates with high Gleason score and advanced stage. Cancer Res 1999;59(17): 4291–6.
15. Bertram J, Peacock JW, Fazli L, et al. Loss of PTEN is associated with progression to androgen independence. Prostate 2006;66(9):895–902.
16. Ayala G, Thompson T, Yang G, et al. High levels of phosphorylated form of Akt-1 in prostate cancer and non-neoplastic prostate tissues are strong predictors of biochemical recurrence. Clin Cancer Res 2004;10(19):6572–8.

17. Kreisberg JI, Malik SN, Prihoda TJ, et al. Phosphorylation of Akt (Ser473) is an excellent predictor of poor clinical outcome in prostate cancer. Cancer Res 2004;64(15):5232–6.
18. Majumder PK, Febbo PG, Bikoff R, et al. mTOR inhibition reverses Akt-dependent prostate intraepithelial neoplasia through regulation of apoptotic and HIF-1-dependent pathways. Nat Med 2004; 10(6):594–601.
19. Morgan TM, Koreckij TD, Corey E. Targeted therapy for advanced prostate cancer: inhibition of the PI3K/Akt/mTOR pathway. Curr Cancer Drug Targets 2009;9(2):237–49.
20. Hermans KG, van Marion R, van Dekken H, et al. TMPRSS2:ERG fusion by translocation or interstitial deletion is highly relevant in androgen-dependent prostate cancer, but is bypassed in late-stage androgen receptor-negative prostate cancer. Cancer Res 2006;66(22):10658–63.
21. Ribeiro FR, Henrique R, Hektoen M, et al. Comparison of chromosomal and array-based comparative genomic hybridization for the detection of genomic imbalances in primary prostate carcinomas. Mol Cancer 2006;5:33.
22. Bethel CR, Faith D, Li X, et al. Decreased NKX3.1 protein expression in focal prostatic atrophy, prostatic intraepithelial neoplasia, and adenocarcinoma: association with Gleason score and chromosome 8p deletion. Cancer Res 2006; 66(22):10683–90.
23. Magee JA, Abdulkadir SA, Milbrandt J. Haploinsufficiency at the Nkx3.1 locus. A paradigm for stochastic, dosage-sensitive gene regulation during tumor initiation. Cancer Cell 2003;3:273–83.
24. Ouyang X, DeWeese TL, Nelson WG, et al. Loss-of-function of Nkx3.1 promotes increased oxidative damage in prostate carcinogenesis. Cancer Res 2005;65(15):6773–9.
25. Song H, Zhang B, Watson MA, et al. Loss of Nkx3.1 leads to the activation of discrete downstream target genes during prostate tumorigenesis. Oncogene 2009;28(37):3307–19.
26. Korkmaz CG, Korkmaz KS, Manola J, et al. Analysis of androgen regulated homeobox gene NKX3.1 during prostate carcinogenesis. J Urol 2004;172(3):1134–9.
27. Cher ML, Bova GS, Moore DH, et al. Genetic alterations in untreated metastases and androgen-independent prostate cancer detected by comparative genomic hybridization and allelotyping. Cancer Res 1996;56(13):3091–102.
28. Freedman ML, Haiman CA, Patterson N, et al. Admixture mapping identifies 8q24 as a prostate cancer risk locus in African-American men. Proc Natl Acad Sci U S A 2006;103:14068–73.
29. Pal P, Xi H, Guha S, et al. Common variants in 8q24 are associated with risk for prostate cancer and tumor aggressiveness in men of European ancestry. Prostate 2009;69(14):1548–56.
30. Pomerantz MM, Beckwith CA, Regan MM, et al. Evaluation of the 8q24 prostate cancer risk locus and MYC expression. Cancer Res 2009;69(13): 5568–74.
31. Sato K, Qian J, Slezak JM, et al. Clinical significance of alterations of chromosome 8 in high-grade, advanced, nonmetastatic prostate carcinoma. J Natl Cancer Inst 1999;91(18):1574–80.
32. Ellwood-Yen K, Graeber TG, Wongvipat J, et al. Myc-driven murine prostate cancer shares molecular features with human prostate tumors. Cancer Cell 2003;4(3):223–38.
33. Gurel B, Iwata T, Koh CM, et al. Nuclear MYC protein overexpression is an early alteration in human prostate carcinogenesis. Mod Pathol 2008;9:1156–67.
34. Tomlins SA, Rhodes DR, Perner S, et al. Recurrent fusion of TMPRSS2 and ETS transcription factor genes in prostate cancer. Science 2005; 310(5748):644–8.
35. Mosquera JM, Perner S, Genega EM, et al. Characterization of TMPRSS2-ERG fusion high-grade prostatic intraepithelial neoplasia and potential clinical implications. Clin Cancer Res 2008; 14(11):3380–5.
36. Attard G, Clark J, Ambroisine L, et al. Duplication of the fusion of TMPRSS2 to ERG sequences identifies fatal human prostate cancer. Oncogene 2008;27(3):253–63.
37. Perner S, Demichelis F, Beroukhim R, et al. TMPRSS2:ERG fusion-associated deletions provide insight into the heterogeneity of prostate cancer. Cancer Res 2006;66(17):8337–41.
38. Darnel AD, Lafargue CJ, Vollmer RT, et al. TMPRSS2-ERG fusion is frequently observed in Gleason pattern 3 prostate cancer in a Canadian cohort. Cancer Biol Ther 2009;8(2):125–30.
39. Gopalan A, Leversha MA, Satagopan JM, et al. TMPRSS2-ERG gene fusion is not associated with outcome in patients treated by prostatectomy. Cancer Res 2009;69(4):1400–6.
40. Attard G, Jameson C, Moreira J, et al. Hormone-sensitive prostate cancer: a case of ETS gene fusion heterogeneity. J Clin Pathol 2009;62(4): 373–6.
41. Tomlins SA, Laxman B, Dhanasekaran SM, et al. Distinct classes of chromosomal rearrangements create oncogenic ETS gene fusions in prostate cancer. Nature 2007;448(7153):595–9.
42. Warburg O. On respiratory impairment in cancer cells. Science 1956;124(3215):269–70.
43. Medes G, Paden G, Weinhouse S. Metabolism of neoplastic tissue. XI. Absorption and oxidation of dietary fatty acids by implanted tumors. Cancer Res 1957;17(2):127–33.

44. Vander Heiden MG, Cantley LC, Thompson CB. Understanding the Warburg effect: the metabolic requirements of cell proliferation. Science 2009; 324(5930):1029–33.
45. Menendez JA, Lupu R. Fatty acid synthase and the lipogenic phenotype in cancer pathogenesis. Nat Rev Cancer 2007;7(10):763–77.
46. Hatzivassiliou G, Zhao F, Bauer DE, et al. ATP citrate lyase inhibition can suppress tumor cell growth. Cancer Cell 2005;8(4):311–21.
47. Wellen KE, Hatzivassiliou G, Sachdeva UM, et al. ATP-citrate lyase links cellular metabolism to histone acetylation. Science 2009;324(5930): 1076–80.
48. Wang C, Xu C, Sun M, et al. Acetyl-CoA carboxylase-alpha inhibitor TOFA induces human cancer cell apoptosis. Biochem Biophys Res Commun 2009;385(3):302–6.
49. Baron A, Migita T, Tang D, et al. Fatty acid synthase: a metabolic oncogene in prostate cancer? J Cell Biochem 2004;91(1):47–53.
50. Migita T, Ruiz S, Fornari A, et al. Fatty acid synthase: a metabolic enzyme and candidate oncogene in prostate cancer. J Natl Cancer Inst 2009; 101(7):519–32.
51. Little JL, Wheeler FB, Fels DR, et al. Inhibition of fatty acid synthase induces endoplasmic reticulum stress in tumor cells. Cancer Res 2007;67(3):1262–9.
52. Fiorentino M, Zadra G, Palescandolo E, et al. Overexpression of fatty acid synthase is associated with palmitoylation of Wnt1 and cytoplasmic stabilization of beta-catenin in prostate cancer. Lab Invest 2008;88(12):1340–8.
53. Siddiqui IA, Malik A, Adhami VM, et al. Green tea polyphenol EGCG sensitizes human prostate carcinoma LNCaP cells to TRAIL-mediated apoptosis and synergistically inhibits biomarkers associated with angiogenesis and metastasis. Oncogene 2008;27(14):2055–63.
54. Kuhajda FP, Pizer ES, Li JN, et al. Synthesis and antitumor activity of an inhibitor of fatty acid synthase. Proc Natl Acad Sci U S A 2000;97(7): 3450–4.
55. Zhuang L, Kim J, Adam RM, et al. Cholesterol targeting alters lipid raft composition and cell survival in prostate cancer cells and xenografts. J Clin Invest 2005;115(4):959–68.
56. Williams TM, Hassan GS, Li J, et al. Caveolin-1 promotes tumor progression in an autochthonous mouse model of prostate cancer: genetic ablation of Cav-1 delays advanced prostate tumor development in tramp mice. J Biol Chem 2005;280(26): 25134–45.
57. Di Vizio D, Sotgia F, Williams TM, et al. Caveolin-1 is required for the upregulation of fatty acid synthase (FASN), a tumor promoter, during prostate cancer progression. Cancer Biol Ther 2007;6(8):1263–8.
58. Polyak K, Hahn WC. Roots and stem: stem cells in cancer. Nat Med 2006;12(3):296–300.
59. Gu G, Yuan J, Wills M, et al. Prostate cancer cells with stem cell characteristics reconstitute the original human tumor in vivo. Cancer Res 2007;67(10): 4807–15.
60. Patrawala L, Calhoun T, Schneider-Broussard R, et al. Highly purified CD44+ prostate cancer cells from xenograft human tumors are enriched in tumorigenic and metastatic progenitor cells. Oncogene 2006;25:1696–708.
61. Collins AT, Berry PA, Hyde C, et al. Prospective identification of tumorigenic prostate cancer stem cells. Cancer Res 2005;65:10946–51.
62. Maitland NJ, Collins AT. Prostate cancer stem cells: a new target for therapy. J Clin Oncol 2008;26: 2862–70.
63. Liu R, Wang X, Chen GY, et al. The prognostic role of a gene signature from tumorigenic breast-cancer cells. N Engl J Med 2007;356:217–26.
64. Hurt EM, Kawasaki BT, Klarmann GJ, et al. CD44+ CD24(−) prostate cells are early cancer progenitor/stem cells that provide a model for patients with poor prognosis. Br J Cancer 2008;98(4):756–65.
65. Klarmann GJ, Hurt EM, Mathews LA. Invasive prostate cancer cells are tumor initiating cells that have a stem cell-like genomic signature. Clin Exp Metastasis 2009;26(5):433–46.
66. Palapattu GS, Wu C, Silvers CR, et al. Selective expression of CD44, a putative prostate cancer stem cell marker, in neuroendocrine tumor cells of human prostate cancer. Prostate 2009;69(7): 787–98.
67. Signoretti S, Loda M. Prostate stem cells: from development to cancer. Semin Cancer Biol 2007; 17(3):219–24.
68. Pomerantz MM, Freedman ML, Kantoff PW. Genetic determinants of prostate cancer risk. BJU Int 2007;100(2):241–3.
69. Lieberfarb ME, Lin M, Lechpammer M, et al. Genome-wide loss of heterozygosity analysis from laser capture microdissected prostate cancer using single nucleotide polymorphic allele (SNP) arrays and a novel bioinformatics platform dChipSNP. Cancer Res 2003;63(16):4781–5.
70. Tørring N, Borre M, Sørensen KD, et al. Genome-wide analysis of allelic imbalance in prostate cancer using the Affymetrix 50K SNP mapping array. Br J Cancer 2007;96(3):499–506.
71. Liu W, Sun J, Li G, et al. Association of a germ-line copy number variation at 2p24.3 and risk for aggressive prostate cancer. Cancer Res 2009; 69(6):2176–9.
72. Ross RW, Oh WK, Xie W, et al. Inherited variation in the androgen pathway is associated with the efficacy of androgen-deprivation therapy in men with prostate cancer. J Clin Oncol 2008;26(6):842–7.

73. Hittelman A, Sridharan S, Roy R, et al. Evaluation of whole genome amplification protocols for array and oligonucleotide CGH. Diagn Mol Pathol 2007;16(4): 198–206.
74. Paris PL, Andaya A, Fridlyand J, et al. Whole genome scanning identifies genotypes associated with recurrence and metastasis in prostate tumors. Hum Mol Genet 2004;13(13):1303–13.
75. Ishkanian AS, Mallof CA, Ho J, et al. High-resolution array CGH identifies novel regions of genomic alteration in intermediate-risk prostate cancer. Prostate 2009;69(10):1091–100.
76. Huang J, Pang J, Watanabe T, et al. Whole genome amplification for array comparative genomic hybridization using DNA extracted from formalin-fixed, paraffin-embedded histological sections. J Mol Diagn 2009;11(2):109–16.
77. Schweiger MR, Kerick M, Timmermann B, et al. Genome-wide massively parallel sequencing of formaldehyde fixed-paraffin embedded (FFPE) tumor tissues for copy-number- and mutation-analysis. PLoS One 2009;4(5):e5548.
78. Golub TR, Slonim DK, Tamayo P, et al. Molecular classification of cancer: class discovery and class prediction by gene expression monitoring. Science 1999;286(5439):531–7.
79. Lapointe J, Li C, Higgins JP, et al. Gene expression profiling identifies clinically relevant subtypes of prostate cancer. Proc Natl Acad Sci U S A 2004; 101(3):811–6.
80. Bibikova M, Chudin E, Arsanjani A, et al. Expression signatures that correlated with Gleason score and relapse in prostate cancer. Genomics 2007; 89(6):666–72.
81. Nakagawa T, Kollmeyer TM, Morlan BW, et al. A tissue biomarker panel predicting systemic progression after PSA recurrence post-definitive prostate cancer therapy. PLoS One 2008;3(5):e2318.
82. Sidransky D. Circulating DNA: what we know and what we need to learn. Ann N Y Acad Sci 2000; 906:1–4.
83. Holdenrieder S, Stieber P, Bodenmüller H, et al. Nucleosomes in serum of patients with benign and malignant diseases. Int J Cancer 2001;95:114–20.
84. Sozzi G, Conte D, Leon M, et al. Quantification of free circulating DNA as a diagnostic marker in lung cancer. J Clin Oncol 2003;21(21):3902–8.
85. Holdenrieder S, Stieber P, von Pawel J, et al. Circulating nucleosomes predict the response to chemotherapy in patients with advanced non-small cell lung cancer. Clin Cancer Res 2004;10(18):5981–7.
86. Stroun M, Maurice P, Vasioukhin V, et al. The origin and mechanism of circulating DNA. Ann N Y Acad Sci 2000;906:161–8.
87. Papadopoulou E, Davilas E, Sotiriou V, et al. Cell-free DNA in plasma as a new molecular marker for prostate cancer. Oncol Res 2004;14:439–45.
88. Boddy JL, Gal S, Malone PR, et al. Prospective study on quantitation of plasma DNA levels in the diagnosis of malignant versus benign prostate diseases. Clin Cancer Res 2005;11:1394–9.
89. Chun FK, Muller I, Lange I, et al. Circulating tumor-associated plasma DNA represents an independent and informative predictor of prostate cancer. BJU Int 2006;98:544–8.
90. Altimari A, Grigioni AD, Benedettini E, et al. Diagnostic role of circulating free plasma DNA detection in patients with localized prostate cancer. Am J Clin Pathol 2008;129(5):756–62.
91. Schwarzenbach H, Alix-Panabières C, Müller I, et al. Cell-free tumor DNA in blood plasma as a marker for circulating tumor cells in prostate cancer. Clin Cancer Res 2009;15(3):1032–8.
92. Schwarzenbach H, Chun FK, Lange I, et al. Detection of tumor-specific DNA in blood and bone marrow plasma from patients with prostate cancer. Int J Cancer 2007;120(7):1465–71.
93. Müller I, Urban K, Pantel K, et al. Comparison of genetic alterations detected in circulating microsatellite DNA in blood plasma samples of patients with prostate cancer and benign prostatic hyperplasia. Ann N Y Acad Sci 2006;1075:222–9.
94. Schwarzenbach H, Chun FK, Müller I, et al. Microsatellite analysis of allelic imbalance in tumour and blood from patients with prostate cancer. BJU Int 2008;102(2):253–8.
95. Pantel K, Brakenhoff RH, Brandt B. Detection, clinical relevance and specific biological properties of disseminating tumour cells. Nat Rev Cancer 2008; 8(5):329–40.
96. Riethdorf S, Wikman H, Pantel K. Review: biological relevance of disseminated tumor cells in cancer patients. Int J Cancer 2008;123(9):1991–2006.
97. Panteleakou Z, Lembessis P, Sourla A, et al. Detection of circulating tumor cells in prostate cancer patients: methodological pitfalls and clinical relevance. Mol Med 2009;15(3–4):101–14.
98. Wood DP Jr, Banerjee M. Presence of circulating prostate cells in the bone marrow of patients undergoing radical prostatectomy is predictive of disease-free survival. J Clin Oncol 1997;15(12):3451–7.
99. Berg A, Berner A, Lilleby W, et al. Impact of disseminated tumor cells in bone marrow at diagnosis in patients with nonmetastatic prostate cancer treated by definitive radiotherapy. Int J Cancer 2007;120(8):1603–9.
100. Köllermann J, Weikert S, Schostak M, et al. Prognostic significance of disseminated tumor cells in the bone marrow of prostate cancer patients treated with neoadjuvant hormone treatment. J Clin Oncol 2008;26(30):4928–33.
101. Kantoff PW, Halabi S, Farmer DA, et al. Prognostic significance of reverse transcriptase polymerase chain reaction for prostate-specific antigen in

men with hormone-refractory prostate cancer. J Clin Oncol 2001;19(12):3025–8.
102. Ross RW, Manola J, Hennessy K, et al. Prognostic significance of baseline reverse transcriptase-PCR for prostate-specific antigen in men with hormone-refractory prostate cancer treated with chemotherapy. Clin Cancer Res 2005;11(14):5195–8.
103. Danila DC, Heller G, Gignac GA, et al. Circulating tumor cell number and prognosis in progressive castration-resistant prostate cancer. Clin Cancer Res 2007;13(23):7053–8.
104. de Bono JS, Scher HI, Montgomery RB, et al. Circulating tumor cells predict survival benefit from treatment in metastatic castration-resistant prostate cancer. Clin Cancer Res 2008;14(19):6302–9.
105. Goodman OB Jr, Fink LM, Symanowski JT, et al. Circulating tumor cells in patients with castration-resistant prostate cancer baseline values and correlation with prognostic factors. Cancer Epidemiol Biomarkers Prev 2009;18(6):1904–13.
106. Olmos D, Arkenau HT, Ang JE, et al. Circulating tumour cell (CTC) counts as intermediate end points in castration-resistant prostate cancer (CRPC): a single-centre experience. Ann Oncol 2009;20(1):27–33.
107. Davis JW, Nakanishi H, Kumar VS, et al. Circulating tumor cells in peripheral blood samples from patients with increased serum prostate specific antigen: initial results in early prostate cancer. J Urol 2008;179(6):2187–91.
108. Attard G, Swennenhuis JF, Olmos D, et al. Characterization of ERG, AR and PTEN gene status in circulating tumor cells from patients with castration-resistant prostate cancer. Cancer Res 2009; 69(7):2912–8.
109. Leversha MA, Han J, Asgari Z, et al. Fluorescence in situ hybridization analysis of circulating tumor cells in metastatic prostate cancer. Clin Cancer Res 2009;15(6):2091–7.
110. Holcomb IN, Grove DI, Kinnunen M, et al. Genomic alterations indicate tumor origin and varied metastatic potential of disseminated cells from prostate cancer patients. Cancer Res 2008;68(14): 5599–608.

Index

Note: Page numbers of article titles are in **boldface** type.

Urol Clin N Am 37 (2010) 143–148
doi:10.1016/S0094-0143(09)00125-6

Q

R

S

T

Printed and bound by CPI Group (UK) Ltd, Croydon, CR0 4YY
03/10/2024
01040351-0018